Dale Hayden
Geneva College
April 1998

PSYCHOANALYTIC DIAGNOSIS

Psychoanalytic Diagnosis

Understanding Personality Structure in the Clinical Process

NANCY McWILLIAMS, Ph.D.

THE GUILFORD PRESS
New York London

A Division of Guilford Publications
72 Spring Street, New York, NY 10012

Printed in the United States of America

This book is printed on acid-free paper.

Last digit is print number: 9 8 7 6 5

Library of Congress Cataloging-in-Publication Data

McWilliams, Nancy.
Psychoanalytic diagnosis: understanding personality structure in the clinical process / Nancy McWilliams.
p. cm.
Includes bibliographical references and index.
ISBN 0-89862-199-2
1. Typology (Psychology) 2. Personality assessment.
3. Personality development. I. Title.
[DNLM: 1. Psychoanalytic Interpretation. 2 Personality Disorders. 3. Psychoanalytic Therapy. WM 460.5.P3 M478p 1994]
RC489.T95M38 1994
616.89'17—dc20
DNLM/DLC
for Library of Congress

94-8549
CIP

In Grateful Memory

Howard Gordon Riley
Millicent Wood Riley
Jane Ayers Riley

Preface

My desire to write a primer on character diagnosis has developed gradually over many years of teaching psychoanalytic conceptualization to aspiring therapists in the Graduate School of Applied and Professional Psychology at Rutgers University. While there are a number of good recent books on assessment, most of them are oriented toward relating clinical material to the available categories in the latest edition of the *Diagnostic and Statistical Manual of Mental Disorders* (DSM) of the American Psychiatric Association, a nosology that has attempted to classify types of psychopathology descriptively rather than according to any particular theory of psychology.

The categories of psychopathology in the two earliest editions of the DSM reflected a distinct, implicit psychoanalytic bias. The change away from an inherently structural nosology to one that seeks to be simply descriptive has offered many benefits to psychotherapists, now that several powerful alternative ways of conceptualizing psychological problems have been developed. But I have found that those of my students who want to understand individual differences according to a psychoanalytic model now have no text that explains the concepts by which analytically oriented therapists understand and treat their clients. When I pass on to them the general psychoanalytic "lore" on the recommended approach to any particular kind of person, they wonder where they can find this lore organized and explicated.

Currently, there is no such source. Fenichel's classic tome (1945) is unduly difficult for therapists in training, especially these days, when undergraduate exposure to analytic thinking tends to consist of one or two lectures on Freud's drive theory, with emphasis on its quaintness, followed by a nod to Erikson. Fenichel's work also suffers from its age, in that significant developments in ego psychology, object relations theory, and self psychology are unrepresented in it. Some psychoanalytically influenced textbooks in Abnormal Psychology cover more traditional diagnostic concepts, but without a stress on character per se, and without much attention to how assessed personality patterns should influence the tone and content of therapeutic work.

In what follows, I hope to present psychoanalytic notions of personality structure in an interesting and sympathetic way, and to demonstrate the clinical utility of a good diagnostic formulation. In this enterprise I am indebted to MacKinnon and Michels, whose book *The Psychiatric Interview in Clinical Practice* (1971) is the only text I know of that represents a project similar to the one I am undertaking here. That has now also become dated, despite its continuing value in illuminating many conditions, in that it does not discuss more recent characterological concepts, such as borderline, masochistic (self-defeating), narcissistic, and dissociative psychologies.

The move away from a psychodynamically biased nosology has left many contemporary students unexposed to important concepts with which previous generations of trainees had at least passing familiarity. The omission of the term "hysterical," for example, from the Personality Disorders section of the third edition of the DSM (DSM-III; American Psychiatric Association, 1980) and later manuals has deprived beginning therapists of a historically significant, clinically valuable, and technically relevant concept. Because this and similar omissions handicap communication between recently trained diagnosticians and those for whom the more traditional labels remain meaningful, they have disadvantaged beginning therapists both practically and educationally.

I have therefore attempted to rectify here a deficiency I have noticed in the education of contemporary students of psychotherapy. For those readers who see themselves as psychodynamically oriented, this book should provide an introduction to psychoanalytic diagnostic thinking that can be elaborated, refined, and revised as they mature as clinicians and confront the complexity of the human condition in general and the idiosyncracy of each individual human being in particular. For those who are not attracted to psychodynamic ways of working, either because they object to some of the assumptions inherent in an analytic perspective or because their chosen area of human relations does not lend itself to reliance on psychoanalytic concepts in any central way, it should foster adequate psychoanalytic literacy, a capacity to understand what their analytically oriented colleagues are talking about.

The intended audience of this text includes graduate students in social work and psychology, physicians in psychiatric rotations or residencies, psychiatric nurses, pastoral counselors, marriage and family therapists, and candidates in analytic institutes. It will please me if it also turns out that I have organized and discussed the following diagnostic concepts and their implications for treatment with enough originality to make the book interesting to more seasoned practitioners.

When I first decided that psychoanalytic psychotherapy was my calling, I made an appointment with Freud's protégé Theodor Reik, who was still practicing in New York City, and asked what advice he would give to a young person embarking on a career as a therapist. "First, you *must* be analyzed," he responded, with indescribably graceful Viennese emphasis. It is the best advice I have ever gotten, and it remains true. The surest way to have a feel for diagnostic issues is to explore all one's own internal areas—borderline and psychotic as well as neurotic ones—and all the hints of processes that can in anyone become locked into character.

This book will be only as useful as the reader's psychology allows. To the extent that one has access to and acceptance of one's personal dynamics, one can have a compassionate, respectful appreciation for those of others. A textbook cannot substitute for a depth of personal insight. Nor can it provide the profound and contagious conviction about the efficacy of treatment that personal psychotherapy can supply. But if I have in this organization of analytic concepts provided a useful structure for making sense of, and drawing inspiration from, the complex affective, intuitive, sensory, and cognitive responses that a sensitive interviewer may have to a suffering stranger, I have accomplished my task.

Acknowledgments

This book is a synthesis of my intellectual background, therapy training, and life experience over the past 30 years as they pertain to learning and teaching about individual personality structure. My debts are therefore extensive and beyond hope of fully reckoning, but they include the following.

Among my teachers, Dorothy Peavey and the late Margaret Fardy, who knew more about individual psychology than most psychologists, began giving me high-quality training in assessing personality when I was still a teenager. Daniel Ogilvie, my dissertation advisor and later my department chair, introduced me to the personological tradition and to object relations theory. George Atwood, my cherished friend, showed me how to approach people with a freshness of inquiry, eschewing formulas and appreciating each person's uniqueness; he also persuaded me to do a doctoral dissertation on characterological altruism, a disposition he exemplifies. The late Silvan Tomkins was an inspiring scholar and thinker. Iradj Siassi provided superior training in formal psychiatric diagnosis.

The faculty of the National Psychological Association for Psychoanalysis endowed psychoanalytic training with integrity, artistry, and wisdom. Michaela Babakin, Emmanuel Hammer, Esther Menaker, Milton Robin, Alan Roland, Henry Sindos, and the late Doris Bernstein were especially talented teachers, and Stanley Moldawsky was a singularly noncontrolling control analyst. My mentor and friend Arthur Robbins taught me, long before relational concepts went mainstream, how to diagnose not only with my cognitive faculties but also with my aesthetic, affective, intuitive, and sensory ones. I apologize for purveying so many of his ideas without attribution; it is hard for me to tell anymore what clinical lore came from whom, but the greater part of what I know derives ultimately from his supervision.

My colleagues at the Institute for Psychoanalysis and Psychotherapy of New Jersey continually feed my mind. I want especially to thank Joseph Braun, Carol Goodheart, Cecele Kraus, Stanley Lependorf, Judith Felton Logue, Peter Richman, Helene Schwartzbach, and Floyd Turner for their friendship and stimulation over 20 years, and Jean Ciardiello for critiquing the entire manuscript on a moment's notice. To Albert Shire I owe much more than I can put into words. I am also grateful to the faculty, staff, and administrators at the Graduate School of Applied and Professional Psychology at Rutgers University, who have accomplished the remarkable feat of collaborating respectfully and creatively despite radically divergent convictions. Sandra Harris, Stanley Messer, Ruth Schulman, and Sue Wright have supported my teaching and professional growth over many years. Jamie Walkup and Louis Sass each critiqued portions of this manuscript, with unusual tact and care. Many students—too many to list—at IPPNJ and GSAPP have been generous and helpful with their comments about this book.

Other colleagues who have contributed directly and indirectly to this enterprise include Hilary Hays, who for over two decades has encouraged me to promote my ideas; Otto Kernberg, who donated his scarce time and abundant intelligence at the outset of this project; Barbara Menzel, whose professional expertise and extra-professional companionship have been equally valuable; Fred Pine, who endorsed this undertaking with his characteristic generosity of spirit; Arthur Raisman and Diane Suffridge, who acquainted me with control–mastery theory in its earliest incarnations; Nicholas Susalis, who shared his impressively compassionate professional knowledge of psychopathy and critiqued Chapter 7; and Thomas Tudor, who reviewed Chapter 15, but more consequentially, introduced me to the literature on clients with dissociative disorders long before most of the mental health community was willing to take this population seriously. I also owe a great deal to those therapists who have come to me for supervision; by exposing their own struggles to be of help to their clients, they continue to advance mine. And to all the mental health groups in New Jersey on whom I test-drove these ideas, thank you.

My editor, Kitty Moore, took the concept of this book and ran with it, always with enthusiasm and good sense. The original reviewers for Guilford did me a great service: Bertram Karon, whose impassioned commitment to help the desperate, underserved, and psychotic has always moved me, felt the manuscript had promise; and David

Wolitzky submitted a detailed and encouraging critique that conquered my resistance to going forward.

As for nonspecific but critical influences, as most of what I know about therapy is deeply experiential rather than intellectual, I credit my analyst, the late Louis Berkowitz, and his successors Edith Sheppard and Theodore Greenbaum, with exemplifying what is truest and most healing in the analytic tradition. Several people in my intimate circle who are not therapists are unfailingly therapeutic to me. My husband, Carey, who introduced me to Freud 30 years ago, has not only given consistent verbal support to my professional ambitions, he has also actively promoted them by being an equal partner and full-time parent. Our daughters Susan and Helen have willingly put up with their mother's strange occupation and hours at the laptop; they have also obligingly taught me more about psychology than any theory could have. Nancy Schwartz sensitively critiqued portions of the manuscript from the viewpoint of an educated reader outside the field. Richard Tormey, who welcomed an improbable friendship with grace and generosity, overcame my resistance to becoming computer literate and, with the cheerfully relentless nagging that only a veteran teacher and coach can carry off, kept me on the job. Cheryl Watkins encouraged me unselfishly at every step, poured champagne at milestones, and made her home a refuge from the burdens of writing.

Finally, the most significant contributors to this book must go unnamed; I hope they have some idea how much they have taught me. To be a psychoanalytic therapist is the closest approximation I have found to gratifying my wish to live more than one life in a single, very short lifetime. Not only have I learned something of what it is like to be alcoholic or depressive or bulimic; I have glimpsed what it is like to be a divorce lawyer, a scientist, a rabbi, a cardiologist, a gay activist, a preschool teacher, a mechanic, a police officer, an intensive-care nurse, a mother on welfare, an actor, a medical student, a politician, an artist, and many other kinds of people.

It has always seemed miraculous to me that one can pursue an enthusiasm that any voyeur would envy, be useful to others in the process, and earn a living at the same time. My patients have been my primary inspirers in this effort to describe one area of psychoanalytic expertise. To those clients who have read and approved publication of the vignettes from their own treatment in the chapters that follow, special thanks for your permission to use accounts of your personal subjectivities in the service of educating others.

Contents

Introduction 1
A Comment on Terminology 1
A Comment on Tone 4

I **CONCEPTUAL ISSUES** 5

1 **Why Diagnose?** 7
Treatment Planning 8
Prognostic Implications 9
Consumer Protection 10
The Communication of Empathy 12
Forestalling Flights From Treatment 14
Fringe Benefits 15
Limits to the Utility of Diagnosis 17
Suggestions for Further Reading 18

2 **Psychoanalytic Character Diagnosis** 19
Classical Freudian Drive Theory 21
Ego Psychology 25
The Object Relations Tradition 29
Self Psychology 34
Other Psychoanalytic Contributions to Personality Assessment 37
Summary 38
Suggestions for Further Reading 38

3 **Developmental Levels of Personality Organization** 40

Historical Context: Diagnosing Level of Character Pathology 42

Kraepelinian Diagnosis: Neuroses Versus Psychoses 43

Ego Psychology Diagnostic Categories: Symptom Neurosis, Neurotic Character, and Psychosis 45

Object Relations Diagnosis: Borderline Psychopathology 49

Specific Dimensions of a Neurotic–Borderline–Psychotic Spectrum 53

Summary 65

Suggestions for Further Reading 65

4 **Clinical Implications of Developmental Levels of Organization** 67

Psychoanalytic Therapy with Neurotic-Level Patients 69

Psychoanalytic Therapy with Psychotic-Level Patients 72

Psychoanalytic Therapy with Borderline Patients 80

Interaction of Maturational and Typological Dimensions of Character 91

Summary 94

Suggestions for Further Reading 94

5 **Primary (Primitive) Defensive Processes** 96

Primitive Withdrawal 100

Denial 101

Omnipotent Control 103

Primitive Idealization (and Devaluation) 105

Projection, Introjection, and Projective Identification 107

Splitting of the Ego 112

Dissociation 114

Summary 115

Suggestions for Further Reading 116

6 **Secondary (Higher-Order) Defensive Processes** 117

Repression 118

Regression 120

Isolation 122
Intellectualization 123
Rationalization 124
Moralization 125
Compartmentalization 127
Undoing 127
Turning Against the Self 129
Displacement 130
Reaction Formation 131
Reversal 133
Identification 135
Acting Out 138
Sexualization (Instinctualization) 140
Sublimation 142
Summary 144
Suggestions for Further Reading 144

II TYPES OF CHARACTER ORGANIZATION 145
Rationale for Chapter Organization 145
Character, Character Pathology, and Situational Factors 147
Limits on Personality Change 148

7 Psychopathic (Antisocial) Personalities 151
Drive, Affect, and Temperament in Psychopathy 152
Defensive and Adaptive Processes in Psychopathy 153
Object Relations in Psychopathy 155
The Psychopathic Self 157
Transference and Countertransference with Psychopathic Patients 159
Therapeutic Implications of the Diagnosis of Psychopathy 160
Differential Diagnosis 165
Summary 167
Suggestions for Further Reading 167

8 Narcissistic Personalities 168
Drive, Affect, and Temperament in Narcissism 171
Defensive and Adaptive Processes in Narcissism 173
Object Relations in Narcissism 174
The Narcissistic Self 177

Transference and Countertransference with Narcissistic Patients 178
Therapeutic Implications of the Diagnosis of Narcissism 181
Differential Diagnosis 184
Summary 187
Suggestions for Further Reading 188

9 **Schizoid Personalities** 189
Drive, Affect, and Temperament in Schizoid Personalities 190
Defensive and Adaptive Processes in Schizoid Personalities 192
Object Relations in Schizoid Conditions 193
The Schizoid Self 195
Transference and Countertransference with Schizoid Patients 197
Therapeutic Implications of the Diagnosis of Schizoid Personality 199
Differential Diagnosis 202
Summary 204
Suggestion for Further Reading 204

10 **Paranoid Personalities** 205
Drive, Affect, and Temperament in Paranoid Personalities 207
Defensive and Adaptive Processes in Paranoia 209
Object Relations in Paranoia 211
The Paranoid Self 214
Transference and Countertransference with Paranoid Patients 216
Therapeutic Implications of the Diagnosis of Paranoia 217
Differential Diagnosis 224
Summary 225
Suggestions for Further Reading 226

11 **Depressive and Manic Personalities** 227
Depressive Personalities 228
Drive, Affect, and Temperament in Depression 229
Defensive and Adaptive Processes in Depression 231
Object Relations in Depression 233
The Depressive Self 237
Transference and Countertransference with Depressive Patients 239

Therapeutic Implications of the Diagnosis of Depression 241
Differential Diagnosis 246
Manic and Hypomanic Personalities 248
Drive, Affect, and Temperament in Mania 248
Defensive and Adaptive Processes in Mania 249
Object Relations in Mania 250
The Manic Self 250
Transference and Countertransference with Manic Patients 251
Therapeutic Implications of the Diagnosis of Mania or Hypomania 251
Differential Diagnosis 253
Summary 255
Suggestions for Further Reading 256

12 Masochistic (Self-Defeating) Personalities 257
Drive, Affect, and Temperament in Masochism 260
Defensive and Adaptive Processes in Masochism 261
Object Relations in Masochism 264
The Masochistic Self 267
Transference and Countertransference with Masochistic Patients 268
Therapeutic Implications of the Diagnosis of Masochism 271
Differential Diagnosis 275
Summary 277
Suggestions for Further Reading 277

13 Obsessive and Compulsive Personalities 279
Drive, Affect, and Temperament in Obsessive and Compulsive Personalities 281
Defensive and Adaptive Processes in Obsessive and Compulsive Personalities 283
Object Relations in Obsessive and Compulsive Personalities 286
The Obsessive Compulsive Self 289
Transference and Countertransference with Obsessive and Compulsive Patients 292
Therapeutic Implications of the Diagnosis of Obsessive or Compulsive Personality 294
Differential Diagnosis 298
Summary 300
Suggestions for Further Reading 300

14 Hysterical (Histrionic) Personalities 301
Drive, Affect, and Temperament in Hysteria 303
Defensive and Adaptive Processes in Hysteria 304
Object Relations in Hysteria 308
The Hysterical Self 310
Transference and Countertransference with Hysterical Patients 313
Therapeutic Implications of the Diagnosis of Hysteria 316
Differential Diagnosis 318
Summary 321
Suggestions for Further Reading 322

15 Dissociative Personalities 323
Drive, Affect, and Temperament in Dissociative Conditions 328
Defensive and Adaptive Processes in Dissociative Conditions 329
Object Relations in Dissociative Conditions 332
The Dissociative Self 334
Transference and Countertransference with Dissociative Patients 336
Therapeutic Implications of the Diagnosis of a Dissociative Condition 338
Differential Diagnosis 342
Summary 346
Suggestions for Further Reading 346

Appendix: Suggested Diagnostic Interview Format 349
Demographic Data 349
Current Problems and Their Onset 349
Personal History 349
Current Presentation (Mental Status) 350
Concluding Topics 350
Inferences 351

References 353

Author Index 381

Subject Index 386

Introduction

Most of what follows is accumulated psychoanalytic wisdom. It will be clear to the knowledgeable reader, however, that it is my own synthesis of that wisdom and reflects my idiosyncratic conclusions, interpretations, and extrapolations. The organization of character possibilities along two axes, for example, which seems to me so clearly inferable from psychoanalytic theories and metaphors, may seem contrived to some analysts, who may visualize the varieties of human personality in other images, along other spectra. I can only respond that this graphic depiction has been of value in my experiences acquainting relatively unprepared students with the welter of analytic concepts that have developed over more than a century.

The main object of this book is to enhance practice, not to resolve any of the conceptual and philosophical problems with which the psychoanalytic literature is replete. I am more interested in being pedagogically useful than in being "right." A recurrent emphasis in the chapters that follow concerns the relationship between psychodynamic formulations and the art of psychotherapy. Beyond conveying certain basic therapeutic attitudes, including curiosity, respect, compassion, devotion, integrity, and the willingness to admit mistakes and limitations, I do not believe in teaching a particular "technique" in the absence of understanding the kind of person to whom one is applying the technique.

A COMMENT ON TERMINOLOGY

A strikingly cyclical effort to sanitize speech has contributed to widespread misunderstanding of the psychoanalytic tradition. Over time, whatever the original intentions of those people who coined any specific psychological term, labels for certain conditions ineluctably come to have a negative connotation. Language that was invented to be simply descriptive—in fact, invented to replace previous value-laden words—develops an evaluative cast and is applied, especially by lay people, in ways that pathologize. Certain topics seem inherently unsettling to human beings, and however carefully we try to talk about them in nonjudgmental language, the words we use to do so attain a pejorative tone over the years.

Today's "antisocial personality," as a case in point, was in 1835 termed "moral insanity." Later it became "psychopathy," then "sociopathy." Each change was intended to give a descriptive, noncensorious label to a disturbing phenomenon. Yet the power of that phenomenon to disturb eventually contaminated each word that was invented to keep the concept out of the realm of moralization. Something similar occurred in the successive transformations of "inversion" to "deviation" to "homosexuality" to being "gay"—recently, I heard a 9-year-old girl disparage an idea because, she noted sneeringly, it was "too gay." Any phenomenon that tends to trouble people, for whatever reason, seems to instigate this futile chasing after nonstigmatizing language. It occurs with nonpsychological terms also; for example, it is endemic in recent controversies about political correctness. One outcome of this doomed project to sanitize language is that the older a particular psychological tradition is, the more negative, judgmental, and quaint its terminology sounds. The swift consumption, distortion, and prejudicial application of psychoanalytic terms, within the mental health professions and outside them, have been a bane of the psychodynamic tradition.

Paradoxically, another burden to the reputation of psychoanalysis has been its appeal. As concepts get popularized, they acquire not only judgmental meanings but also simplistic ones. I assume it would be hard for a psychoanalytically naive reader to come upon the adjective "masochistic," for instance, without reacting to the label as a judgment that the person so depicted loves pain and suffering. Such a reaction is understandable but ignorant; the history of the psychoanalytic concept of masochism abounds with humane, insightful, useful, nonreductionistic observations about why some people repeatedly involve themselves in activities painful to them despite often heroic conscious efforts to do otherwise. The same can be said for many other terms that have been grabbed up by both nonanalytic clinicians and the literate public, and then bruited about with glib or condescending conviction about their meaning.

Concepts also get watered down as they come into common use. The term "trauma," as popularly used, has lost its catastrophic overtones, and it can frequently be heard meaning "discomfort" or "injury." "Depression" has come to be indistinguishable from brief periods of the blues. The term "panic disorder" had to be invented in order to restore to our ear the connotations of the older, perfectly useful phrases "anxiety neurosis" and "anxiety attack" once the word anxiety had been applied to everything from how one feels at a business lunch to how one would feel in front of a firing squad.

Given all this, I have struggled over how to present some of the material in this book. On a personal level, I try to observe the current preferences of minority groups as to how they should be identified. With patients who have sensitivities to the use of certain diagnostic labels (e.g., people who feel that "bipolar" is a less objectionable term than "manic–depressive"), I respect their sensibilities. But at a scholarly level, it seems an exercise in futility to continue to rename things rather than to use their existing names. Substituting "self-defeating" for "masochistic" or "histrionic" for "hysterical" may be understandably preferred by nonanalytic practitioners who want to avoid terms that contain psychodynamic assumptions, but such changes make less sense for those of us who think analytically and assume the operation of unconscious processes in character formation.

My somewhat ambivalent conclusion about the language to be used in this book has been to employ mostly traditional psychoanalytic nomenclature, alternating occasionally, in the hope of reducing the clanking weight of professional jargon, with more recent, roughly equivalent terms. Since I am trying to raise the consciousness of my audience about the rationale for each label that has come to denote a character attribute, I will generally rely on familiar psychoanalytic language and try to make it user-friendly.* To the reader without a psychodynamic background, this may lend an anachronistic or even inferred judgmental tone to the text, but I can only ask such a person to try to suspend criticism temporarily and give the analytic tradition the benefit of the doubt while trying to consider the possible utility of the concepts covered.

*I should also note that I use the term "patient"—a word shunned by many nonmedical practitioners as implying a contemptuous objectification of suffering people—interchangeably with the often-preferred "client," with no hidden significance attached to either term. I use "character" as a synonym for "personality," despite the useful distinctions some (e.g., Kupperman, 1991; Brody & Siegel, 1992) have made between those concepts; and I do not differentiate "psychoanalytic" from "psychodynamic" (see Westen, 1990), especially when discussing theory rather than technique.

A COMMENT ON TONE

Nearly everything one can say about individual character patterns and meanings, even in the context of accepting a general psychoanalytic approach, is disputable. Many concepts central to analytic thinking have not only not been systematically researched and validated, they are inherently so resistant to being operationalized and manipulated that it is difficult to imagine how they even *could* be empirically tested (see Fisher & Greenberg, 1985). Many scholars prefer to place psychoanalysis within the hermeneutic rather than the scientific tradition, partly because of this resistance of the subject matter to investigation by the scientific method as it has come to be defined by contemporary philosophers of science (see, e.g., Grünbaum, 1979).

With a concept as abstract and complex as character, much of what we think we know derives from the accretion of comparable and shared clinical experiences by people who speak the same metapsychological language. I am keenly aware of the reputation of psychoanalysts for insisting arrogantly on their formulations in the absence of "hard" evidence, or even in the presence of contradictory data; consequently, I have tried to avoid a tone of smug or condescending certainty. On the other hand, extensive clinical agreement exists about much of what follows, and I would prefer not to have to burden the reader with a list of disclaimers, equivocations, exceptions, and caveats each time I generalize.

I have therefore erred in the direction of oversimplifying rather than obfuscating, of stating some ideas in perhaps a more sweeping way than many thoughtful researchers and experienced professionals would consider warranted. I hope I have at least done so with appropriate humility. This text is aimed at beginning practitioners. I have no wish to increase the anxiety that inevitably suffuses the process of becoming a therapist by introducing endless complexity. All of us learn soon enough, from the unpredictable nuances of each therapy relationship into which we extend ourselves, just how pale are even our most elegant and satisfying formulations next to the mystery that is human nature. Hence, I trust my readers to outgrow my constructions.

I
CONCEPTUAL ISSUES

The following six chapters comprise a rationale for character diagnosis, a review of the major psychoanalytic orientations and their respective contributions to models of personality structure, an exploration of those differences in personality that reflect differing developmental issues, commentary on the therapeutic import of such issues, and an exposition of the psychoanalytic concept of defense and the role of defenses in defining character. Together they constitute a way of thinking about the consistencies in an individual that we think of as his or her personality.

This section culminates in the representation of diagnostic possibilities along a biaxial grid. Such a schema is both arbitrary and oversimplified, but I have found it useful in introducing therapists to central dynamic formulations and their clinical utility. To my knowledge, this graphic representation of character possibilities does not appear elsewhere in the analytic literature, though I believe it to be implicit throughout it.*

Other analysts have provided other visual representations of diagnostic possibilities (e.g., Kohut, 1971, p. 9; G. Blanck & R. Blanck, 1974, pp. 114–117; Greenspan, 1981, pp. 234–237; Kernberg, 1984, p.

*After I had finished the early drafts of this book, my colleague Gene Nebels called my attention to a similar but three-dimensional illustration in M. Stone's (1980) book *The Borderline Syndromes* (Stone included an axis for genetic predisposition). That an analyst of Stone's breadth has generated a kindred model supports my belief that this kind of diagnostic imagery is the unstated, possibly sometimes even unconscious, visual substrate of most contemporary analytic writing on personality diagnosis.

29; Horner, 1990, p. 23). In some ways my diagram incorporates their thinking; in others it does not. My aim is not to dispute other organizations of developmental, structural, and temperamental concepts but to offer a synthesized and streamlined image for newcomers to this confusing field.

❖ 1 ❖

Why Diagnose?

For many people, including some therapists, diagnosis is a dirty word. We have all seen the misuse of psychodiagnostic formulations: The complex person gets flippantly oversimplified by the interviewer who is anxious about uncertainty; the anguished person gets linguistically distanced by the clinician who cannot bear to feel the pain; the troublesome person gets punished with a pathologizing label. Racism, sexism, heterosexism, classism, and numerous other prejudices can be (and have been) handily fortified by nosology. Currently, when insurance companies and managed care groups dictate specific consequences of many diagnostic categories, often in defiance of a therapist's judgment, the assessment process is especially subject to corruption. The abuse of psychodiagnostic language is thus easily demonstrated. That something can be abused, however, is not a legitimate argument for discarding it. All kinds of evil can be wreaked in the name of worthy ideals—love, patriotism, Christianity, whatever—through no fault of the original vision but because of its perversion. The important question is: Does the careful, nonabusive application of psychodiagnostic concepts increase a client's chances of being helped?

There are at least five interrelated advantages of the diagnostic enterprise when pursued sensitively and with adequate training: (1) its utility for treatment planning, (2) its implicit information about prognosis, (3) its contribution to protecting consumers of mental health services, (4) its value in enabling the therapist to communicate empathy, and (5) its role in reducing the probability that certain easily frightened people will flee from treatment. In addition, there are fringe benefits to the diagnostic process that indirectly facilitate therapy.

By the diagnostic process, I mean that except in crises the initial sessions with a new client should be spent gathering information of the sort traditional in analytically influenced psychiatric training (see Appendix).* In enigmatic cases, psychological testing or structured interviewing may be carried out. I am not convinced that allowing a relationship to develop will create a climate of trust in which all pertinent material will eventually surface. Once the patient feels close to the therapist, it may become *harder* for him or her to bring up certain aspects of personal history or behavior. Alcoholics Anonymous (AA) meetings are full of people who spent years in analysis, or consulted a bevy of professionals, without ever having mentioned *or been asked about* substance abuse. For those who associate a diagnostic session with images of authoritarianism and holier-than-thou detachment, let me stress that there is no reason an in-depth interview cannot be conducted in an atmosphere of sincere respect and egalitarianism. Patients are usually grateful for professional thoroughness. One woman I interviewed who had seen several previous therapists made the comment, "No one has ever been this interested in me!"

TREATMENT PLANNING

Treatment planning is the traditional rationale for diagnosis. It assumes a parallel between psychotherapeutic "treatment" and medical treatment, and in medicine the relationship between diagnosis and therapy is (ideally) straightforward. This parallel sometimes obtains in psychotherapy, and sometimes it does not. It is easy to see the value of a good diagnosis for those conditions in which there is some specific, consensually endorsed treatment approach. Examples include the diagnosis of an alcohol or drug problem (treatment implication: Individual therapy is likely to be useful only if the chemical dependency is dealt with directly by a detoxification program), an organic condition (treatment implication: Address the organicity if possible, and educate the patient and others about handling its effects), bipolar illness (treatment implica-

*I usually devote the first meeting with a patient to the details of the presenting problem and its background. At the end of that session I check out the person's overall reaction to me and comfort with the prospect of our working together. Then I explain that I can understand more fully if I can see the problem in a broader context, and I get agreement to take a complete personal history during our next meeting. At the second session I reiterate that I will be asking lots of questions, I request permission to take confidential notes, and I say that if I ask about anything the client does not yet feel ready to talk about, he or she may simply put me off (no one ever does, but it seems to relieve people to understand that I will not demand premature disclosure).

tion: Individual therapy should be supplemented with medication), or multiple personality disorder (treatment implication: The therapeutic process must emphasize the acknowledgment of all alter personalities and the remembering of a traumatic history).

But for personality problems of a less specific and more complicated nature, no "treatment plan" is usually suggested other than long-term individual therapy or analysis. Hence, the argument has been made that careful diagnostic formulations are unnecessary: If anyone who seeks character change should undergo intensive, open-ended individual psychotherapy, all kinds of character pathologies warrant an identical "prescription." Why diagnose if you already know what the treatment will be? People within as well as outside the psychoanalytic community have made this point. Self psychologists, for example, have been particularly sensitive to the potential misuse of labels and to their possible detraction from the therapist's empathy. Some have contended that the only way to get a true reading of a person's central issues is to establish a therapy relationship and see what develops.

I disagree on the grounds that long-term individual therapy or analysis is not a uniform procedure applied inflexibly regardless of the patient's individual personality. Even the most classical analyst will be more careful of boundaries with a hysterical patient, more pursuant of affect with an obsessional person, more tolerant of silence with a schizoid one, and so forth. Efforts by the therapist to be empathic do not guarantee that such discriminations will automatically be made. Advances in the psychoanalytic understanding of people with psychotic disorders (e.g., Karon & VandenBos, 1981) and borderline conditions (e.g., Kernberg, 1975) have led to treatment approaches that may not be classical analysis but nonetheless are solidly psychodynamic. To use them, one must first recognize one's client as, respectively, essentially psychotic or characterologically borderline. Psychoanalysis and analytic psychotherapies are not monolithic activities foisted in a procrustean way on whatever hapless person comes through the office door. A good diagnostic formulation will inform the therapist's choices in the crucial areas of style of relatedness, tone of interventions, and topics of initial focus.

PROGNOSTIC IMPLICATIONS

The practitioner who expects from a patient with an obsessive *character* the same rate of progress achievable with a person who suddenly developed an intrusive obsession is riding for a painful fall. An appreciation of differences in depth and extensivity of personality problems benefits the clinician as well as the patient. The categories in the *Diagnostic and Statistical Manual of Mental Disorders* (DSM) of the American Psychiatric Assocation sometimes contain implications about the gravity and eventual prognosis of a particular condition—the organization of information along axes was a move in this direction—but sometimes they simply allow for consensually accepted classification with no implicit information about what one can expect from the therapy process.

One of the main themes in this book is the futility of making a "diagnosis" based on the manifest problem alone. A phobia in someone with a depressive or narcissistic personality is a very different phenomenon from a phobia in a characterologically phobic person. One reason psychodiagnosis has a bad name in some quarters is that it has been done badly; people have simply attached a label to the patient's presenting complaint. It is also impossible to do good statistical research on different diagnostic entities if they are being defined strictly by their manifest appearance. As any computer hacker can testify, if garbage goes in, garbage comes out.

One of the strengths of the psychoanalytic tradition is its appreciation of personality structure (see, e.g., Horner, 1990).* To illustrate, at the risk of belaboring a point, if one is working with a bulimic woman who developed her eating disorder when she went away to college and who recognizes her behavior as driven and self-destructive, one holds different expectations from those one would have of a borderline woman who has had binge–purge cycles since elementary school and who regards her behavior as reasonable given social pressures on women to be thin. One may expect to provide lasting help to the first client within a few weeks, while with the second a realistic goal for therapy would be that after a couple of years the patient would clearly see the price her bulimia has extracted and have come to trust the therapist enough to begin trying in earnest to change.

CONSUMER PROTECTION

Conscientious diagnostic practices also encourage ethical communication between practitioners or clinics and their potential clients. This function amounts to a kind of mental health "truth in advertising." On the basis of a careful assessment, one can tell the patient something

*This was not always true. Freud seems originally to have made few distinctions between characterological hysterics and people of other types who had a hysterical reaction, or between what would now be considered an obsessive character at a borderline level of functioning and a person with an obsessional neurosis.

about what to expect and thereby avoid promising too much or giving glib misdirection. I have found that few people are upset upon being told, for example, that given their history and current circumstances, psychotherapy can be expected to take a long time before yielding dependable, internally experienced change. Mostly clients seem encouraged that the therapist appreciates the depth of their problem and is willing to make a commitment to travel the distance. Margaret Little (1990) felt relief when an analyst to whom she had gone for a consultation commented to her, "But you're very ill!" For those few clients who demand a miracle cure and lack the desire or ability to make the commitment it would take to make genuine change, honest feedback from the therapist after the diagnostic period allows them to withdraw gracefully and not waste their own and the practitioner's time looking for magic.

Therapists, whether practicing independently or for a clinic, have an obligation to spell out for their customers what their options are. It is dubiously ethical to say, for instance, "I do psychoanalysis, and if you want to try that, let's start on Monday." Instead, one might say,

> "If you want to work in a problem-solving way on some of the issues in your marriage, I would recommend couples therapy. It seems to me, though, that some of your own personality patterns contribute to your marital difficulties, and if you are willing to go through the long, demanding experience of psychoanalytic treatment, you can reasonably expect to change your part in the scenario permanently. You might want to start with a couples approach; if you find that personality issues of a deeper, more stubborn nature keep coming up, you could come back and consider psychoanalysis."

Therapists working in agencies that are forced by economic necessity to provide only short-term therapy can be tempted to believe and to convey to their patients that because brief therapy is the only kind the facility can provide it must be the treatment of choice. Short-term therapy is, in fact, sometimes preferable for genuinely therapeutic reasons, but one must guard against the human tendency to make a virtue out of a necessity. A good assessment will give the interviewer information about how likely it is that a short-term approach will significantly help a particular person. It is honest, though painful to both parties, to say to a client,

> "I think ideally you would profit from working over a long time period on this problem. It doesn't really admit of quick solutions.

> Unfortunately, this agency does not have the resources to give you what you need. It can offer the following options, some of which may be of some use, but to get the result you want is impossible in our circumstances."

The alternative, to make oneself and/or the client believe that one can do effective therapy with anyone despite obvious institutional limitations, contributes to self-blame in both participants ("What's the matter with me that significant progress, which I was led to believe should be possible with limited treatment, has not yet taken place?").

Converse clinical situations are also easy to find. In the the era some refer to as the golden age of psychoanalysis, many people stayed in therapy for years when they might have been better off at a drug treatment center or in a support group or with therapy and medication. A careful diagnostic evaluation reduces the likelihood that someone will spend years in a professional relationship from which he or she is deriving little or no benefit.

THE COMMUNICATION OF EMPATHY

The term "empathy" has been watered down to virtual uselessness in recent times. Still, there is no other existing word that gets at the quality of "feeling *with*" rather than "feeling *for*" that constituted the original reason for distinguishing between empathy and sympathy (or compassion, pity, concern, interest, and similar terms that imply a degree of defensive distancing from the suffering person). "Empathy" is regularly misused to mean warm, accepting, sympathetic reactions to the patient no matter what he or she is communicating emotionally. I want to stress that I use the term in this section and throughout this book in its literal sense of the capacity to feel emotionally what the client is feeling.

I have often heard my patients who are also therapists express brutal self-criticism about their "lack of empathy" when they are having a hostile or frightened reaction to one of their clients. What they mean is that they wish they did not feel such powerful negative affects; it is unpleasant to acknowledge the extent to which the therapeutic enterprise can include primitive levels of hatred and misery that no one warned us about when we decided to go into the business of helping people. Therapists in this condition may be regarded as suffering from a high rather than a low degree of empathy, for if they are really feeling *with* their patient, they are feeling his or her hostility, terror, misery, and other wretched states of mind. Affects of people in therapy can be intensely negative, and they induce in others anything but a warm response.

That one should not *behave* in accordance with such emotional reactions is obvious even to a completely untrained person. That such reactions are potentially of the greatest value is less obvious, but true. When observed in the self, they are essential contributants to making a good diagnosis, on the basis of which one can choose a way of addressing a client's unhappiness that will be received as genuinely empathic rather than as rote compassion, professionally dispensed irrespective of the unique identity of the person in the other chair.

For example, someone who is experienced by an interviewer as manipulative may have an essentially hysterical character or may be sociopathic, among other possibilities. Therapeutic communication would depend on the clinician's diagnostic hypothesis. For the hysterical client, one would be helpful by showing understanding of the degree of fear and the sense of powerlessness that pervade his or her emotional experience. With the sociopath, one would want to convey a wry appreciation for his or her skills as a con artist, along with the implication that one has not been taken in. If the therapist has not gone beyond the label "manipulative," with no more sophisticated diagnostic context in which to understand the phenomenon, it is unlikely that he or she will be able to offer the client any deep hope of being understood. If one overgeneralizes—seeing all manipulative clients as hysterics, or, alternatively, as sociopaths—one will make therapeutic contact only part of the time. A hysterically organized person may feel devastated to be misunderstood as executing a cynical power play when he or she feels desperately in need of comfort for the frightened child within; a sociopathic person will have nothing but contempt for the therapist who misses the centrality of his or her need to "get over" on others.

Another example of the utility of diagnosis in enabling the therapist to convey empathy can be found in the common situation of a borderline patient's calling or coming to an emergency service with a threat of suicide. Emergency mental health workers are ordinarily trained in a generic crisis-intervention model of response rather than in an explicitly diagnostic one, and in most circumstances, the crisis-intervention model serves them well. But in the case of borderline patients, it does not, as is evidenced by the gnawing frustration emergency personnel readily express when interviewed about this portion of their clientele (Shinefield, 1989).

For most people who threaten suicide, the best response is the one suggested by generic crisis-intervention strategies: Assess suicidality by inquiring about the plan, means, and lethality of the means (Litman &

Farberow, 1970). People with borderline personality organization, however, tend to talk suicide not when they actually want to die but when they are feeling what Masterson (1976) has aptly called "abandonment depression." They need to counteract their panic and despair with the sense that someone cares about how bad they feel. Typically, they learned in their families of origin that no one pays attention to your feelings unless you are threatening mayhem. Assessment of suicidal intent only exasperates them, since the interviewer is, in terms of the patients' not-very-conscious subjective experience, distracted by the *content* of their threat when they feel desperate to talk about its *context*.

A clinician's effort to follow standard crisis-intervention procedures (e.g., Kalafat, 1984) without a diagnostic sensibility can be countertherapeutic, even dangerous, since it can frustrate such a patient to the point of feeling that he or she must *demonstrate* rather than discuss suicide in order to be heard. It also leaves the therapist hating the patient, since the person seems to be asking for help and then rejecting the helper's earnest efforts to give it (Frank et al., 1952). Emergency clinicians trained in identifying borderline clients become adept at responding to the painful affects behind the suicidal threat rather than doing an immediate suicide inventory; paradoxically, they probably prevent more self-destructive acts than colleagues who automatically evaluate suicidality. They may also have fewer demoralizing experiences of hating clients for "not cooperating" or "not being truthful."

FORESTALLING FLIGHTS FROM TREATMENT

An issue related to conveying empathy involves keeping the skittish patient in treatment. Many people seek out professional help and then become frightened that attachment to the therapist represents a grave danger. The hypomanic person, for example, tends to bolt from relationships as soon as they stimulate dependency longings because early experiences of depending on others came out disastrously. Counterdependent people, whose self-esteem requires denial of their need for care from others, will also tend to rationalize running from treatment when an attachment forms because they feel humiliated when implicitly acknowledging the emotional importance of another person.

Experienced diagnosticians generally know by the end of the initial interview whether they are dealing with a person whose character presses for flight. It is not only reassuring to the hypomanic or counterdependent person for the therapist to comment on how hard it will be for him or her to find the courage to stay in treatment, since the emotional understanding in such a statement rings true, but it also increases the probability that the patient will resist the temptation to flee.

FRINGE BENEFITS

People are much more comfortable when they sense that their interviewer is at ease. A therapeutic relationship is likely to get off to a good start if the client feels the clinician's curiosity, relative lack of anxiety, and conviction that the appropriate treatment can begin once the patient is better understood. A therapist who feels pressure to begin *doing therapy* before having come to a good provisional understanding of the patient's dynamics and character structure is, like a driver with some sense of direction but no road map, going to suffer needless anxiety.* The patient will feel it and will wonder about the practitioner's competence. This self-replicating cycle can lead to all sorts of basically iatrogenic problems.

Perhaps one source of some therapists' discomfort with diagnosis is the fear of misdiagnosis. Fortunately, a clinician's original formulation does not have to be "right" to provide many of the benefits mentioned here. A diagnostic hypothesis has a way of grounding the interviewer in a focused, low-anxiety activity whether or not it turns out to be supported by later clinical evidence. Moreover, the professional can consider a formulation tentatively, with no loss to the process. The patient will often be grateful for the practitioner's avoidance of pretension and demonstration of care in considering different possibilities.

The diagnostic enterprise also gives both participants in the process something to do before the client knows the therapist well enough to open up spontaneously without the comforting structure of being questioned. Therapists tend to underestimate the importance of this "settling in" process. Often, it allows the therapist to get information that will become hard for the patient to share later in treatment, when the development of strong transference reactions may

*Of course, one *is* doing therapy during a diagnostic evaluation; the process itself contributes to a working alliance without which "treatment" is an empty ritual. But the formal agreement about how the parties will proceed, what the boundaries and respective responsibilities of the participants will be, and so on, should derive from a diagnostic formulation.

inhibit the free expression of some topics. For example, most adults can answer questions about their sexual practices with relative frankness when talking to a professional who is still a stranger. But once the therapist has started to feel like one's prudish mother or moralistic father, the words flow anything but easily. Later in treatment when the transference has heated up, the client may be comforted to remember that in one of the first meetings with this person whose condemnation is now feared, the client had talked about all kinds of intimate matters without incurring either shock or disapproval. The patient's contrasting experiences of the therapist during the diagnostic phase and later accentuates the fact that the transference *is* a transference (i.e., not a fully accurate reading of the therapist's personality). This insight is crucial to the eventual success of a psychoanalytic therapy.

Finally, a positive side effect of diagnostic work is its contribution to the therapist's ability to maintain his or her self-esteem by pursuing realistic goals. To do effective psychotherapy, one must first of all stay in business. Among the occupational hazards of a career in mental health are feelings of fraudulence, worries about treatment failures, and eventual burnout. These processes are greatly accelerated by unrealistic expectations. Practitioner demoralization and emotional withdrawal have far-reaching implications not only for affected clinicians but also for patients who have come to depend on them.

If one knows, say, that one's depressed patient is a borderline rather than a neurotic-level depressive, one will not be surprised if during the second year of treatment he or she makes a suicide gesture. Once depressed clients with borderline structure start to have real hope of change, they often panic and become suicidal in an effort to protect themselves from the devastation that would ensue if they let themselves hope and then were traumatically disappointed by yet another important person. Issues surrounding this kind of suicidal preoccupation can be interpreted, providing emotional relief for both client and therapist (possible interpretative foci include the felt dangers of hope and disappointment just mentioned, guilt toward original love objects over the transfer of emotional investment from them to the therapist, and related magical fantasies that one must expiate such guilt by a ritual attempt to die).

Over many years of consulting with colleagues, I have regretfully noted the frequency with which basically competent, devoted, and intuitively gifted therapists lose confidence and find rationalizations for getting rid of ostensibly suicidal borderline patients at precisely the moment in treatment when the person is expressing, in an identifiably provocative borderline way, how important and effective the treatment is becoming. Typically, the session preceding the suicide gesture was one in which the patient expressed trust or hope for the first time, and the therapist became excited after so many months of arduous work with a difficult, oppositional client. Then with the suicide gesture the therapist's own hopes crumple. He or she decides that the excitement was illusory and self-serving, and that the patient's deterioration is evidence that the therapeutic prospects are nil after all. (Examples of therapist thoughts at this juncture are: Maybe my Psych 101 teacher was right: Psychoanalytic therapy is a waste of time. Maybe I should transfer this person to a therapist of the other sex. Maybe I should ask a psychiatrist with pharmacological enthusiasms to take over the case. Maybe I should transfer the patient to the Chronic Group.) Therapists, who are themselves often rather depressive people, are quick to turn any apparent treatment setback into an opportunity for self-censure. Sufficient diagnostic facility can make enough of a dent in this propensity to allow reason to prevail and keep one in the clinical trenches.

LIMITS TO THE UTILITY OF DIAGNOSIS

For clinicians doing predominantly long-term or open-ended psychoanalytic therapy, the value of careful assessment is greatest in two instances: (1) at the very beginning of treatment, for the reasons given above, and (2) at times of crisis or stalemate, when a rethinking of the kind of personality structure one faces may hold the key to effective changes in technique. Once the therapist has a good "feel" for the person he or she is working with, and the work is going well, the disposition to think diagnostically should recede. A therapist who stays preoccupied with getting just the right diagnostic handle on his or her patient will burden the therapeutic relationship with an intellectualized atmosphere.

Finally, I should mention that people exist for whom the existing developmental and typological categories of personality are at best a poor fit. When any label obscures more than it illuminates, the practitioner is better off discarding it and relying on common sense and human decency, like the lost sailor who throws away a useless navigational chart and reverts to orienting by a few familiar stars. And even when an official psychoanalytic category is a good match to a particular patient, there are such wide disparities among people on dimensions other than their developmental level and defensive style that empathy and healing may be best pursued via attunement to some of these. A deeply religious person of any personality type will need first for the therapist to demonstrate respect for his or her depth of conviction (see Lovinger, 1984); diagnosis-influenced interventions will be of value, but only secondarily. Similarly, it is sometimes more important, at least in the early phases of developing a therapeutic relationship, to consider the emotional implications of a person's age, race, ethnicity, class background, physical disability, political attitudes, or sexual orientation than it is to appreciate his or her appropriate diagnostic category.

Assessment of character structure is always provisional and never definitive; an ongoing willingness to reassess one's initial diagnosis in the light of new information is part of being optimally therapeutic. As treatment proceeds with any individual human being, the oversimplification inherent in our diagnostic concepts becomes startlingly clear. People are much more complex than our categories admit. Hence, even the most sophisticated personality assessment can become an obstacle to the therapist's perceiving critical nuances of the patient's unique material. Notwithstanding the advantages of the diagnostic process, it should not be applied beyond its usefulness.

SUGGESTIONS FOR FURTHER READING

My favorite book on interviewing, mostly because of its tone, is Harry Stack Sullivan's (1954) *The Psychiatric Interview*. Another classic work that is full of useful background and wise technical recommendations is *The Initial Interview in Psychiatric Practice* by Gill, Newman, and Redlich (1954). I have already mentioned my admiration for the work of MacKinnon and Michels (1971), whose basic premises are similar to the ones informing this text. Gabbard (1990), in *Psychodynamic Psychiatry in Clinical Practice*, has accomplished a masterful integration of dynamic and structural diagnosis and the *Diagnostic and Statistical Manual of Mental Disorders*, third edition (DSM-III-R; American Psychiatric Assocation, 1987). Kernberg's (1984) *Severe Personality Disorders* contains a short but comprehensive section on diagnosis and, in particular, on the structural interview. Most beginning therapists find Kernberg hard to read, but this section is lucidly written and seamlessly fills in the gap between the classic texts above and more contemporary psychoanalytic theorizing about personality structure.

2

Psychoanalytic Character Diagnosis

Classical psychoanalytic conceptualization approached the study of character or personality in two very different ways, each deriving from an early theoretical model of individual development. In the era of Freud's original *drive theory*, an attempt was made to understand personality on the basis of fixation (at what early developmental phase is this person psychologically stuck?). Later, with the development of *ego psychology*, character was conceived as expressing the operation of particular styles of defense (what are this person's typical ways of avoiding anxiety?). This second way of understanding character was not in conflict with the first; it provided a different set of ideas and metaphors for comprehending what was meant by a type of personality, and it added to the concepts of drive theory certain assumptions about how we each develop our characteristic adaptive and defensive patterns.

An appreciation of these two approaches is at the center of my own visualization of character possibilities. I shall also try to show how the more recent developments in British object relations theory (and its American cousin, interpersonal psychoanalysis) and in the self psychology movement can illuminate aspects of character organization. In addition, my own understanding of personality and diagnosis has been enriched by less clinically influential psychodynamic formulations such as Henry Murray's "personology" (e.g., 1938), Silvan Tomkins's (1992) "script theory," and the ideas developed by Weiss and Sampson and the Mount Zion Psychotherapy Research Group (e.g., 1986), sometimes under the label of "control–mastery" theory.

The discerning reader may note that I am applying to the diagnostic enterprise several different models and theories within psychoanalysis that are held by some scholars to be mutually exclusive or essentially contradictory in nature. Because this book is intended for therapists, and because I am temperamentally more of a synthesizer than a critic or distinction maker, I have not addressed the question of which analytic model is most scientifically or heuristically or metapsychologically defensible. In this position I owe a substantial intellectual debt to Fred Pine (1985, 1990), whose efforts to integrate drive, ego, object, and self theories have been of incalculable clinical value. I am not minimizing the importance of critically evaluating competing theories. My decision not to do so derives from the specifically *clinical* purpose of this book and from my observation that most therapists seek to assimilate a diversity of models and metaphors, whether or not they are controversial or conceptually problematic in some way. Every new development in psychoanalytic theory offers practitioners a fresh way of trying to communicate to troubled people their wish to understand and help. Effective psychodynamic therapists—and I am assuming that effective therapists and brilliant theorists are overlapping but not identical samples—seem to me more often to draw freely from many psychoanalytic sources than to become ideologically wedded to one or two favored theories. They mistrust those whose professional identity centers on the defense of one way of thinking and working. Adherence to dogma is found in some analysts, but its existence has not enriched our clinical theory, nor has it contributed to the esteem in which our field is held by those who value humility about the extent of contemporary understanding and who appreciate ambiguity and complexity (cf. Goldberg, 1990b).

Different clients have a way of making different theories or models relevant: One person stimulates in the therapist thoughts of concepts promulgated by Kernberg; another sounds like a type of person described by Horney; still another has an unconscious fantasy life so classically Freudian that the therapist starts to wonder if the patient boned up on early drive theory before entering treatment. Stolorow and Atwood (1979) have shed considerable light on the emotional processes that contribute to the development of a theory of personality, and they have made a persuasive case that the central character themes in the theorist's life become the issues emphasized in that person's theories of general psychology, personality formation, psychopathology, and psychotherapy. Considered in this light, it is not surprising that we have so many alternative conceptions. And even if some of them are *logically* at odds with one another, I would argue that they are not *phenomenologically* so, and that they apply differentially to different kinds of people.

Having stated my own biases and predilections, I now offer a brief and necessarily oversimplified summary of diagnostically significant models within the psychoanalytic tradition. They are covered in order to give the student with minimal exposure to psychoanalytic theory some basis for comprehending the categories that are second nature for analytically trained therapists. I will also specify some underlying assumptions inherent in these models before applying them more or less uncritically to various personality constellations.

CLASSICAL FREUDIAN DRIVE THEORY

Freud's original theory of personality development was a biologically derived model that stressed the centrality of instinctual processes and construed human beings as passing through an orderly progression of bodily preoccupations from oral to anal to phallic and genital concerns. It was theorized that in infancy and early childhood, the person's natural dispositions concern basic survival issues, which were experienced at first in a deeply sensual way via nursing and the mother's other activities with the infant's body and later in the child's fantasy life about birth and death and the sexual tie between its parents.

Babies, and therefore the infantile aspects of self that live on in adults, were seen as uninhibited seekers of instinctual gratification, with some individual differences in the strength of the drives. Appropriate caregiving was construed as oscillating sensitively between, on the one hand, sufficient gratification to create emotional security and pleasure and, on the other, developmentally appropriate frustration such that the child would learn in titrated doses how to replace the *pleasure principle* ("I want all my gratifications, including mutually contradictory ones, right now!") with the *reality principle* ("Some gratifications are problematic, and the best are worth waiting for"). Freud talked little about the specific contributions of his patients' parents to their psychopathology. But when he did, he saw parental failures as involving either excessive gratification of drives, such that nothing had impelled the child to move on developmentally, or excessive deprivation of them, such that the child's capacity to absorb frustrating realities was overwhelmed. Parenting was thus a balancing act between indulgence and inhibition—an intuitively resonant model for most mothers and fathers, to be sure.

Drive theory postulated that if a child was either overfrustrated or overgratified at an early psychosexual stage (as per the interaction of the child's constitutional endowment and the parents' responsiveness), he or she would become "fixated" on the issues of that stage. Character was seen as expressing the long-term effects of this fixation: If an adult man had a depressive personality, it was theorized that he had been either neglected or overindulged in his first year and a half or so (the oral phase of development); if he was obsessional, it was inferred that there had been problems between roughly $1^{1}/_{2}$ and 3 (the anal phase); if he was hysterical, he had met either rejection or overstimulating seductiveness, or both, between about 3 and 6, when the child's interest has turned to the genitals and sexuality (the "phallic" phase, in Freud's male-oriented language, the later part of which came to be known as the "oedipal" phase because the sexual competition issues and associated fantasies characteristic of that stage parallel the themes in the ancient Greek story of Oedipus). It was not uncommon in the early days of the psychoanalytic movement to hear someone referred to as having an oral, anal, or phallic character, depending on which issues seemed central to him or her. Later, as the theory became more sophisticated, analysts would specify whether it was oral dependent or oral aggressive (sucking versus biting aspects of orality being seen as preponderant, respectively), anal retentive or anal expulsive, early or late oral, anal, or phallic, and so forth.

Lest this oversimplified account sound entirely fanciful, I should stress that the theory did not spring full-blown from Sigmund Freud's fevered imagination; there was an accretion of data that influenced and supported it, collected not only by Freud but by his colleagues as well. In Wilhelm Reich's (1933) *Character Analysis*, the drive theory approach to personality diagnosis reached its zenith. Although the language of that book sounds archaic to most contemporary students, it is full of fascinating insights about character types, and its observations still frequently strike a chord in the sympathetic reader. Ultimately, the effort to understand character entirely on the basis of instinctual fixation proved disappointing. Freud's colleague Karl Abraham devoted his formidable intellect to the task of correlating psychological phenomena with particular stages and substages, yet he failed eventually to achieve a satisfactory set of conclusions about such relationships. Although the drive-based fixation model has never been rejected by most psychoanalysts as completely misconceived, it has been supplemented with other ways of understanding character that have more explanatory power.

One way in which the original drive theory model is retained or echoed to some degree is in the tendency of psychodynamic practitioners to continue to think in terms of maturational stages and to understand psychopathology in terms of developmental arrest or conflict at a particular phase. Although few analysts now reduce all phenomena to classical drive categories, most assume a basic stage theory of development. Efforts like those of Daniel Stern (1985) to rethink the whole concept of predictable developmental phases have met with respectful interest, but these new ways of thinking do not seem to have deterred many clinicians from construing their patients' problems in terms of some unfinished developmental task, the normal source of which is seen as a certain phase of early childhood.

In the 1950s and 1960s, Erik Erikson's reformulation of the psychosexual stages according to both the interpersonal and intrapsychic tasks of each phase received a great deal of attention. Although Erikson's work (e.g., 1950) is usually seen as prototypical of the ego psychology tradition, his stage theory echoes many assumptions in Freud's drive model of development. One of Erikson's most appealing additions to Freudian theory (Erikson saw his conceptualization as supplementing rather than replacing Freud's) was the renaming of the early stages in the interest of modifying Freud's biologism.

The oral phase became understood by its condition of total dependency, in which the establishment of *basic trust* (or the lack thereof) was the specific outcome of the gratification or deprivation of the oral drive. The anal phase was conceptualized as involving the attainment of *autonomy* (or, if poorly navigated, of shame and doubt). The prototypical struggle of this phase might be the mastery of toilet functions, as Freud had stressed, but it also involved a vast range of issues relevant to the child's learning self-control and coming to terms with the expectations of the family and the larger society. The oedipal phase was seen as a critical time for developing a sense of basic *efficacy* ("initiative versus guilt") and a sense of pleasure in *identification* with one's love objects. Erikson extended the idea of developmental phases and tasks throughout the life span. He also broke down the earliest phases into subdivisions (oral-incorporative, oral-expulsive; anal-incorporative, anal-expulsive).* In the 1950s, Harry Stack Sullivan (e.g., 1953) offered another stage theory, one that stressed communicative achievements like speech and play rather than drive satisfaction.

*For some reason, probably including its muting of Freud's emphasis on our animal nature, Erikson's theory got into academic curricula, unlike much subsequent analytic work of comparable quality. The isolation of analysts in freestanding training institutes has been convenient for them in some ways, but, overall, the estrangement between psychoanalysis and academic psychology has been a great misfortune. Most university-based psychologists, even those who routinely teach Freud, Jung, Adler, and Erikson, are unfamiliar with the last 40 years of psychoanalytic theory. And analysts have been deprived of the stimulation and discipline of working in the company of diverse and skeptical colleagues, many of whom are interested in questions of some relevance to analytic theory.

Like Erikson, he believed that personality continues to develop and change well beyond the first 6 or so years that Freud had stressed as the bedrock of adult character.

Margaret Mahler's work (e.g., Mahler, 1968, 1972a, 1972b; Mahler, Pine, & Bergman, 1975) on the phases and subphases of the separation–individuation process, a task that reaches its initial resolution by about the age of 3, was a further step in conceptualizing processes that are relevant to eventual personality structure. Her theory is generally placed within the object relations area, but its implicit assumptions of fixation owe a debt to Freud's developmental model. As Erikson subdivided the oral phase, Mahler broke down what were to Freud the first two stages, oral and anal, and looked at the infant's movement from a state of relative unawareness of others (the autistic phase, lasting about 6 weeks) to one of symbiotic relatedness (lasting over the next 2 or so years—this period itself subdivided into "hatching," "practicing," "rapprochement," and "on the way to object constancy" subphases) to a condition of relative psychological separation and individuation.

These contributions were greeted eagerly by therapists. With the post-Freudian advances in stage theories, they had fresh ways of understanding how their patients had gotten "stuck." They could now also offer interpretations and hypotheses to their self-critical clients that went beyond speculations about their having been weaned too early or too late, or toilet trained too harshly or with too much laxity, or seduced or rejected during the oedipal phase. Rather, patients could be told that their predicaments reflected family processes that had made it difficult for them to feel security or autonomy or pleasure in their identifications (Erikson), or that fate had handed them a childhood devoid of the crucially important preadolescent "chum" (Sullivan), or that their mother's hospitalization when they were 2 had overwhelmed the rapprochement process normal for that age and necessary for optimal separation (Mahler). For therapists, such alternative models were not just interesting intellectually, they provided ways of helping people to understand and find compassion for themselves—in contradistinction to the usual internal explanations that human beings generate about their more incomprehensible qualities (viz., "I'm bad," "I'm ugly," "I'm lazy and undisciplined," "I'm just inherently rejectable," "I'm dangerous," etc.).

Many contemporary commentators have said at one time or another that our propensity to construe problems in developmental terms smacks of reductionism and is only questionably supported by clinical and empirical evidence (e.g., Kernberg, 1984). Others have pointed to different patterns and stages of psychological development in non-Western cultures (e.g., Roland, 1988). Still, the tendency of therapists to see psychological phenomena as residues of problems at a particular maturational phase persists. Perhaps this persistence reflects the fact that the general developmental model has about it both a kind of elegant simplicity and an overall humanity that appeals to the mental health community. There is a generosity of spirit, a kind of "There but for fortune go I" quality, to believing there is one archetypal, progressive, universal pattern of development, and that under unfortunate circumstances, any of us could have gotten stymied at any of its phases. It may not be a *sufficient* explanation for personality types or psychopathology, but it feels to most practitioners like a necessary *part* of the picture. As readers may note in the Chapters 3 and 4, one of the axes on which I have aligned diagnostic data contains this developmental bias, in the form of symbiotic (psychotic), separation–individuation (borderline), and oedipal (neurotic) levels of personality organization and psychopathology.

EGO PSYCHOLOGY

With the publication of *The Ego and the Id* (1923), Freud introduced his structural model, and a new theoretical era began. Analytic investigators shifted their interest from the *contents* of the unconscious to the *processes* by which those contents were kept out of consciousness. Arlow and Brenner (1964) have argued cogently for the greater explanatory power of the structural theory, with its emphasis on understanding ego processes, but there were also practical clinical reasons for therapists to welcome the changes of focus from id to ego operations and from deeply unconscious material to those wishes, fears, and fantasies that were closer to consciousness and accessible if one worked with the defensive functions of a patient's ego. A crash course in the structural model and its associated assumptions follows, with apologies to sophisticated readers for the brevity with which complicated concepts are covered.

The *id* was the term Freud used for the part of the mind that contains primitive drives, impulses, prerational strivings, wish–fear combinations, and fantasies. It seeks only immediate gratification and is totally "selfish" in the lay sense, operating according to the pleasure principle. Cognitively, it is preverbal, expressing itself in images and symbols. It is also prelogical, having no concept of time, mortality, limitation, or the impossibility that opposites can coexist. Freud called this primitive kind of cognition, which survives in the language of dreams, jokes, and hallucinations, *primary process thought.*

The id is entirely unconscious. Its existence and power can, however, be inferred from *derivatives*, such as thoughts, acts, and emotions. In Freud's time, it was a common cultural conceit that modern, "civilized" human beings were rationally motivated creatures who had moved beyond the sensibilities of the "lesser" animals and of non-Western "savages." (Freud's emphasis on our animality, including the dominance of sex as a motivator, was one reason for the degree of outrage that his ideas provoked in the Victorian and post-Victorian eras.)

The *ego* was Freud's name for a set of functions that adapt to life's exigencies, finding ways that are acceptable within one's family to handle id strivings. It develops continuously throughout one's lifetime but most rapidly in childhood, starting in earliest infancy (cf. Hartmann, 1958). The ego operates according to the reality principle and is the seedbed of *secondary process thought* (sequential, logical, reality-oriented types of cognition). It thus mediates between the demands of the id and the constraints of reality and ethics. It has both conscious and unconscious aspects. The conscious ones are similar to what most of us mean when we use the term "self" or "I," while the unconscious aspects include defensive processes like repression, displacement, rationalization, and sublimation. With the structural theory, analytic therapists had a new language for making sense of some kinds of character pathology; namely, that everyone develops ego defenses that are adaptive within his or her childhood setting but may turn out to be maladaptive later in the adult world beyond the family.

One important aspect of this model for both diagnosis and therapy is the portrayal of the ego as having a range of operations, from deeply unconscious (e.g., primitive feeling reactions to events, counteracted by a powerful defense like denial) to fully conscious. During the process of psychoanalytic treatment, it was noted, the "observing ego," the part of the self that is conscious and rational and can comment on emotional experience, makes an alliance with the practitioner to understand the total self together, while the "experiencing ego" holds a more visceral sense of what is going on in the therapy relationship. This "therapeutic split in the ego" (Sterba, 1934) was seen as a necessary condition of effective analytic therapy. If the patient was unable to talk from an observing position about less rational, more "gut-level" emotional reactions, the first task of the therapist was to help the patient develop that capacity. The presence or absence of an observing ego became of paramount diagnostic value, since the existence of a symptom or problem that was dystonic (alien) to the observing ego was found to be treatable much faster than a similar-looking problem that the patient had never regarded as noteworthy. This insight persists among analytic diagnosticians in the language of whether a problem or personality style is "ego alien" or "ego syntonic."

The basic role of the ego in perceiving and adapting to reality is the source of the useful psychoanalytic phrase "ego strength," meaning the person's capacity to acknowledge reality, even when it is extremely unpleasant, without resorting to more primitive defenses like denial. Over the years of the development of psychoanalytic clinical theory, a distinction emerged between the more archaic and the more mature defenses, the former characterized by the psychological avoidance or radical distortion of disturbing facts of life, and the latter involving more of an accommodation to reality.

Another important clinical assumption that flowed from the ego psychology movement was the belief that psychological health involved not only having *mature* defenses but also being able to use a *variety* of defensive processes (cf. Shapiro, 1965). In other words, it was recognized that the person who habitually reacts to every stress with, say, projection, or with rationalization, is not as well off psychologically as the person who uses different ways of coping, depending on circumstances. Concepts like "rigidity" of personality and "character armor" (W. Reich, 1933) express this idea that mental health has something to do with emotional flexibility.

Freud coined the term *superego* for the part of the self that oversees things, especially from a moral perspective.* Roughly synonymous with "conscience," the superego is the part of the self that congratulates us for doing our best and criticizes us when we fall short of our own standards. It is a part of the ego, although it is experientially felt as separate from it. Freud believed that the superego was formed mainly during the oedipal period, through identification with parental values, but most contemporary analysts regard it as originating much earlier in primitive infantile notions of good and bad.

The superego is, like the ego to which it belongs, partly conscious and partly unconscious. Again, the assessment of whether an inappropriately punitive superego was experienced by the patient as ego alien or ego syntonic was eventually understood to have important prognostic implications. The client who announces that she is evil because she has had bad thoughts about her father is a very different kind of person from the one who reports that a part of her seems to *feel* she is evil when she entertains such thoughts. Both may be depressive,

*Note that Freud wrote in simple, non-jargon-laden language: Id, ego, and superego translate as "it," "me," and "above me." Few contemporary psychoanalytic theorists, it is sad to note, write with anything like his grace and stylistic simplicity.

self-attacking people, but the magnitude of the first woman's problem is so much greater than that of the second that it warrants a different level of classification.

Again, there was a lot of clinical benefit to the development of the concept of the superego. Therapy went beyond simply trying to make the patient's unconscious conscious; the practitioner could view the therapeutic task as also involving the modification of the client's superego. A common therapeutic aim, especially throughout the first half of the 20th century, when adults in the middle and upper-middle classes tended to have been reared in ways that produced unreasonably harsh superegos, was helping one's patients reevaluate overly stringent moral standards (e.g., antisexual strictures or internal chastisement for thoughts, feelings, and fantasies that were universal). Psychoanalysis as a movement—and Freud in particular—was emphatically not hedonistic, but the modification of inhumanly harsh superegos was one of its frequent goals. In practice, this tended to encourage more rather than less ethical behavior by patients, since people with condemnatory superegos frequently behave in defiance of them, especially in states of intoxication or in situations in which acting out can be rationalized. Efforts to expose the operations of the id, to bring a person's unconscious life into the light of day, had little therapeutic benefit if the patient reacted to such illumination as revealing evidence of his or her depravity.

Ego psychology's achievement in describing processes that are now subsumed under the general rubric of "defense" is centrally relevant to character diagnosis. Just as we may attempt to understand people in terms of the developmental phase that exemplifies their current struggle, we can sort them out according to their characteristic modes of handling anxiety. The idea that a primary function of the ego was to defend the self against anxiety arising from either powerful instinctual strivings (the id), upsetting reality experiences (the ego), or guilt feelings and associated fantasies (the superego) was most elegantly elaborated in Anna Freud's (1936) *The Ego and the Mechanisms of Defense.*

Sigmund Freud's original ideas had included the notion that anxious reactions were *caused* by defenses, most notably repression (motivated forgetting). Bottled-up feelings were seen as causing inner tension that pressed for discharge, experienced as anxiety. When Freud made the shift to the structural theory he reversed himself, deciding that repression was a *response* to anxiety, and that it was only one of several ways in which human beings try to avoid an unbearable sense of irrational fear. He began construing psychopathology as a state in which a defensive effort had not worked, where the anxiety was felt despite the operation of one's habitual means of handling it, or where the behavior that masked the anxiety was self-destructive.

In Chapters 5 and 6 I shall cover the defenses, the ones identified by Sigmund and Anna Freud as well as by others, including some preverbal, archaic processes first elucidated by Melanie Klein. This summary will provide enough background for the subsequent portrayal of different character types.

THE OBJECT RELATIONS TRADITION

As the ego psychologists were mapping out a theoretical understanding of patients whose psychological processes were illuminated by the structural model, some theorists in Europe, especially in England, were looking at different kinds of unconscious processes and their manifestations. Some, like Klein (e.g., 1932, 1957), worked both with children and with patients whom Freud had regarded as too disturbed to be suitable for analysis.* These representatives of the "British School" of psychoanalysis were finding that they needed another language to describe the processes they observed. Their work was controversial for many years, partly due to the personalities, loyalties, and convictions of those involved, and partly because it is hard to write persuasively about inferred primitive phenomena. Object relations theorists struggled with how to put preverbal, prerational processes into words governed by reason. Although their respect for the power of unconscious dynamics made them clearly analytic, they disputed Freud on certain central issues.

W. R. D. Fairbairn (e.g., 1954), for example, rejected Freud's biologism outright, proposing that people do not seek drive satisfaction so much as they seek relationships. In other words, a baby is not so much focused on *getting mother's milk* as it is on having the experience of *being nursed*, with the sense of warmth and attachment that is part of that experience. Psychoanalysts influenced by Sandor Ferenczi (such as Michael and Alice Balint, sometimes referred to as belonging to the "Hungarian School" of psychoanalysis) pursued the study of primary experiences of love, loneliness, creativity, and integrity of self that do not fit neatly within the confines of the structural theory. People in this orientation put their emphasis not so much on what drive had been mishandled in a person's childhood, or on what developmental

*Freud was more conservative than many of his successors about the power of analytic therapy to effect significant changes, especially in those suffering from psychotic illnesses.

phase had been poorly negotiated, or on what ego defenses had predominated. Rather, the emphasis was on what the main objects* in the child's world had been like, how they had been experienced,† how they and felt aspects of them had been internalized, and how internal images and representations of them lived on in the unconscious lives of adults. In the object relations tradition, oedipal issues loom less large than themes of separation and individuation. Interestingly, the work of Otto Rank (e.g., 1929, 1945) presaged much of the object relations work that came after his time. However, because Rank left the analytic mainstream after his painful break with Freud, many of his most important observations had to be rediscovered (Menaker, 1982).

Freud's own work was not inhospitable to the development and elaboration of object relations theory. His appreciation of the importance of the child's actual and experienced infantile objects comes through in his concept of the "family romance," in his recognition of how different the oedipal phase could be for the child depending on the personalities of the parents, and also in his increasing emphasis on relationship factors in treatment. Richard Sterba, one of the last analysts who knew Freud well, has commented (1982) on how much object relations theory has enriched Freud's original observations, implying that Freud would have welcomed this direction in psychoanalysis.

By the middle of the 20th century, object relational formulations from the British and Hungarian schools were paralleled to a striking degree by developments among therapists in the United States who

*The term "object relations" is unfortunate, since "object" in psychoanalese usually means "person." It derives from Freud's early explication of instincts as having a *source* (some bodily tension), an *aim* (some kind of biological satisfaction), and an *object* (typically a person, since the drives Freud saw as central to one's psychology were the sexual and aggressive ones). This phrase remains in use despite its unattractive, mechanistic connotations because of this derivation and also because there are instances in which an important "object" to someone is a nonhuman attachment (e.g., the American flag to a patriot; footwear to a shoe fetishist) or is *part* of a human being (the mother's breast, the father's smile, the sister's voice, etc.).

†The reason analysts distinguish between actual objects and the child's experience of them is that children, especially infants, may misperceive important family figures and their motives, and retain an internalization of the misperception. For example, a girl whose father goes off to war when she is 2 years old will inevitably experience him as having rejected and abandoned her, and she may later cling internally to the belief that she was not very important to him. Alternatively, a boy may see a grandmother as a virtual saint because she was warm to him, yet the same grandmother may realistically be a destructive person who acted out her competition with her daughter in ways that undermined the boy's mother and foiled the mother's attempts to attach affectionately to her son. His internal objects will include a loving grandmother and a cold rejecting mother.

identified themselves as "interpersonal psychoanalysts." These theorists, who included Harry Stack Sullivan, Erich Fromm, Karen Horney, Clara Thompson, Otto Will, Frieda Fromm-Reichmann, and others were, like their European colleagues, trying to work psychodynamically with more seriously disturbed patients. They differed from object relations analysts across the Atlantic mainly in the extent to which they emphasized the internalized nature of early object relations: The American-based therapists tended to put less stress on the stubbornly persisting unconscious images of early objects and aspects of objects.

Freud had made a shift toward an interpersonal theory of treatment when he stopped regarding his patients' transferences as distortions to be explained away and began seeing them as offering the emotional context necessary for healing: "It is impossible to destroy anyone *in absentia* or *in effigie*" (1912, p. 108). The conviction that the emotional connection between therapist and client constitutes the most vital curative factor in therapy is widely held by contemporary practitioners who identify themselves as relational in orientation. It is also supported by considerable empirical work on psychotherapy outcome (Strupp, 1989).

Relational concepts allowed therapists to extend their empathy into the subtle area of how their clients experienced interpersonal connection. They might be in a state of psychological fusion with another person, in which self and object are emotionally indistinguishable. They might be in a dyadic space, where the object was felt as either for them or against them. Or they might see others as fully independent of themselves. The child's movement from experiential symbiosis (early infancy) through me-versus-you struggles (age 2 or so) through more complex identifications (age 3 and up) became more salient in this theory than the oral, anal, and oedipal preoccupations of those stages. The oedipal phase was appreciated as a *cognitive* developmental milestone, not just as a psychosexual one, in that it is a substantial leap—a victory over infantile egocentrism—to be able to understand that two other people (one's parents, in the classical paradigm) might be relating *to each other* in a way that had little to do with the self.

The appearance of concepts from the European object relations theorists and from the interpersonalists in the United States heralded significant advances in treatment because the psychologies of many clients, especially those suffering from more debilitating kinds of psychopathology, are not easily construed in terms of id, ego, and superego. Instead of having an integrated ego with a self-observing function, such persons seem to have different "ego states," conditions of mind in which they feel and behave one way, often contrasting with the way they feel and behave at other times. In the grip of these states, they appear to have no capacity to think objectively about what is going on in themselves, and they may insist that their current emotional experience is natural and inevitable given their situation.

Clinicians trying to help these difficult patients learn that treatment goes better if one can figure out which internal parent or other important early object is being activated at any given time, rather than trying to relate to them as if there is a consistent "self" with mature defenses that can be engaged. Thus, the arrival of the object relations point of view had significant implications for extending the scope and range of treatment (see L. Stone, 1954). Therapists could now listen for the attitudes of "introjects," those internalized others who had influenced the child and lived on in the adult, and from whom the client had not yet achieved a satisfactory psychological separation.

Within this formulation, character could be seen as reasonably predictable patterns of behaving like, or unconsciously inducing others to behave like, the experienced objects of early childhood. The "stable instability" of the borderline personality (Kernberg, 1975) had become more theoretically comprehensible and hence more clinically addressable. With the metaphors and models of object relations theory, filtered through the therapist's internal images and emotional reactions to the patient's communications, a practitioner now had additional means of understanding what was happening in therapy, especially when an observing ego could not be accessed. For example, when a disturbed patient would launch a paranoid diatribe, the therapist could make sense of it as a recreation of the patient's having felt relentlessly and unfairly criticized as a child.

A new appreciation of *countertransference* evolved in the psychoanalytic community, reflecting therapists' accumulating clinical knowledge and exposure to the work of relational theorists writing about their internal responses to patients. In the United States, Harold Searles distinguished himself for frank depictions of normal countertransference storms, as in his 1959 article on efforts of psychotic people to drive therapists crazy. In Britain, D. W. Winnicott was one of the bravest self-disclosers, as in his justly famous 1949 article "Hate in the Countertransference." Freud had regarded strong emotional reactions to patients as evidence of the analyst's incomplete self-knowledge and inability to maintain an affectively positive, physicianly attitude toward the other person in the room. In gradual contrast to this appealingly rational position, analysts working with psychotic clients and with those we would now consider borderline were finding that one of their best vehicles for comprehending these overwhelmed, disorganized, desperate, tormented people was their own intense countertransferential response to them.

In this vein, Heinrich Racker (1968), a South American analyst influenced by Klein, offered the clinically invaluable categories of *concordant* and *complementary countertransferences*. The former term refers to the therapist's feeling (empathically) what the patient as a child had felt in relation to an early object; the latter connotes the therapist's feeling (unempathically, from the viewpoint of the client) what the object had felt toward the child.

For example, one of my patients once seemed to be going nowhere for several sessions. I noticed that every time he mentioned someone, he would attach a sort of verbal "footnote" to his commentary, such as "Marge is the secretary on the third floor that I eat lunch with on Tuesdays"—even if he had often talked about Marge before. I commented on this habit of his, wondering whether someone in his family had not listened to him very carefully: He assumed I didn't remember any of the important figures in his current life.

He protested angrily. His parents were *very* interested in him—especially his mother, he volunteered. He then commenced a long defense of her, during which I began, without even really noticing it, to get very bored. Suddenly, I realized I had not heard a thing he had said for several minutes. I was off in a fantasy about how I would present my work with him as a case study to some eminent colleagues, and how my account of this treatment would impress them with my skill. As I pulled myself out of this narcissistic reverie and started listening again, I was fascinated to hear that he was saying, in the context of defending his mother against the charge of lack of attentiveness, that every time he was in a play in elementary school, she would make the most elaborate costume of any mother in the grade, would rehearse every line of dialogue with him over and over, and would sit in the front row on the day of the performance, radiating pride.

In my fantasy, I had become startlingly like the mother of his childhood years, interested in him mainly as a potential enhancer of my own reputation. Racker would call this countertransference complementary, since my emotional state paralleled that of one of the patient's significant childhood objects. If instead I had found myself feeling, presumably like the client as a child, that I was not really being attended to but was valued by him mainly for the ways I enhanced his self-esteem (an equally possible outcome of the emotional atmosphere between us), then my countertransference would be considered concordant.

This process of unconscious induction of attitudes comparable to those assimilated in earliest infancy can sound rather mystical. But there are ways of looking at such phenomena that may make them more comprehensible. Consider that in the initial one to two years of life, most communication between infant and others is nonverbal.

People relating to babies figure out what they need largely on the basis of intuitive, emotional reactions. Nonverbal communication can be remarkably powerful, as anyone who has ever taken care of a newborn, or been moved to tears by a melody, or fallen inexplicably in love can testify. Analytic theory assumes that we draw on our early infantile knowledge in all the realms of making contact that both predate and transcend the formal, logical interactions we find easy to put into words. The phenomenon of *parallel process* (Ekstein & Wallerstein, 1958), which draws from the same emotional and preverbal sources, has been extensively documented in the clinical literature on supervision.

This transformation of countertransference from obstacle to asset is one of the most significant contributions of object relations theory (see Ehrenberg, 1992). Over time, countertransference information has also become increasingly recognized as critical to an accurate assessment of personality structure. The diagnostic use of the interviewer's emotional responses to the client has not been stressed in most textbooks on diagnosis (with the pioneering exception of MacKinnon & Michels, 1971); there is still some squeamishness in the field about acknowledging the extent to which an attunement to "irrational" countertransference reactions should inform diagnosis. It is an aspect of assessment that I have tried to give its deserved amount of attention here.

SELF PSYCHOLOGY

Theory not only influences practice, it is also influenced by it. When enough therapists come up against aspects of psychology that do not seem to be adequately addressed by prevailing models, the time is ripe for a paradigm shift (Kuhn, 1970; Spence, 1987). By the 1960s, practitioners were reporting that their patients' problems were not always well described in the language of any of the then current analytic models; that is, the central complaints of many people seeking treatment were not reducible to either a problem managing an instinctual urge and its inhibitors (drive theory), or to the inflexible operation of particular defenses against anxiety (ego psychology), or to the activation of internal objects from which the patient had inadequately differentiated (object relations theory). Such processes might be inferable, but they lacked both the economy of explanation and the extent of explanatory power one would want from a good theory.

Rather than seeming full of stormy, primitive introjects, as object relations theory described so well, these people reported feeling empty—devoid of internal objects rather than beleaguered by them. They lacked a sense of inner direction and dependable, orienting values, and they came to therapy to find some meaning in life. On the surface, they might look very self-assured, but internally they were in a constant search for reassurance that they were acceptable or admirable or valuable. Even among clients whose reported problems lay elsewhere, a sense of inner confusion about self-esteem and basic values could be discerned.

With their chronic need for mirroring from outside sources, such patients were regarded by analytically oriented people as essentially narcissistic, even when they did not fit the stereotype of the "phallic" narcissistic character (arrogant, vain, charming) that Reich had delineated. They induced a countertransference noteworthy not for its intensity, but for its boredom, impatience, and sense of vague irritation and futility in the interviewer. People treating such clients reported that they felt insignificant, invisible, and either devalued or overvalued by them. They could not feel appreciated as a real other person trying to help, but instead seemed to be regarded as a replaceable source of their clients' emotional inflation or deflation.

The disturbance of such people seemed to center in their sense of who they were, what their values were, and what maintained their self-esteem. They would sometimes say they did not know who they were or what really mattered to them, beyond getting reassured that they mattered. They often did not appear flagrantly "sick" from a traditional standpoint (they had impulse control, ego strength, interpersonal stability, etc.), but they nevertheless felt little pleasure in their lives and in who they were. Some analytic practitioners considered them untreatable, since it is a much more monumental task to help someone develop a self than it is to help him or her repair or reorient one that already exists. Others worked at finding new constructs through which these patients' suffering could be better conceptualized and hence more sensitively treated. Some stayed within existing psychodynamic models to do so (e.g., Erikson and Rollo May within ego psychology, Kernberg and Masterson within object relations); others went elsewhere. Carl Rogers (1951, 1961) went outside the psychoanalytic tradition altogether to develop a theory and therapy that made affirmation of the client's developing self and self-esteem its hallmark.

Within psychoanalysis, Heinz Kohut formulated a new theory of the self: of its development, possible distortion, and treatment. He emphasized processes like the normal need to idealize and the implications for adult psychopathology when one grows up without objects that can be initially idealized and then gradually and nontraumatically deidealized. Kohut's contributions (e.g., 1971, 1977, 1984) proved valuable not only to those who were looking for new ways to understand and help narcissistically impaired clients; they also furthered a general reorientation toward thinking about people in terms of self-structures, self-representations, self-images, and how one comes to depend on internal processes for self-esteem. An appreciation of the emptiness and pain of those without a reliable superego began to coexist with the compassion that analysts already felt for those whose superegos were excessively strict.

Kohut's work, its influence on other writers (e.g., Alice Miller, Robert Stolorow, George Atwood, Arnold Goldberg, Sheldon Bach, Paul and Anna Ornstein, Ernest Wolf), and the general tone it set for rethinking psychological issues had important diagnostic implications—despite the fact that among many self psychologists, as noted earlier, the traditional assessment–interview process is viewed with suspicion. This new way of conceptualizing clinical material added to analytic theory the language of self and encouraged evaluators to try to understand the dimension of self-experiences in people. Therapists began observing that even in patients not notable for their overall narcissism, one could see the operation of processes oriented toward supporting self-esteem, self-cohesion, and a sense of self-continuity—functions that had not been stressed in most earlier literature. Defenses were reconceptualized as existing not only to protect a person from anxiety about id, ego, and superego dangers but also to sustain a consistent, positively valued sense of self (Goldberg, 1990a). Interviewers could understand patients more completely by asking, in addition to the traditional questions about defense ("Of what is this person afraid? When afraid, what does this person do?" [Waelder, 1960]), "How vulnerable is this person's self-esteem? When it is threatened, what does he or she do?"

A clinical example may show why this addition to theory is useful. Two persons may be clinically depressed, with virtually identical vegetative signs (sleep problems, appetite disturbance, tearfulness, psychomotor retardation, etc.), yet have radically disparate subjective experiences. One is a man who feels *bad*, in the sense of morally deficient or evil. He is contemplating suicide because he believes that his existence only aggravates the problems of the world and that he would be doing the planet a favor by removing his corrupting influence from it. The other is a man who feels not morally bad but internally *empty*, defective, ugly. He also is considering suicide, not to improve the world, but because he sees no point in living. The former feels a piercing guilt, the latter a diffuse shame (cf. Blatt, 1974). In object relations terms, the first man is too full of internalized others telling him he is bad; the second is too empty of internalizations that could give him any direction.

The diagnostic discrimination between the former kind of depression, once referred to in the psychoanalytic literature as "melancholia," and the second, a more narcissistically depleted state of mind, is a critical one for very practical reasons. The first kind of depressive client will not respond well to an overtly sympathetic, supportive tone in the interviewer; he will feel misunderstood as a person more deserving than *he* knows he really is, and he will get more depressed. The second kind of depressive man will be greatly relieved by the therapist's direct expression of concern and support; his emptiness will be temporarily filled, and the agony of his shame will be mitigated. I will have more to say about these kinds of discriminations later, but the point at hand is that the appearance of self psychology and its categories of analysis has had significant diagnostic value.

OTHER PSYCHOANALYTIC CONTRIBUTIONS TO PERSONALITY ASSESSMENT

In addition to drive, ego psychology, object relations, and self orientations, there are several other theories within a broad psychoanalytic framework that have affected our conceptualizations of character. They include, but are not limited to, the ideas of Jung, Adler, and Rank; the "personology" of Murray; the "modern psychoanalysis" of Spotnitz; the "transactional analysis" of Berne; the "script theory" of Tomkins; the "control–mastery" theory of Sampson and Weiss; and the evolutionary biology model of Slavin and Kriegman (1990). Many therapists draw from these perspectives as well as from the more general ones depicted above. I shall occasionally refer to some of these paradigms in subsequent chapters. By the time this book sees print, there will no doubt be an application of chaos theory to the field, providing another useful set of images and constructs to illuminate personality development, structure, function, and malfunction.

In concluding this chapter, I want to stress the importance of dynamic processes in character. Psychoanalytic theories emphasize dynamisms, not traits. It is the appreciation of oscillating patterns that makes analytic notions of character richer and more clinically germane than the lists of static attributes one finds in most assessment instruments and in compendia like the DSM. People become organized on *dimensions* that have significance for them, and they typically show characteristics expressing both polarities of any salient dimension.

Philip Slater (1970) captured this idea succinctly in a footnote commentary on contemporary literary criticism and biography:

> Generations of humanists have excited themselves and their readers by showing "contradictions" and "paradoxes" in some real or fictional person's character, simply because a trait and its opposite coexisted in the same person. But in fact traits and their opposites always coexist if the traits are of any intensity, and the whole tradition of cleverly ferreting out paradoxes of character depends upon the psychological naivete of the reader for its impact. (pp. 3n–4n)

Thus, people with conflicts about closeness can get upset by both closeness and distance. People who crave success the most hungrily are often the ones who sabotage it the most wrecklessly. The manic person is psychologically more similar to the depressive than to the schizoid individual; a compulsively promiscuous man has more in common with someone who resolved a sexual conflict by celibacy than with someone for whom sexuality is not problematic. People are complicated, but their intricacies are not random. Analytic theories offer us ways of helping our clients to make sense out of seemingly inexplicable ironies and absurdities in their lives, and to transform their vulnerabilites into strengths.

SUMMARY

I have briefly described the major current paradigms within psychoanalysis: drive theory, ego psychology, object relations theory, and self psychology approaches to understanding people. Their respective implications for conceptualizing character were emphasized, with attention to the clinical inferences that can be drawn from seeing people through these different lenses. I also noted other influences on dynamic ideas about character structure and their associated therapeutic approaches. This review could only hit the highlights of over a hundred years of intellectual ferment, controversy, and theory development.

SUGGESTIONS FOR FURTHER READING

For those who have never read him, the best way to get a sense of Freud, and of nascent drive theory, is to peruse *The Interpretation of*

Dreams (1900), skipping over the parts where he addresses contemporary controversies or develops grand metaphysical schemes. His "Outline of Psychoanalysis" (1938) gives a synopsis of his later theory, but I find it too condensed and dry; *Freud and Man's Soul* (Bettelheim, 1983) is a good corrective. Brenner's (1955) *An Elementary Textbook of Psychoanalysis* is comprehensive but authoritarian to the contemporary ear; I prefer Hall (1954).

Several more recent books give historical reviews of psychoanalytic clinical theory. The Blancks' (G. Blanck & R. Blanck, 1974) *Ego Psychology: Theory and Practice* has a particularly good one. Guntrip's (1971) *Psychoanalytic Theory, Therapy, and the Self*, a model of psychoanalytic humanitarianism, puts object relations theory in context, as does Symington's (1986) well-written study. Hughes (1989) has gracefully explicated Klein, Winnicott, and Fairbairn. Fromm-Reichmann (1950) and Levenson (1972) are excellent spokespeople for the American interpersonalists. Greenberg and Mitchell (1983) discerningly contrast drive–conflict models and relational ones.

For self psychological sources, Kohut's (1971) *The Analysis of the Self* is almost impenetrable to beginners, but *The Restoration of the Self* (1977) is easier going. Chessick's (1985) review and critical interpretation of the self psychology movement is quite helpful. Stolorow and Atwood's (1992) *Contexts of Being* is a readable introduction to the intersubjective view.

For an introduction to control–mastery theory, consider *How Psychotherapy Works* by Joseph Weiss (1993). The most concise and clear recent review of developments in psychoanalytic personality theory is probably Westen's (1990) essay in the *Handbook of Personality Theory and Research*. For integrationists, both of Fred Pine's recent books (1985, 1990) are outstanding.

❖3❖

Developmental Levels of Personality Organization

This chapter will focus on the maturational issues that may organize a person's character, the aspect of personality structure that has usually been referred to, following Freud, as *fixation*. I shall explore the implications of inferred fixation at three possible levels of psychological development. At this point, let me set out the major diagnostic premise of this text: *The essential character structure of any human being cannot be understood without an appreciation of two distinct and interacting dimensions: developmental level of personality organization and defensive style within that level.* The first dimension conceptualizes a person's extent of individuation or degree of pathology (psychotic, borderline, neurotic, "normal"); the second identifies his or her type of character (paranoid, depressive, schizoid, etc.).

A close friend of mine, a man with no experience in psychotherapy, who cannot imagine why anyone would go into a field where one spends hour upon hour listening to other people's problems, was trying to understand my interest in writing this book. "It's simple for me," he commented. "I have just two categories for people: (1) Nuts and (2) not nuts." I responded that in psychoanalytic theory, which assumes that everyone is irrational to some degree, we also have two basic attributions: (1) How nuts? and (2) nuts in what particular way? As I summarized briefly in the section on classical drive theory in Chapter 2, although most analytic diagnosticians now conceive the relevant stages through which young children pass in less drive-defined ways than Freud did, psychoanalysis has never seriously questioned three of his main convictions: (1) current psychological preoccupations reflect infantile precursors; (2) interactions in our earliest years set up the template for how we later assimilate experience, making that experience comprehensible unconsciously according to categories that were salient in childhood; and (3) identifying a person's developmental level is a critical part of understanding him or her. Interestingly, regardless of revision, the same three phases of infantile* psychological organization keep reappearing in psychoanalytic developmental theory: (1) the first year and a half to 2 years (Freud's oral phase), (2) the period from 1½ or 2 to about 3 (Freud's anal phase), and (3) the time between 3 or 4 and about 6 (Freud's oedipal period). The approximateness of these ages reflects individual differences in children; the sequence is always the same even if a child is precocious or late blooming.

Many theorists have discussed aspects of the tasks of these phases, whether with an emphasis on drive and defense, on ego development, or on images of self and other that characterize them. Some have stressed the behavioral issues of the stages, others the cognitive ones, still others the affective maturation of the child. Some, like Daniel Stern (1985), have subjected prevailing stage theories to an extensive critique in light of recent research on infant development. Nevertheless, the clinical relevance of some concept of psychological stages most likely guarantees their survival in our conceptual formulations. Gertrude and Rubin Blanck (1974, 1979, 1986) have been particularly adept at translating maturational concepts into tailored therapeutic applications. Phyllis and Robert Tyson's (1990) recent synthesis of psychoanalytic developmental theory covers this territory with scholarly comprehensiveness. For purposes of an introductory text like this one, I shall mostly be synthesizing the ideas of Erik Erikson and Margaret Mahler, who investigated the child's maturing ego competencies and parallel experiences of self and object.

It has never been demonstrated to my satisfaction—and I am in good company (see Masling's research [1986])—that people with a lot of "oral" qualities have more severe degrees of psychopathology than those with features that analysts would regard as either anal or oedipal, even though Freud's naming of the first three stages of development by these inferred drive concepts has a lot of intuitive appeal and correlates to some degree with *type* of personality (depressive people of any level of health or pathology tend to manifest orality; compulsive people are notoriously anal in their preoccupations, whether or not their compul-

*The reader should note that psychoanalytic habit has established the word "infantile" as referring to the whole preschool period of childhood emotional, cognitive, behavioral, and sensory maturation.

sivity presents major problems to them). I mentioned earlier the failure of Karl Abraham's effort to correlate degree of psychopathology with type of drive organization, and no one since Abraham has convincingly made the case either.

Yet there *is* substantial clinical evidence, and some empirical research as well (e.g., L. Silverman, Lachmann, & Milich, 1982), supporting a correlation between one's level of ego development and self–other differentiation, on the one hand, and the health or pathology of one's personality organization, on the other. To a certain extent this correlation is definitional and therefore tautological—that is, assessing primitive levels of ego development and object relations in an interviewee is like saying that he or she is "sick," whereas regarding someone as obsessive or schizoid is not necessarily assigning pathology. But this way of conceptualizing psychological robustness versus disturbance according to categories from ego psychology, object relations theory, and self psychology has profound clinical implications across different character types. A brief history of psychoanalytic attempts to make diagnostic distinctions between people based on the extent or "depth" of their difficulties rather than their *type* of personality follows.

HISTORICAL CONTEXT: DIAGNOSING LEVEL OF CHARACTER PATHOLOGY

Before the advent of descriptive psychiatry in the 19th century, certain forms of mental disturbance that occurred with any frequency among people in what was considered the "civilized world" were recognized, and most observers presumably made distinctions between the sane and the insane, much as my nonpsychological friend distinguishes between "nuts" and "not nuts." Sane people agreed more or less about what constituted reality; insane people deviated from this consensus.

Men and women with hysterical conditions, phobias, obsessions, compulsions, and manic and depressive tendencies of less than what we would now consider psychotic intensity were understood to have psychological difficulties that fell short of complete insanity. People with hallucinations, delusions, and thought disorders were regarded as insane. People we would today call antisocial were judged to be exhibiting "moral insanity" (Prichard, 1835) but were considered mentally in touch with reality. This rather crude taxonomy survives in the categories of our legal system, which puts emphasis on whether the person accused of a crime was able to assess reality at the time of its commission.

KRAEPELINIAN DIAGNOSIS: NEUROSES VERSUS PSYCHOSES

Emil Kraepelin (1856–1926) is usually cited as the father of contemporary diagnostic classification in that he tried to observe carefully those who suffered from mental and emotional disturbances, with the aim of identifying general syndromes that share common characteristics. In addition, he developed theories about their etiology, at least to the extent of regarding their origins as either exogenous and treatable or endogenous and incurable (Kraepelin, 1913). Interestingly, he put manic–depressive psychosis in the former category and schizophrenia—then known as "dementia praecox" and believed to be an organic deterioration of the brain—in the latter. The "lunatic" began to be understood as a person afflicted with one of several possible documented illnesses.

Freud accepted many Kraepelinian terms describing mental and emotional difficulties but went beyond description and simple levels of inference into more speculative theoretical formulations. Among other contributions, Freud's developing theory posited complex epigenetic explanations as preferable to Kraepelin's simple internal/external versions of causality. Still, Freud tended to regard psychopathology by the categories then available. For example, if a man was troubled by obsessions (e.g., Freud's patient the "Wolf Man" [Freud, 1918; Gardiner, 1971]), he would have described him as having an obsessive compulsive neurosis. By the end of his career, Freud began to discriminate between a condition of obsession in an otherwise nonobsessive person and an obsession that was part of an obsessive compulsive character. But it was later analysts (e.g., Eissler, 1953; Horner, 1990) who made the distinctions that are the subject of this chapter, that is, the distinctions among (1) the obsessive person who is essentially delusional and using ruminative thoughts to ward off total psychotic decompensation, (2) the person whose obsessing is part of an overall borderline personality structure (as in the "Wolf Man"), and (3) the obsessive person with a neurotic-to-normal personality organization.

Before the category of "borderline" emerged in the middle of the 20th century, analytically influenced therapists followed Freud in differentiating only between neurotic and psychotic levels of pathology, the former being distinguished by a general appreciation of reality and the latter by a loss of contact with it. A neurotic woman knew at some level that her problem was in her own head; the psychotic one believed it was the world that was out of kilter. When Freud developed the structural model of the mind, this distinction took on the quality of a comment on a person's psychological infrastructure: Neurotic people were viewed as suffering because their ego defenses were too automatic and inflexible, cutting them off from id energies that could be put to creative use; psychotic ones suffered because their ego defenses were too weak, leaving them helplessly overwhelmed by primitive material from the id.

The neurotic-versus-psychotic distinction had important clinical ramifications, some of which are still being taught in their most simplistic forms in some mental health facilities. The gist of the clinical effects of such a nosology, once it coexisted with Freud's structural model of the mind, was that therapy with a neurotic person should involve weakening the defenses and getting access to the id so that its energies may be released for more constructive activity. In contrast, therapy with a psychotic person should aim at strengthening defenses, covering over primitive preoccupations, influencing realistically stressful circumstances so that they are less upsetting, encouraging reality testing, and pushing the bubbling id back into unconsciousness. It was as if the neurotic person were like a pot on the stove with the lid on too tight, making the therapist's job to let some steam escape, while the psychotic pot was boiling over, necessitating that the therapist get the lid back on and turn down the heat.

Many trainees have heard a supervisor recommend that one should attack the defenses with healthier patients and support them with schizophrenics and other psychotic people. With the advent of antipsychotic drugs, this formulation lent itself to a widespread tendency not only to medicate—often the compassionate response to psychotic levels of anxiety—but also to assume that medication would do the covering over and would be needed on a lifetime basis. One would not want to do any therapy that might be "uncovering" with a potentially psychotic person: That might disturb the patient's fragile defenses and send him or her over the edge again. In general, this way of conceptualizing degree of pathology is not without usefulness; it has opened the door to the development of different therapeutic approaches for different kinds of difficulties. But it falls short of a comprehensive and clinically nuanced ideal. Any theory oversimplifies, but this neurotic-versus-psychotic division, even with Freud's elegant structural underpinnings and their therapeutic implications, offered only a start at a useful inferential diagnosis. The model is too gross to permit a sensitive practitioner to derive from it any specific ideas about what kinds of human relatedness will be therapeutic to what kinds of human beings.

EGO PSYCHOLOGY DIAGNOSTIC CATEGORIES: SYMPTOM NEUROSIS, NEUROTIC CHARACTER, AND PSYCHOSIS

In the psychoanalytic community, in addition to a distinction between neurosis and psychosis, differentiations of extent of maladaptation, not simply type of psychopathology, gradually began to appear *within* the neurotic category. The first clinically important one was a discrimination between "symptom neuroses" and "character neuroses" (W. Reich, 1933). From professional experience, therapists learned that it was useful to distinguish between a person with a discrete neurosis and one with a character permeated by neurotic patterns. (This distinction continues to be reflected in the DSM, in which conditions labeled "disorder" tend to be those that analysts have typically called neuroses, and conditions labeled "personality disorder" resemble the old analytic concept of neurotic character.)

To assess whether they were dealing with a symptom neurosis or a character problem, therapists were trained to pursue the following kinds of information when interviewing a person with neurotic-level complaints:

1. Is there an identifiable precipitant of the difficulty, or has it existed to some degree as long as the patient can remember?
2. Has there been a dramatic increase in the patient's anxiety, especially pertaining to the neurotic symptoms, or has there been only an incremental worsening of the person's overall state of feeling?
3. Is the patient self-referred, or did others (relatives, friends, the legal system, or some other source) send him or her for treatment?
4. Are the person's symptoms ego alien (seen by him or her as problematic and irrational) or are they ego syntonic (regarded as the only and obvious way the patient can imagine reacting to current life circumstances)?
5. Is the person's capacity to get some perspective on his or her problems (the "observing ego" in analytic jargon) adequate to develop an alliance with the therapist against the problematic symptom, or does the patient seem to regard the interviewer as either a potentially hostile or magically rescuing outsider?

The former alternative in each of the above possibilities was presumptive evidence of a symptom problem, the latter of a character problem (see Nunberg, 1955). The significance of this distinction lay in its implications for treatment and prognosis. If it was a symptom neurosis that the client suffered, then one would assume that something in the person's current life had activated an unconscious infantile conflict and that the patient was now using maladaptive mechanisms to cope with it—methods that may have been the best available solution in childhood but which were now creating more problems than they were solving. The task in such a case involved determining the conflict, helping the patient process the emotions connected to it, and developing new solutions to cope with it. The prognosis would be favorable, and treatment would not necessarily involve years of work (cf. Menninger, 1963). One could also expect a climate of mutuality in the process of therapy, one in which strong transference (and countertransference) reactions might appear, but usually in the context of an even stronger degree of realistic cooperation.

If the patient's difficulties were more aptly conceptualized as expressing a character or personality problem, then the therapeutic task would be more complicated, demanding, and time-consuming, and the prognosis more guarded. This is only common sense, of course, in that setting out to change an individual's personality obviously poses more challenges than helping him or her to get rid of a maladaptive response to a particular stress. But analytic theory went beyond common sense in specifying the ways in which work on a person's basic character would differ from work with a symptom not embedded in one's personality.

First, one could not take for granted that what the patient wanted (immediate relief from suffering) and what the therapist saw as necessary for the patient's eventual recovery and resistance to future difficulties (restructuring of personality) could be seen by the patient as compatible. Under circumstances when the patient's aims and the analyst's conception of how to pursue realistically achievable objectives were at variance, the analyst's *educative role* became much more critical to the outcome of the therapeutic relationship. It became the job of the therapist first of all to convey to the patient how the therapist saw the problem. Psychoanalytic lingo for this process is "making ego alien what has been ego syntonic."

For example, a 30-year-old accountant once came to me looking to "achieve more balance" in his life. Raised to be the hope of his family, with a mission to compensate for his father's failed ambitions, he was hardworking to the point of drivenness. He feared that he was missing precious years with his young children, whom he might enjoy if only he could stop pushing himself relentlessly to produce at work. He wanted me to develop a "program" with him in which he agreed to spend a certain amount of time per day exercising, a certain amount playing with his kids, a certain amount working on a hobby, and so forth. The proposed program included designated space for volunteer work, watching television, cooking, doing housework, and making love to his wife.

In the meeting that followed our initial interview, he brought in a sample schedule detailing such changes. He felt that if I could get him to put this program into effect, his problems would be solved. My first task was to try to show him that this solution was part of the problem: He approached therapy with the same drivenness he was complaining about and pursued the serenity he knew he needed as if it were another job to do. I told him he was very good at *doing*, but he evidently had had little experience with just *being*. While he grasped this notion intellectually, he had no emotionally salient memory of a less compulsive approach to life, and he regarded me with a mixture of hope and skepticism. Although simply telling his story to someone else had provided some short-term relief of his depression, I saw him as having to get used to the fact that to avoid this kind of misery in the future, he would need to bring into conscious awareness and to rethink some of the major premises of his life.

Second, in working with someone whose fundamental character was neurotic, one could not take for granted the prompt appearance of a "working alliance" (Greenson, 1967). Instead, one would have to create the conditions under which it could develop. The concept of the *working* or *therapeutic alliance* refers to the collaborative dimension of the work between therapist and client, the level of cooperation that endures in spite of the strong and often negative emotions that may surface during treatment. While its status as a metapsychological construct has been questioned (see Rawn, 1991), the concept of the working alliance is experientially meaningful to most psychoanalytic clinicians, and it is very useful for evaluating what is going on between them and their various clients.

People with symptom neuroses feel on the side of the therapist in opposing a problematic *part* of the self; there is no need for a long period in which a joint perspective is developed. In contrast, with those who are learning a completely new way of thinking about their whole personality, their problem is so much a part of their whole self that they easily feel alone and under attack by the therapist. Distrust is inevitable, and it must be patiently endured by both parties until the therapist has earned the client's confidence. With some patients, this process of building an alliance can take more than a year. Obviously, the therapy approach is quite different when one is creating an alliance from how one works when one is assuming that it exists.

Third, the content of the therapeutic endeavor in the case of a person with a character rather than a symptom problem could be expected to be less exciting, less surprising, less dramatic. Whatever the therapist's and patient's respective fantasies about unearthing spectacular repressed memories or unconscious conflicts, they would have to content themselves with a much more prosaic process, the painstaking unraveling of all the threads that had created the emotional knot that the patient had up to now believed was just the way things had to be, and the slow working out of some different ways of thinking and handling feelings in a human relationship.

In the development of personality disorders, as opposed to the appearance of neurotic reactions to particular stresses, there are long patterns of identification, learning, and reinforcement. Where the etiology is traumatic, there are instances of repeated trauma rather than the one unassimilated, unmourned injury that Hollywood's early portrayals of psychoanalytic therapy would have had us believe.* As a consequence, one could expect that in the therapy of character neuroses, both parties would have to deal with occasional boredom, impatience, irritability and demoralization—the patient by expressing them without fear of criticism and the therapist by using them to increase empathy for the patient's struggle with such a difficult and protracted task.

This distinction between neurotic symptoms and neurotic personality still has significant applicability. David Shapiro's (1989) *Psychotherapy of Neurotic Character* is a good example of the contemporary and disciplined explication of the concept of character pathology and of what one can expect in conducting a systematic treatment of it. It continues a long psychoanalytic tradition, one that began with Reich and continued through Fenichel and others, of looking at character in the context of ego psychology and using its concepts to help people with mature but inflexible defenses to loosen up and develop more creative and effective ways of responding to life's challenges.

For a long time, the categories of symptom neurosis, character neurosis, and psychosis constituted the main constructs by which diagnosticians understood personality differences among people on the dimension of severity of disorder. A neurosis was the least serious

*Psychoanalysis was for a short while a great boon to the motion picture industry; see, for example, the classic Hitchcock thriller *Spellbound*.

condition, a personality disorder more serious, and a psychotic disturbance quite grave. These formulations maintained the old distinction between sane and insane, with the sane category including two possibilities: neurotic reactions and neurotically structured personalities. Over time, however, it became apparent to the mental health community that such an overall scheme of classification was both incomplete and misleading.

One drawback of this taxonomy is its implication that all character problems are by definition more pathological than all neuroses. One can still discern such an assumption, in fact, in the DSM, in which the criteria for diagnosing most syndromes in the Personality Disorders section include significant impairments in functioning. Experienced therapists will attest that some stress-related neurotic-level reactions are much more crippling to a person's capacity to cope than, say, some hysterical and obsessional personality disorders.

To complicate the issue still further, there is also a problem in the other direction: Some character disturbances seem to be much *more* severe and primitive in quality than anything that could reasonably be called "neurotic." One can see that there is no way in such a linear, three-part system of classification to differentiate between distortions of character that are mildly incapacitating and those that involve fairly grievous consequences. A problem can be characterological and of any level of severity. The line between benign personality "traits" and mild personality "disorders" is quite blurry; and on the other end of the continuum, some character disorders have been for a long time understood as involving such substantial deformities of the ego that they are closer to psychosis than neurosis. Both sociopathy and what would today be considered the more severe degrees of narcissistic pathology, for example, have been recognized for some time as variants of human individuality, but until fairly recently, both have tended to be considered as special cases of abnormality somewhat outside the scope of possible therapeutic intervention and not easily placed on a neurotic–character disordered–psychotic continuum.

OBJECT RELATIONS DIAGNOSIS: BORDERLINE PSYCHOPATHOLOGY

Even in the later part of the 19th century, some psychiatric observers were finding that they had patients who seemed to inhabit a psychological "borderland" between sanity and insanity (Rosse, 1890), and by the middle of the twentieth century other ideas about personality organization suggesting some middle ground between neurosis and psychosis began to appear. Helene Deutsch (1942), for example, proposed the concept of the "as-if personality" for a subgroup of people we would now regard as seriously narcissistic, and Hoch and Polatin (1949) made a case for the category of "pseudoneurotic schizophrenia."

By the middle 1950s, the general mental health community had followed these innovators in their discomfort with the limitations of the neurosis-versus-psychosis model. Numerous analysts began complaining about clients who seemed character disordered, but in a peculiarly chaotic way. Because they rarely or never reported hallucinations or delusions, they could not clearly be considered psychotic, but they also lacked the stability and predictability of neurotic-level patients, and they seemed to be miserable on a much grander and less comprehensible scale than neurotics. In psychoanalytic treatment, they sometimes would become temporarily psychotic, yet outside the consulting room there was an odd stability to their instability. In other words, they were too sane to be considered crazy, and too crazy to be considered sane.

Therapists began suggesting new diagnostic labels that captured the quality of these people who lived on the border between neurotic and psychotic character disturbance. In 1953, Knight published a thoughtful essay about "borderline states." In the same decade, T. F. Main (1957) was referring to similar pathology as simply "The Ailment." Frosch (1964), responding to comparable clinical phenomena, suggested the diagnostic category of "psychotic character."

In 1968, Roy Grinker and his colleagues (Grinker, Werble, & Drye, 1968) did a seminal study that provided empirical support for the existence of a "borderline syndrome," inhering in personality, with a range of severity from the border with the neuroses to the border with the psychoses. Gunderson and Singer (e.g., 1975) developed programs of controlled investigation that continued to subject the concept to empirical scrutiny, and eventually, via both research and clinical findings, and thanks to the elucidation of writers like Kernberg (e.g., 1975, 1976), Masterson (e.g., 1976), and M. Stone (e.g., 1986), the concept of a borderline level of personality organization attained widespread acceptance in the psychoanalytic community.

Although one still sometimes hears the term "borderline" used (confusingly) to refer to someone regarded as at significant risk of a psychotic break, and although it covers such a broad range of symptoms that it can be misused as a wastebasket category for any "difficult" patient that one does not want to take the trouble to diagnose carefully, the label is now widely understood as denoting a type of personality structure graver in its implications than neurosis yet not vulnerable to lasting psychotic decompensations. In 1980, the term had become sufficiently legitimate to appear in the DSM, third edition (DSM-III; American Psychiatric Association, 1980) as a type of personality disorder.*

The development of the object relations viewpoint in psychoanalysis made theoretical sense out of a lot of these clinical observations, and by the second half of the 20th century, most analytically oriented clinicians struggling to help clients that we now understand as borderline found themselves drawing inspiration and confirmation from the writings of people in the American interpersonal group and the British object relations movement, who looked at key figures in childhood and their internalized representations. Specifically, these theorists emphasized understanding the patient's experience of relationship, of attachment and separation: Was the person preoccupied with symbiotic issues, separation–individuation themes, or highly individuated competitive and identificatory motifs? Erikson's (1950) reworking of Freud's three infantile stages in terms of the child's *interpersonal* task, not just his or her drive concerns, also influenced therapists in midcentury, in that patients could be conceptualized as fixated at either primary dependency issues (trust vs. mistrust), secondary separation–individuation issues (autonomy vs. shame and doubt), or more advanced levels of identification (initiative vs. guilt). These concepts of stages of psychological development made sense of the differences therapists were noticing among psychotic, borderline, and neurotic-level patients: People in a psychotic state seemed fixated at a fused, preseparation level in which they could not differentiate between what was inside and what was outside themselves; people in a borderline condition were construed as fixated in dyadic struggles between total enmeshment, which they

*For analytic therapists, this was a meaningful milestone, since recognition of the general category of borderline personality organization affirmed a concept of central analytic significance. As the diagnosis has been listed in the Personality Disorders section of the DSM-III and subsequent editions, however, there is no way the reader can know that this label represents a *level* rather than a *type* of pathology. One can be a borderline hysteric, a borderline obsessive compulsive, a borderline narcissistic personality, and so on; one can be organized narcissistically at a neurotic, borderline, or psychotic level. The listing of "borderline" alongside personality labels like histrionic, obsessive compulsive, and narcissistic, as if it is parallel to them, mixes apples and oranges—or more aptly, mixes a more specific label like "apples" with a more generic one like "fruit." (Among analytic theorists, some disagreement also exists about whether the term should identify a level or a type of personality structure, with Kernberg, among others, propounding the former and Gunderson proposing the latter; I have followed Kernberg here on the grounds that his model has had more influence on clinical practice.)

feared would obliterate their identity, and total isolation, which they equated with traumatic abandonment; and people with neurotic difficulties were understood as having accomplished separation and individuation but as having run into conflicts between, for example, things they wished for and things they feared, the prototype for which was the oedipal drama. This way of thinking made sense of numerous puzzling and demoralizing clinical challenges, and it accounted for why one woman with phobias seemed to be clinging to sanity by a thread, while another was oddly stable in her phobic instability, and yet a third woman was, despite having a phobia, overall a paragon of mental health.

There is at this point, both within the psychoanalytic tradition and outside it, a vast literature on borderline psychopathology, showing a bewildering divergence of professional beliefs about its etiology. Some investigators (e.g., M. Stone, 1977) have emphasized constitutional and neurological predispositions; some (e.g., Masterson, 1972, 1976; G. Adler, 1985) have focused on developmental failures, especially in the separation–individuation phase described by Mahler (1971); some (e.g., Kernberg, 1975) have conjectured about aberrant parent–child interaction at an earlier phase of infantile development; some (e.g., Mandelbaum, 1977; Rinsley, 1982) have pointed to poor boundaries between members in dysfunctional family systems; some (e.g., McWilliams, 1979; Westen, 1993) have made sociological speculations. Recently, considerable evidence has emerged that trauma, especially incest, plays a much bigger role in the development of borderline dynamics than had previously been suspected (e.g., Wolf & Alpert, 1991).

Whatever the etiology of borderline personality organization, and it is probably highly complex and different from person to person, clinicians of diverse perspectives have attained a surprisingly reliable consensus on the clinical manifestations of problems in the borderline range. Especially when an interviewer is trained in what information, subjective as well as objective, should be observed and pursued, the diagnosis of borderline level of character structure may be readily confirmed or disconfirmed (e.g., through Kernberg's [1984] "structural interview").

Currently, dynamically oriented therapists tend to make an overall assessment, as early as possible in a therapy transaction, as to whether a person's character structure is essentially neurotic, borderline, or psychotic. Once that primary distinction is made, the clinician may proceed to understand *what kind* of neurotic, borderline, or psychotic personality will be the object of therapeutic intent. There is a rough consensus to the effect that, despite its gross oversimplification, the following formula has clinical utility: *People with a vulnerability to psychosis may be understood as psychologically fixated on the issues of the early symbiotic phase; people with borderline personality organization are comprehensible in terms of their preoccupation with separation–individuation themes; and those with neurotic structure can be usefully construed in more oedipal terms.* The reasons why this formula has evolved and why it has clinical relevance will be covered in the next section and the next chapter, respectively.

SPECIFIC DIMENSIONS OF A NEUROTIC–BORDERLINE–PSYCHOTIC SPECTRUM

In the following sections, I shall differentiate among neurotic, borderline, and psychotic levels of character structure in a number of areas (favored defenses, level of identity integration, adequacy of reality testing, capacity to observe one's pathology, nature of one's primary conflict, and transference and countertransference potential), giving specifics about how these abstractions manifest themselves as discernible behaviors and communications in the context of either an initial interview or an ongoing treatment. In Chapter 4, I will explore some implications of these discriminations for the conduct of therapy and the expectations of clinician and client.

Characteristics of Neurotic-Level Personality Structure

It is one of the ironies of contemporary psychoanalytic parlance that the term "neurotic" is now reserved for people so emotionally healthy that they are considered rare and unusually gratifying clients. In Freud's time, the word was applied to most nonorganic, nonschizophrenic, nonpsychopathic, and non-manic–depressive patients—that is, to a large class of people with emotional distress short of psychosis. Many of the people Freud referred to as having (symptom) neuroses had borderline character organizations, and some had periods of psychotic decompensation (hysteria was understood to include hallucinatory experiences that clearly crossed the border into unreality). The more we have learned about the depth of certain problems, and their stubborn enmeshment within the matrix of a person's character, the more we currently reserve the term "neurotic" to denote a very high level of capacity to function despite some emotional suffering.

People whose personalities would contemporarily be described by psychoanalytic observers as organized at an essentially neurotic level rely primarily on the more mature or second-order defenses. While they also use primitive defenses, these are not nearly so prominent in their overall functioning and are evident mostly in times of unusual stress. *While the presence of primitive defenses does not rule out the diagnosis of neurotic level of character structure, the absence of mature defenses does.* It has been particularly noted in the psychoanalytic literature that healthier people use repression as their basic defense, in preference to more indiscriminate solutions to conflict such as denial, splitting, projective identification, and other archaic mechanisms.

Myerson (1991) has described how empathic parenting in the early years allows a child to experience strong feelings and primitive affect states without having to hang on to infantile ways of dealing with them. As the child grows up, these powerful and often painful states of mind are put away and forgotten rather than continually reexperienced and then denied, split off, or projected. They may reemerge in long-term, intensive treatment, when analyst and analysand together, under the conditions of safety that evoke a "transference neurosis," peel back layers of repression; but ordinarily, primitive affects and archaic ways of handling them are not characteristic of persons in the neurotic range. And even in deep psychoanalytic treatment, the neurotic-level client maintains some more rational, objective capacities in the middle of whatever affective storms and associated distortions occur.

People with healthier character structure also have an integrated sense of their identity (Erikson, 1968). Their behavior shows some consistency, and their inner experience is of continuity of self through time. When asked to describe themselves, they are not at a loss for words, nor do they respond one-dimensionally; they can usually delineate their overall temperament, values, tastes, habits, convictions, virtues, and shortcomings with a sense of their long-range stability. When asked to describe important others, such as their parents or lovers, their characterizations tend to be multifaceted and appreciative of the complex yet coherent set of qualities that constitutes anyone's personality.

Neurotic-level people are ordinarily in solid touch with what most of the world calls "reality." Not only are they strangers to hallucinatory or delusional misinterpretations of experience (except under conditions of chemical or organic influence, or posttraumatic flashback), they also strike the interviewer or therapist as having comparatively little need to misunderstand things in order to assimilate them. Patient and therapist live subjectively in more or less the same world. Typically, the therapist feels no compelling emotional pressure to be complicit in seeing life through a distorted lens. Some portion of what has brought a neurotic patient for help is seen by him or her as odd; in other words, much of the psychopathology of neurotically organized people is ego alien or capable of being addressed so that it becomes so.

People in the neurotic range show early in therapy a capacity for what Sterba (1934) called the "therapeutic split" between the observing and the experiencing parts of the self. Even when their difficulties are somewhat ego syntonic, neurotic-level people do not seem to demand the interviewer's implicit validation of their neurotic ways of perceiving. For example, a paranoid person who is organized neurotically will be willing at least to consider the possibility that his or her suspicions derive from some *internal* disposition to emphasize the destructive intent of others. Contrastingly, paranoid patients at the borderline or psychotic level will put intense pressure on the therapist to confirm their conviction that their difficulties are external in origin, for example, for the therapist to acknowledge that others may be out to get them. Moreover, without such validation, they will worry that they are not safe with the therapist.*

Similarly, compulsive people in the neurotic range will complain that their repetitive rituals are crazy but that they feel anxiety if they neglect them; compulsive borderline and psychotic people sincerely believe themselves to be protected in some elemental way by acting on their compulsions and have often developed elaborate rationalizations for them. In the former instance, the patient will understand a therapist's assumption that the compulsive behaviors are in some realistic sense unnecessary, but in the latter, the patient may privately worry that the practitioner who minimizes the importance of observing such rituals is deficient in either common sense or moral decency.

As a case in point, a neurotic woman with a housecleaning compulsion will be embarrassed to admit how frequently she launders the sheets, while a borderline or psychotic one will feel that anyone who washes the bedding less regularly is unclean. Sometimes years can go by in treatment before a borderline or psychotic person will even mention a compulsion or phobia or obsession—there is nothing unusual about it from the patient's point of view. I worked with one borderline client for more than 10 years before she casually mentioned an elaborate, time-consuming morning ritual to "clear her sinuses" that she considered part of ordinary good hygiene. Another borderline

*The important differences between borderline and psychotic patients on this dimension will be explored below. In short, borderline clients show more conflict between primitive and reality-based ways of interpreting events.

woman, who had never mentioned bulimia in her abundance of even more distressing symptoms, dropped the comment, after 5 years in therapy, "By the way, I notice I'm not puking anymore." She had not previously thought to regard that part of her behavioral repertoire as consequential.

One other important aspect of the differential diagnosis between neurotic and less healthy people is the nature of their difficulties. Their histories and their behavior in the interview situation, as noted previously, give evidence of their having more or less successfully achieved the respective outcomes of Erikson's first two stages, basic trust and basic autonomy, and of their having made at least some progress toward the third, the attainment of a sense of identity and initiative. They tend to seek therapy because of problems not in essential security or sense of agency, but because they keep running into conflicts between what they want and obstacles to attaining it that they suspect are of their own making. Freud's contention that the proper goal of therapy is the removal of inhibitions against love and work applies to this group; some neurotic-level people are also looking to expand their capacity for solitude and play.

The experiential accompaniments of being in the presence of a person at the healthier end of the continuum of character pathology are generally benign. The counterpart of the patient's possession of a sound observing ego is the therapist's experience of a sound working alliance. Often from the time of the very first session, the therapist of a neurotic client feels that he or she and the patient are on the same side and that their mutual antagonist is a problematic *part* of the patient. The sociologist Edgar Z. Friedenberg (1959) compared this alliance to the experience of two young men tinkering with a car, one the expert, the other an interested learner. In addition, whatever the valence of the therapist's countertransference, positive or negative, it will not feel overwhelming. The neurotic-level client engenders in the listener neither the wish to kill nor the compulsion to save.

Characteristics of Psychotic-Level Personality Structure

At the psychotic end of the spectrum, people are of course much more internally desperate and disorganized. Interviewing a deeply disturbed patient can range from being a participant in a pleasant, low-key discussion to being the recipient of a homicidal attack. Especially before the advent of antipsychotic drugs in the 1950s, few therapists had the natural intuitive talent and emotional stamina to be significantly therapeutic to those in psychotic states. One of the great achievements of the psychoanalytic tradition has been its inference of some order in the apparent chaos of people who are easy to dismiss as hopelessly and incomprehensibly crazy, and consequently its offer of a way of understanding and helping the severely mentally disabled.

It is not difficult to diagnose those patients who are in an overt state of psychosis: They demonstrate hallucinations, delusions, ideas of reference, and illogical thinking. There are many people walking around, however, who are at a psychotic level of organization characterologically whose basic internal confusion does not surface conspicuously unless they are under considerable stress. The knowledge that one is dealing with a "compensated" schizophrenic, or a currently nonsuicidal depressive who nonetheless is subject to periodic delusional yearnings to die, can make the difference between preventing and precipitating someone's death. In this section I shall try to sensitize the reader to some of the characteristic features of people with such fragile psychologies that they are chronically vulnerable to psychotic breaks or to severe mental and emotional deterioration.*

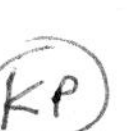

First, it is important to understand the defenses that the psychotic person uses. These processes will be described in detail in Chapter 5; for purposes of this discussion I will simply list them: withdrawal, denial, omnipotent control, primitive idealization and devaluation, primitive forms of projection and introjection, splitting, and dissociation. These defenses are preverbal and prerational; they protect the psychotic person against a level of abject dread so overwhelming that even the frightening distortions that the defenses themselves often create are a lesser evil.

Second, people whose personalities are organized at an essentially psychotic level have grave difficulties with identity—so much so that they are not fully sure *that* they exist, much less whether their existence is satisfying. They are deeply confused about who they are, and they usually struggle with such basic issues of self-definition as body concept, age, gender, and sexual orientation. "How do I know who I am?" or even "How do I know that I exist?" are not uncommon questions for psychotically organized people to ask in earnest. They cannot depend

*It is my firm conclusion, based on many years of following some extremely difficult cases over the long term, that devoted therapists do a great deal of prevention with such people. We preempt psychotic breaks, prevent suicides and homicides, and keep people out of hospitals. Unfortunately, these critical effects of psychotherapy go completely undocumented, since no one can ever prove that he or she prevented a disaster, and it is common for critics of analytic therapy to argue that if one claims to have prevented a psychotic break, the patient was not really psychosis prone in the first place.

experience others as having continuity of self either. When asked to describe themselves or other important people in their lives, they tend to be vague, tangential, concrete, or observably distorting.

Often in rather subtle ways, one feels that a patient with an essentially psychotic personality is not anchored in reality. Although most people have vestiges of magical beliefs (e.g., the idea that God decided to make it rain because I forgot my umbrella), careful investigation will reveal that such attitudes are not ego alien to psychotic individuals. They are often quite confused by and estranged from the assumptions about "reality" that are conventional within their culture. Although they may be preternaturally attuned to the underlying affect in any situation, they often do not know how to interpret its meaning and may assign highly self-referential significance to it.

For example, a very paranoid patient I have worked with for a long time, whose sanity has often been at risk, has an uncanny feel for my emotional state. She reads it accurately but then attaches to her perception of it the primitive preoccupations she has about her own essential goodness or badness, as in, "You look irritated. It must be because you think I'm a bad mother." Or "You look bored. I must have offended you last week by leaving the session 5 minutes early." It took her many years to transform the conviction "Evil people are going to kill me because they hate my lifestyle" into "I feel guilty about some aspects of my life."

In people with a potential for psychotic breakdown, there is a marked incapacity to stand aside from their psychological problems and regard them dispassionately. Cognitively, this deficit may be related to the well-documented difficulties that diagnosed schizophrenic people have with abstraction (Kasanin, 1944). Even those psychotic-level people whose mental health history has given them enough jargon to *sound* like good self-observers (e.g., "I know I tend to overreact" or even "I'm not always oriented to time, place, and person") will reveal to a sensitive interviewer that in an effort to reduce anxiety they are compliantly parroting what they have heard about themselves. One patient of mine had had so many intake experiences at psychiatric hospitals during which she had been asked to give the meaning of the proverb* "A bird in the hand is worth two in the bush" that she had asked an acquaintance what it meant and memorized the answer (she

*Asking clients to abstract by giving them proverbs to interpret is a traditional and useful means of detecting psychotic processes. People who are essentially psychotic but not overtly hallucinatory or delusional will demonstrate a *thought disorder*, the cognitive dimension of psychosis, when abstract thinking is requested.

proudly offered this explanation when I commented in an interested way on the automatic quality of her response).

Early psychoanalytic formulations about the difficulties that psychotic people have in getting perspective on their realistic troubles stressed energic aspects of their dilemma, that is, that they were expending so much energy just fighting off existential terror that none was left over to use in the service of reality assessment. Ego psychology models emphasized the psychotic person's lack of internal differentiation between id, ego, and superego, and between observing and experiencing aspects of the ego. Students of psychosis influenced by interpersonal, object relations and self psychology theories referred to boundary confusion between inside and outside experience, and to deficits in basic trust that made it subjectively too dangerous for the psychotic person to enter the same assumptional world as the interviewer. Again, the full explanation of the lack of an "observing ego" in psychotic people probably includes all these elements and several others, including constitutional, biochemical, situational, and traumatic aspects. The most important thing to understand for someone wishing to help them is that very close to the surface of potentially or actively psychotic people, one can always find both mortal fear and dire confusion.

The nature of the primary conflict in people with a potential for psychosis is literally existential: life versus death, existence versus obliteration, safety versus terror. Their dreams are full of stark images of death and destruction. "To be or not to be" is their recurrent theme. Laing (1965) eloquently depicted them as suffering "ontological insecurity." Psychoanalytically influenced studies of the families of schizophrenic people in the 1950s and 1960s consistently reported patterns of emotional communication in which the psychotic child received subtle messages to the effect that he or she was not a separate person but an extension of someone else (Singer & Wynne, 1965a, 1965b; Mischler & Waxler, 1968; Bateson, Jackson, Haley, & Weakland, 1969; Lidz, 1973). Although the discovery of the major tranquilizers has diverted attention from more strictly psychological investigations of processes involved in psychosis, no one has yet presented evidence controverting the observation that the psychotic person is deeply unconvinced of his or her right to a separate existence, or may even be unfamiliar with the sense of existing at all.

Oddly enough, with patients who are structurally in the psychotic range, the therapist's countertransference is often quite positive. The nature of this good feeling is different from that which characterizes countertransference reactions to neurotic-level clients: One ordinarily has more subjective omnipotence, parental protectiveness, and deep has more subjective omnipotence, parental protectiveness, and deep soul-level empathy toward psychotic people than toward neurotic ones. The phrase "the lovable schizophrenic" was for a long time in vogue as an expression of the solicitous attitude that mental health personnel often feel toward their most severely troubled patients. (The implicit contrast group here, as will be discussed below, is the borderline population.) Psychotic people are so desperate for basic human relatedness and for hope that someone can relieve their misery that they are apt to be deferential and grateful to any therapist who does more than classify and medicate them. Their gratitude is naturally touching.

People with psychotic tendencies are particularly appreciative of sincerity in the therapist. A recovered schizophrenic woman once explained to me that she could forgive even serious failings in the therapist if she deemed them to be "honest mistakes." Psychotic patients also appreciate educative efforts, responding with relief to the normalization or reframing of their preoccupations. These dispositions, combined with their propensity for primitive fusion and idealization, can make the therapist feel strong and benevolent.

The down side of their poignant dependence on the therapist's care is the burden of psychological responsibility they inevitably impose. In fact, the countertransference with psychotic people is remarkably like normal maternal feelings toward infants under a year and a half: They are wonderful in their attachment and terrifying in their needs. They are not yet oppositional and irritating, but they also tax one's resources to the limit. I should not work with a schizophrenic, a supervisor once told me, unless I was prepared to be eaten alive.

This "consuming" feature of their psychology is one reason for the preference of many therapists not to work with schizophrenics and other psychotically organized people. In addition, as Karon (1992) has persuasively argued, the access of the psychotic person to deeply upsetting realities that the rest of us would prefer to ignore is often too much for us. (Other reasons for their relative unpopularity as patients despite their appealing qualities probably include therapists' lack of adequate training in psychotherapy with psychotics, economic pressures that breed rationalizations about limited approaches or "management" instead of therapy, and personal dispositions not to work toward relatively modest treatment goals in contrast to what can be achieved with a neurotic-level person.) But as I will stress in the next chapter, it can be effective and rewarding to work with psychotically inclined clients if one is realistic about the nature of their psychological difficulties.

Characteristics of Borderline Personality Structure

One of the most striking features of people with borderline personality organization is their use of *primitive defenses*. Because they rely on such archaic and global operations as denial, projective identification, and splitting, when they are regressed they can be hard to distinguish from psychotic patients. One important difference between borderline and psychotic people in the area of defense is that when a therapist interprets to a borderline patient the operation of a primitive mode of experiencing, he or she will show at least a temporary responsiveness. When the therapist makes a similar interpretation to a psychotically organized person, he or she will become further agitated.

To illustrate, let us take the defense of primitive devaluation, since being devalued is a familiar experience of any therapist and since this unconscious strategy is fairly easy to appreciate without the explication of the following chapter. The interpretation of such a defense might go something like, "You certainly love to cherish all my defects. Maybe that protects you from admitting that you might need my expertise. Perhaps you would be feeling 'one down' or ashamed if you weren't always putting me down, and you're trying to avoid that feeling." A borderline patient might scorn such an interpretation, or grudgingly admit it, or receive it silently, but in any event, he or she would give some indications of reduced anxiety. A psychotic person would react with *increased* anxiety, since to someone in existential terror, devaluation of the power of the therapist might be the only psychological means by which he or she felt protected from obliteration. The therapist's discussing it as if it were optional would be extremely frightening.

Borderline patients are also both similar to and different from psychotic people on the dimension of *identity integration.* Their experience of self is likely to be full of inconsistency and discontinuity; when asked to describe their personalities, they may, like psychotics, be at a loss. Similarly, when asked to describe important people in their lives, borderline patients respond with anything but three-dimensional, evocative descriptions of recognizable human beings. "My mother? She's just a regular mother, I guess" is a typical response. They often give global and minimizing descriptions like, "An alcoholic. That's all." Unlike psychotic patients, they never sound concrete or tangential to the point of being bizarre, but they do tend to dismiss the therapist's interest in the complex nature of themselves and others.

Borderline clients are also apt to deal with their limitations in the area of identity integration with a hostile defense. One of my patients flew into a full-blown fury at a questionnaire she was given as a standard intake procedure in a mental health clinic. It had a sentence-completion section in which the client was asked to fill in blanks like "I am the kind of person who ________________." "How can anybody know what to do with this shit?" she raged. (Some years and countless sessions later she mused, "Now I could fill in that form. I wonder why I went ballistic about it.")

In two ways, the relation of borderline patients to their own identity is different from that of psychotic people, despite their commonality in lacking identity integration. First, the sense of inconsistency and discontinuity that borderline people suffer lacks the degree of existential terror of the schizophrenic. Borderline patients may have identity confusion, but they know they exist. Second, people with psychotic tendencies are much less likely than borderline patients to react with hostility to questions about identity of self and others. They are too worried about losing their sense of being altogether, consistent or not, to resent the interviewer's focus on that problem.

Despite the distinctions between borderline and psychotic people just mentioned, it is fair to say that both groups, unlike neurotics, rely heavily on primitive defenses and suffer a basic defect in the sense of self. The dimension of experience on which the two groups differ radically is *reality testing.* Borderline clients, when interviewed sensitively, demonstrate an appreciation of reality no matter how crazy or florid their symptoms may seen. It used to be standard psychiatric practice to assess the degree of the patient's "insight into illness" in order to discriminate between psychotic and nonpsychotic people. This issue has been discussed in somewhat different language in the preceding sections, where neurotic-level people were contrasted with those at the psychotic end of the scale. Kernberg (1975) has proposed that "adequacy of reality testing" be substituted for that criterion, since a borderline patient may relentlessly deny psychopathology yet still show a level of discrimination about what is real or conventional that distinguishes him or her from a psychotic peer.

To make a differential diagnosis between borderline and psychotic levels of organization, Kernberg advises investigating the person's appreciation of conventional reality by picking out some unusual feature of his or her self-presentation, commenting on it and asking if the patient is aware that others might find that feature peculiar (e.g., "I notice that you have a tattoo on your cheek that says 'Death!' Can you understand how that might seem unusual to me or others?"). The borderline person will acknowledge that the feature is unconventional and that outsiders might not understand its significance. The psychotic person is likely to become frightened and confused because the sense that he or she is not understood is deeply disturbing. These differing reactions, which Kernberg and his coworkers (e.g., Kernberg, Selzer, Koenigsberg, Carr, & Appelbaum, 1989) have documented on the basis of both clinical experience and empirical research, make sense in the context of psychoanalytic assumptions about the symbiotic nature of psychosis and the centrality of separation–individuation issues for people with borderline pathology.

As noted above, the capacity of a borderline person to observe his or her own pathology—at least the aspects of it that impress an external observer—is quite limited. People with borderline character organization come to therapy for specific complaints such as panic attacks or depression or illnesses that a physician has insisted is related to "stress," or they arrive at the therapist's office at the urging of an acquaintance or family member, but they do not come with the agenda of changing their personalities in the direction that outsiders readily see as advantageous. Having never had any other kind of character, they lack an emotional concept of how it would feel to have identity integration, mature defenses, the capacity to defer gratification, a tolerance for ambivalence and ambiguity, and so forth. They just want to stop hurting, or to get some critic off their back.

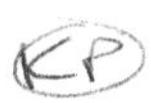

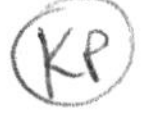

In nonregressed states, because their reality testing is fine and because they can often present themselves in ways that compel a therapist's empathy, they do not look particularly "sick." Sometimes it is only after psychotherapy has proceeded a while that a therapist realizes that a particular patient has an underlying borderline structure. Usually the first clue is that interventions intended by the therapist to be helpful are received as attacks. In other words, the therapist keeps trying to access an observing ego, and the patient does not have one. He or she knows only that some aspect of the self is being criticized. The therapist keeps trying to forge the kind of working alliance that is possible with neurotic-level patients and keeps coming to grief in the effort.

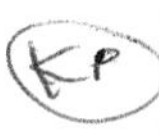

Eventually, whether or not the clinician is diagnostically astute, he or she learns that the first task of therapy will be just to weather the storms that seem to keep happening with this person, and to try to behave in a way that will be experienced by the patient as different from whatever influences have created and supported such a troubled and help-resistant person. Only after therapy has brought about some significant structural change—which in my experience takes roughly 2 years—will the patient be different enough to understand what the therapist was trying to work toward characterologically. In the meantime, many symptoms of emotional distress may have been relieved, but the work will typically have been tumultuous and frustrating to both parties.

Masterson (1976) has vividly depicted, and others with different viewpoints report similar observations, how borderline clients seem caught in a dilemma: When they feel close to another person, they panic because of fears of engulfment and total control; when they feel separate, they feel traumatically abandoned. This central conflict of their emotional experience results in their going back and forth in relationships, including the therapy relationship, in which neither closeness nor distance is comfortable. Living with such a basic conflict, one that does not respond immediately to interpretive efforts, is exhausting for borderline patients, their friends, their families, and their therapists. They are famous among emergency psychiatric service workers, at whose door they frequently appear talking suicide, for manifesting "help seeking–help rejecting behavior."

Masterson sees borderline patients as fixated at the rapprochement subphase of the separation–individuation process (Mahler, 1972b), in which the child has attained a degree of autonomy yet still needs reassurance that the parent remains available and powerful. This drama unfolds in youngsters around the age of 2, when children typically alternate between rejecting mother's help ("I can do it myself!") and dissolving in tears at her knees. Masterson believes that in their individual histories, borderline patients have had the bad luck to have mothers who either discouraged them from separating in the first place or who refused to be there for them when they needed to regress after attaining some independence. Whether or not his ideas about etiology are correct, his observations about the borderline person's entrapment in dilemmas of separation and individuation help to make sense of the changing, demanding, and often confusing qualities of borderline patients. In Chapter 4 I will discuss implications for treatment that derive from this separation–individuation predicament.

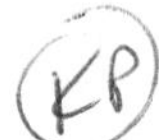

Transferences in borderline clients are strong, unambivalent, and resistant to ordinary kinds of interpretation. The therapist may be perceived as all good or all bad. If a well-intentioned but clinically naive therapist tries to interpret transference as one would with a neurotic person (e.g., "Perhaps what you're feeling toward me is something you felt toward your father"), he or she will find that no relief or helpful sense of insight follows; in fact, often the client will simply agree that the therapist is actually behaving like the earlier object. Also, it is not uncommon for a borderline person in one state of mind to perceive the therapist as godlike in power and virtue, and in another (which may appear a day later) as weak and contemptible.

As the reader may imagine, countertransference reactions with borderline clients tend to be strong and upsetting. Even when they are not negative (as in instances where the therapist feels deeply sympathetic to the desperate child in the borderline person and has fantasies of saving and rescuing the patient), they may have a disturbing, consuming quality. Many analysts in hospital settings (e.g., G. Adler, 1973; Kernberg, 1981) have noted how mental health workers tend either to be oversolicitous toward borderline patients (construing them as deprived, weak individuals who need love to grow) or to be unnecessarily punitive toward them (construing them as demanding, manipulative people who need limits). Staff members in inpatient units frequently find themselves divided into opposing camps when treatment plans for borderline patients are discussed (Gunderson, 1984). Individual practitioners doing outpatient treatment may move internally between one position and the other, mirroring each side of the conflict in the client at different times. It is not unusual for the therapist to feel like the exasperated mother of a 2-year-old who will not accept help yet collapses in frustration without it.

SUMMARY

This chapter has given a cursory overview of evolving efforts to discriminate between different maturational levels of character organization. From Kraepelinian distinctions between the sane and insane, through early psychoanalytic conceptions of symptom versus character neuroses, to current nosologies that emphasize either neurotic-level, borderline, or psychotic-level structure, therapists have sought to account for the varying reactions of their individual clients to their efforts to be of help. I have argued that the assessment of a person's *central preoccupations* (security, autonomy, or identity), *characteristic experience of anxiety* (annihilation anxiety; separation anxiety; or more specific fears of punishment, injury, and loss of control), *primary developmental conflict* (symbiotic, separation–individuation, or oedipal), *object relational capacities* (monadic, dyadic, or triadic), and *sense of self* (overwhelmed, embattled, or responsible) constitutes one comprehensive dimension of analytic psychodiagnosis.

SUGGESTIONS FOR FURTHER READING

On general psychoanalytic developmental theory, the recent contribution of the Tysons (1990) is helpful. For connections between developmental theory and diagnosis, two books by the Blancks (G. Blanck & R. Blanck, 1979, 1986) have sections on this topic. A slightly more difficult but stimulating source on the developmental understanding of psychopathology is Giovacchini's (1986) *Developmental Disorders*.

For a scholarly exegesis of the difference between neurotic symptom and neurotic character, I recommend the chapter entitled "Character Disorders" in Fenichel's (1945) classic volume. A less intimidating and highly readable introduction to analytic ideas about psychopathology is Nemiah's (1973) introductory text. Josephs (1992) and Akhtar (1992) have both recently published integrative books that pursue at a more advanced level some of the characterological issues introduced here.

Over the last decade New York University Press has put out excellent collections of papers on character neurosis (Lax, 1989), psychosis (Buckley, 1988), and borderline conditions (M. Stone, 1986). For conveying a phenomenological appreciation of psychosis, Laing's (1965) *The Divided Self* is still unmatched. Eigen's (1986) *The Psychotic Core* is difficult but rewarding. The literature on borderline conditions is so diverse and abundant as to be overwhelming, but Meissner's (1984) compendious review and Hartcollis's (1977) collection of seminal papers would be good places to start reading in this area.

4

Clinical Implications of Developmental Levels of Organization

Like politics, psychotherapy is the art of the possible. The greatest advantage to the therapist of conceptualizing each client developmentally is that one can derive a sense of what is reasonably expectable, with optimal treatment, for each one. Just as a physician expects a healthy person to recover faster and more completely from an illness than a sickly one or a teacher assumes that an intelligent student will master more material than a slow one, a therapist should have different expectations for people with different levels of character development. Realistic goals protect patients from demoralization and therapists from burnout.

It used to be commonly heard, at least in academic psychology circles, that psychoanalytic therapy was unsuited to anyone but the not-very-troubled, wealthy offspring of white, middle-class families. The kernel of truth in this argument is that classical psychoanalysis lends itself well to the treatment of articulate neurotic-level patients with the ambitious goal of character change. The arrangements and understandings that define classical analysis have generally been found to be less well suited to other kinds of patients, although early in the psychoanalytic movement, analysis was attempted with all kinds of people. Modified approaches had not yet been reported, and the general feeling was that one should at least try out analysis in case it helped. Also, the session frequency that Freud had recommended (originally six, then five times a week; later he felt that three or four might be sufficient) made analysis affordable only by people of some means.*

That psychoanalytic therapy works faster and goes further with already advantaged people than it does with those who have graver emotional handicaps is no different from the phenomenon of healthy people responding to medical care or bright people pursuing an education. Moreover, a similar situation obtains for nonpsychoanalytic treatment: Family systems therapies, rational–emotive therapy, behavioral treatments, humanistic counseling, and pharmacological management all work better with cooperative, relatively undamaged people than they do with the most disturbed and difficult clinical groups. Although it is true that it is harder to do good analytically informed therapy with more troubled people, it is not true that psychoanalytic theory is of little use in understanding and helping the seriously disturbed.

I assume that some of the readers of this book have run into the argument that analytic theory is irrelevant to the problems of the deeply distressed, multiproblem people, minorities, addicts, the poor, and others. If this chapter succeeds in conveying the richness and particularity of psychoanalytically informed therapies, it will correct that misconception. I can by no means cover all the subtleties of different psychodynamic approaches for patients of different developmental organization, but I hope to present enough aspects of the major distinctions among uncovering, supportive, and expressive therapies that the importance of a good diagnostic formulation is underscored.

What follows is a description of and theoretical rationale for some of the specific adaptations a good analytic therapist makes to different levels of character organization. The ultimate goal is to assist each person with the task that is developmentally compelling for him or her—whether that task is the full flowering of the person's creativity or the attainment of some minimal awareness that one exists and deserves to stay alive.

*The phrase "classical psychoanalysis" (or "classical analysis") in the context of this chapter refers to the technical arrangements of that activity and not to the theory that informs it. Specifically, the term refers to a session frequency of three or more times a week, the use of the couch, the direction to the patient to free associate, and the relative confinement of the analyst's activity to interpretations, particularly those concerning the transference. The phrase does not denote therapeutic relationships that are understood mainly or exclusively according to drive–defense models.

PSYCHOANALYTIC THERAPY WITH NEUROTIC-LEVEL PATIENTS

For a variety of reasons, it is easier to do psychoanalytic therapy with healthier patients, at least in the early phases of the work, than with borderline and psychotically structured ones. In Eriksonian terms, one can assume basic trust, a high degree of autonomy, and a reliable sense of identity. The goals of treatment rightfully include the removal of unconscious obstacles to full gratification in the areas of love, work, and play. Freud equated psychoanalytic "cure" with freedom, and in the Platonic tradition, he believed that it was truth that ultimately made one free. A search for difficult truths about the self is possible for neurotic-level people because their self-esteem is resilient enough to tolerate some unpleasant discoveries. Accordingly, Theodor Reik (1948) used to say that the primary requisite to conduct or undergo analysis was moral courage. For lack of a better term, and in deference to the many differences of opinion about what is centrally curative in psychoanalytic therapy with healthier people (interpretation? reconstruction? empathy? "holding?"), I will simply refer to long-term or open-ended therapies with people of neurotic-level diagnoses as "conventional" analytic treatment, with the understanding that any such treatment may be informed by drive, ego, relational, or self concepts—or a combination of these.

Conventional Modes of Therapy with Healthier Patients

The neurotic patient quickly establishes with the therapist a working alliance in which the clinician and the observing part of the client are allies in uncovering previously unconscious defenses, feelings, fantasies, beliefs, conflicts, and strivings. If the patient is looking to have a thorough understanding of his or her personality, with the goal of the greatest possible degree of growth and change, *intensive analysis* should be considered. Contemporarily, students in psychoanalytic training constitute the majority of patients willing at the outset to make the three-or-four-sessions-per-week commitment that analysis dictates (usually because their training institute requires it!), but it is a common experience of analysts that their neurotic-level patients not in the mental health field decide after a period of less intensive therapy that they want to "go deeper" and move from analytically oriented treatment (twice a week or less) into analysis.

The fact that psychoanalysis takes years does not obviate the fact that, perhaps especially with healthier persons, symptomatic and behavioral improvement may happen as quickly as with other therapies. People have a natural feel for the difference between behavior change that is possible in spite of one's psychology and behavior change that has come to feel congruent with one's insides. To move from the first to the second condition is one reason patients often choose to stay in analytic treatment for the long haul. An analogy would be the difference that a man addicted to alcohol feels between early sobriety, during which he struggles minute by minute to resist the temptation to drink, and later recovery, when he no longer feels the urge. The *behavior* of not drinking is the same in early and late sobriety, but the underpinnings of it change. It may have taken years of AA meetings and unremitting discipline to alter old patterns, habits, and beliefs, but to the recovering alcoholic the shift from a barely controlled compulsion to an indifference toward alcohol is a priceless achievement.

For those people who are unable or unwilling to take on the commitment of time, money, and emotional energy involved in intensive analysis, *psychoanalytic therapy* may be of considerable help. What most lay people think of as psychotherapy developed as a modification of classical analysis in the direction of being more specifically problem focused. This translates into patient and therapist meeting for fewer than three sessions a week, usually face-to-face. The therapist is less encouraging of emotional regression, less facilitative of the development of a transference neurosis, and more active in pointing out themes and emphases that in more intensive treatment would await patient identification. In Greenson's (1967) classic text on psychoanalysis there is careful attention to the issue of "analyzability"—by 1967 it had become evident that classical analysis was appropriate for only a portion of people seeking mental health services.

Other Approaches with Healthier Patients

Another attribute of patients in the neurotic range is their suitability for short-term analytic therapies—approaches developed by Malan (1963), Mann (1973), Bellak and Small (1978), Davanloo (1978, 1980), Sifneos (1992), and others. Aggressive focusing on a conflict area can be overwhelming to someone with a borderline or psychotic structure; in contrast, it may be experienced as stimulating and productive by a person of neurotic-level character. In parallel fashion, higher-functioning clients do well in analytically informed group and family modes of treatment, while borderline and psychotic people often do not. (These lower-functioning clients absorb so much of the emotional energy of the group or family unit that the other parties get hopelessly torn between resentment at their always being center stage and guilt about that resentment, since the more troubled person is obviously suffering more.)

In fact, as implied above, virtually any approach to therapy, not just the psychodynamic ones, will be helpful to most clients in the neurotic range. They have had enough experiences with loving people that they assume benevolence in the therapist and try to cooperate with his or her efforts. They are, understandably, popular patients. One of the reasons for the prestige that seems to go with doing classical analysis may be that people with the internal requisites to be analysands are readily responsive to and hence appreciative of their treatment. They are good advertisements for their analysts,* unlike borderline people, for example, who may—even though they may be improving in therapy—disparage their therapists ruthlessly to outsiders or idealize them in such a cloying way that everyone in their circle of friends thinks they have been taken in by a master charlatan.

Most psychodynamic writers feel that intensive psychoanalysis offers neurotically organized people the greatest ultimate benefits and that anyone with the resources to undergo in-depth, high-frequency treatment, especially someone in young adulthood with years ahead to reap the psychological rewards, would be well advised to do so. I share this opinion, having benefitted all my adult life from a good early classical analysis. It is also true, however, that a person in the neurotic range can benefit from all sorts of different experiences and can extract psychological growth even from some conditions that others might find disabling.

Readers who feel they have not been given enough information about analytic therapy with the healthier diagnostic group will find more on that topic in the next two sections. In discussing supportive and expressive therapies, I shall contrast them with more traditional approaches, and in the process the contrast group will be better illuminated.

*Some of the arrogance for which analysts who do exclusively classical treatment are justly known is comprehensible in light of the fact that they tend to work with the easiest patients, utilizing a modality that everyone with wide therapeutic experience agrees is the easiest kind of therapy to do. In other words, they have gotten spoiled. Fortunately for the reputation of the psychoanalytic tradition, their number is small, since most analysts stay in the trenches with a range of patients, and as a result do not lose empathy with the overworked agency-employed professional who interviews one self-destructive, addicted, overwhelmed borderline or psychotic person after another.

PSYCHOANALYTIC THERAPY WITH PSYCHOTIC-LEVEL PATIENTS

The most important thing to understand about people at the symbiotic level of functioning, even if they are not overtly psychotic, is that they are scared. It is no accident that the drugs that are helpful for schizophrenic conditions are major antianxiety agents; the person with a vulnerability to psychotic disorganization lacks a basic sense of security in the world and is always ready to believe that annihilation is imminent. Adopting any approach that permits a lot of ambiguity, as does traditional analytic therapy with neurotics, is like throwing gasoline into the flame of psychotic-level terror. Consequently, the treatment of choice with such patients is usually *supportive psychotherapy*.

Supportive Technique: Providing Psychological Safety

All therapy is supportive, but in the analytic tradition the phrase has a narrower meaning, reflecting the experience of several decades of psychodynamic work with more deeply disturbed people (Klein, 1940, 1945; Rosenfeld, 1947; Fromm-Reichmann, 1950; Segal, 1950; Federn, 1952; Sullivan, 1962; Searles, 1965; Jacobson, 1967; Lidz, 1973; Arieti, 1974; Karon & VandenBos, 1981; Little, 1981; Eigen, 1986; Rockland, 1992).* The first aspect of supportive work I should mention is the therapist's *demonstration of trustworthiness*. The fact that psychotic-level people are often compliant does not mean that they trust. In fact, their compliance means quite the opposite: It expresses their fear that authorities will kill them for being separate, for having their own will. The therapist can never forget the primary goal of confirming that he or she differs from the primitive images of hostile and omnipotent authority with which psychotic-level people are tormented.

To prove that one is a safe object is not so easy. With a neurotic-level person in a paranoid state, it is usually enough to interpret the transference, that is, to comment on how the patient is mixing one up with some negative person from the past or some projected negative part of the self. Interpretation of this sort is useless

*Some analysts, notably Rosenfeld and Segal in the above list, contend that effective therapy of psychotic people does not differ qualitatively from the analysis of neurotic patients. In both cases, insight is sought, the transference is analyzed, resistances are worked through, and so on. But even in their reported work, the analyst's general tone and stance sound to me different enough from the usual style with neurotic clients to warrant calling attention to the special ways therapists must meet the challenges posed by psychotic patients.

with severely disturbed people; in fact, they are likely to consider it a diabolical evasion. Instead, one must repeatedly *act* different from the patient's most frightening expectations. A facial expression that conveys respect is enough to make a neurotic-level patient comfortable, but with a person at risk for psychosis, one must demonstrate much more actively one's acceptance of the patient as a morally equal human colleague. This might include simple communications such as asking such clients to tell you if it gets too warm or too cold in the office, asking their opinions about a new painting, creating opportunities for them to demonstrate areas of personal expertise, or commenting on the creative and positive aspects of even their most bizarre symptoms. In this context, Karon (1989) has provided a pertinent example:

> Therapeutically, it is often useful to tell the patient, "That is a brilliant explanation." The patient is generally startled that any professional would take his or her ideas seriously.
>
> "You mean you think it is right?"
>
> If, as is usually the case, the therapist believes that the patient can tolerate it, the therapist might usefully say, "No, but that is because I know some things about the human mind which you don't know yet, and I'll tell you if you're interested. But given what you do know, that is a brilliant explanation." With such a nonhumiliating approach to the patient, it is often possible to get the most suspicious paranoid to consider what might be going on and its real meaning as an attempt to solve the terrifying dilemmas of his or her symptoms and life history. (p. 180)

Another aspect of demonstrating that one is trustworthy is behaving with unwavering emotional honesty. Anyone experienced with schizophrenics can attest to their attunement to affective nuance and their need to know that their therapist is emotionally truthful. Psychotic-level people require much more emotional self-disclosure than other patients, and without it they will only stew in their fantasies. This is an area where the technique of supportive therapy is diametrically opposite that of uncovering therapy. With healthier people, one avoids emotional revelations so that the patient can notice and explore what his or her fantasies are about the therapist's affective state. With more troubled clients, one must be willing to be known.

Take irritation, for example. It is natural for the therapist to feel irritated with any patient at various points during treatment, especially when the person seems to be behaving self-destructively. A perception that one's therapist looks annoyed would be upsetting to any client, but it is mortally terrifying to more deeply troubled ones. If a neurotic-level person asks, "Are you mad at me?" one helpful response would be something along the lines of, "What are your thoughts and feelings about what it would mean if I were mad at you?" If the same query is made by a potentially psychotic patient, the therapeutic reply is something like, "You're very perceptive. I guess I *am* feeling a little irritation—as much with myself as with you. I'm a bit frustrated that I can't seem to help you as fast as I would like. What was your reason for asking?"

Notice that with the supportive approach, one still invites the patient to explore his or her perceptions, but only after a potentially inhibiting apprehension has been directly counteracted by specific information. In the example above, the therapist has also explicitly expressed respect for the patient's accurate perception, thus contributing to his or her realistically based self-esteem, and has implicitly counteracted primitive fantasies of the therapist's dangerous omnipotence by connecting anger with ordinary human limitation rather than with talionic destruction. No one who finds it uncomfortable to admit to baser human motives should work with people in the psychotic range; they can smell hypocrisy, and it literally makes them crazy.

Along these lines, it is important with a psychotic-level patient to give explicit rationales for one's way of working, rationales that will make emotional sense to the person. Higher-functioning people are often therapy-savvy, and if any arrangement does not seem reasonable to them, they will usually ask about it. Take the fee, for example. With neurotic patients, regardless of how many fantasies they have about what money means to you and to them, there is rarely a need to go into why one charges what one does. It was part of the original contract, and the reasonable part of the healthier patient understands that this is a relationship where a fee is charged for services rendered.

Psychotically vulnerable people, in contrast, can have all kinds of secret and very peculiar ideas about the meaning of money exchange—not in the form of fantasies that coexist with more rational notions, but as their private conviction. One of my more psychotically organized patients told me after several months that he believed that if I really wanted to help him, I would see him for free, and that any other basis for our relationship was corrupt. He was cooperating with me, he explained, because maybe if he could work his way enough into my affections, I would treat him simply out of love and thereby heal his deep conviction of unlovability. This kind of thinking in symbiotically preoccupied people is far from rare and has to be addressed directly. "Analyzing" it as one would do with a neurotic-level person will not be helpful because the belief is syntonic, not a buried vestige of infantile forms of thought.

Hence, if one is asked about the fee by this kind of patient, one should say something like, "I charge what I do because this is the way I earn my living, helping people with emotional problems. Also, I have learned that when I charge less than this, I find myself resenting my patient, and I don't believe I can be fully helpful to someone I'm privately resenting." This is not only useful education about how the world works and about the essentially reciprocal nature of psychotherapy—which is in itself corrective to the more fused, enmeshed conceptions of relationship held by more disturbed people—but it is also emotionally honest and will consequently be received with relief even if the patient still thinks the fee is unnecessary or too high.

My own style with most psychotic-level people is quite self-disclosing. I have been known to talk about my family, my personal history, even my opinions—anything to put the person at ease with me as an ordinary human being. Such an approach is controversial, partly because not every therapist is temperamentally comfortable with disclosure and also because it has certain hazards, not the least of which is that some aspect of the therapist's revealed person will incite a psychotic response in the patient. Again, the rationale lies in the contrast between symbiotically organized people and more individuated ones. The former have such total, encompassing transferences that they can only learn about their distortions of reality when reality is painted in stark colors in front of them, while the latter have subtle and unconscious transferences that surface only when the therapist is carefully opaque.

The terror of the patient that he or she is in the hands of a powerful, distant, and perhaps persecutory Other is so great that the benefits of being more open may outweigh the risks. And if some revelation about the therapist provokes a psychotic response, it can be addressed; nondisclosure certainly provokes its share anyway. In fact, occasional disasters are inevitable in work with more disturbed people and cannot be avoided by the "right" technique. Once I sent a paranoid young man into a full-scale delusion about my intent to murder him because I absentmindedly swatted a bug ("You killed a living thing!") in his presence.

Another way one may have to demonstrate basic concern, and thereby trustworthiness, when treating someone in the psychotic range, is by extending oneself to help in a more specific, problem-solving way than would be warranted in psychotherapy with healthier persons. Karon and VandenBos (1981) have discussed in this context the value of practical advice to the patient about counteracting insomnia. Another is a willingness to take a position on the patient's behalf on certain matters. For instance, "I think it's important that you go to your sister's funeral. I know it won't be easy, but I'm afraid if you avoid it you'll always fault yourself, and you won't have another chance. I'll be here afterward to help you cope with any upset you feel." Offering direction is ordinarily out of place with healthier people, as it implicitly infantilizes a person who has psychological autonomy.

I should note that both self-disclosure and advice giving are aspects of supportive therapy that make it "irreversible." If one has misdiagnosed the patient in the direction of underestimating his or her health, one cannot become more invisible again. Therapy can shift from an uncovering style to a more expressive one, or from expressive to more supportive treatment (when an initial diagnosis was too optimistic), but one cannot restore a potential to analyze transference when one has been more "real."

The reader will have picked up by now that with psychotic-level people one must relate in a much more authoritative (not authoritarian) way than with higher-functioning patients. By acting as a human equal but a professional expert, the therapist makes frightened clients feel safer. Naturally, the issues on which one takes an authoritative stand must be ones in which the therapist is genuinely confident. Eventually, as they progress in treatment, even very disturbed people will develop enough security in the relationship to express a difference of opinion, and the therapist can take pride in having fostered the evolution of some genuine psychological independence.

Supportive Technique: Educating the Patient

A second, and related, aspect of supportive therapy that I want to stress is the therapist's *educative role*. People in the psychotic range have areas of great cognitive confusion, especially about emotions and fantasies. If researchers into family dynamics in schizophrenia have been accurate (Singer & Wynne, 1965a, 1965b; Mischler & Waxler, 1968; Bateson et al., 1969; Lidz, 1973), these clients grew up in systems in which very baffling and paralyzing emotional language was used. Family members may have talked about love while acting hatefully, claimed to represent the patient's feelings while unwittingly distorting them, and so forth. As a result, psychosis-prone people often need explicit education about what feelings are, how they are natural reactions, how they differ from actions, how everyone weaves them into fantasies, and how universal are the concerns that the psychotically organized person believes constitute his or her idiosyncratic and warped drama.

One component of the educative role is normalization. The active solicitation of all the client's concerns, and the reframing of them as natural aspects of being an emotionally responsive human being, are critical to helping a symbiotically fixated person. For example, one of my patients became very agitated on finding herself admiring my legs as I opened a window; she worried that this meant she was a lesbian. With a healthier person, I would simply have encouraged her to associate along that train of thought, assuming that her anxiety about sexual orientation was tolerable and would lead to interesting discoveries about disowned aspects of herself. With this manic–depressive woman, however, I remarked warmly that I felt complimented (because she looked frightened, as if expecting me to be horrified by the prospect of her attraction), and I went on to say that as far as I could tell on the basis of her history she is not essentially a lesbian, although everyone has some sexual feelings toward people of both genders, and that the only way she might differ from others in having noticed this idea in herself is that some people have a knack for automatically keeping such perceptions unconscious. I recast her worry as being another instance of her greater sensitivity to her inner life and to emotional subtlety than most people have, and I reiterated that my role with her includes my trying to help her become comfortable with the fact that she is often in touch with aspects of universal human psychology that many people keep out of awareness.

In this enterprise, one draws on accumulated psychoanalytic wisdom, generalizing to the patient what therapists have learned about human psychology. Early conceptions of psychosis as a state of defenselessness, contrasting with the overdefendedness of neurotic people, contributed to the development of this difference in technique. (We now understand psychotic-level people as having defenses, but very primitive ones that cannot be analyzed without making the client feel bereft of one of his or her few means of feeling less frightened.) Psychotically inclined people become traumatically overstimulated by primary process material and can only reduce their upset from that material by having it normalized.

For example, a young man I treated briefly for a psychotic reaction to his father's death confessed that he sometimes believed that he had *become* his father: His self had died, and his father had taken over his body. He was having recurrent dreams in which monsters pursued him, turned into his father, and tried to kill him; and he was genuinely terrified that the dead man, who had been a difficult and punitive parent in life, was capable of invading his body from the grave. I assured him that this was a natural though not always conscious fantasy that people have after bereavement, told him he could expect to lose that feeling as the mourning period progressed, and explained that his belief that his father inhabited his body was expressing numerous natural responses to the death of a parent. First, it indicated denial that his father was dead—a normal phase of grief; second, it expressed his own survivor guilt, handled by the fantasy that he rather than his father had died; third, it was an attempt to reduce anxiety, in that if his father was in his body, he was not somewhere else planning to murder his son for the sin of outliving him.

This kind of active, educative stance is vital to the emotional equilibrium of a psychotically anxious person because it mitigates the terror that he or she harbors about going crazy. It also welcomes the client into a world of greater psychological complexity and implicitly invites him or her to "join the human race." Most people with psychotic–symbiotic personality structure have been placed since early childhood in the sick role, first by their families and later by other social systems that define them as oddballs; consequently, they come to treatment expecting that a therapist will be similarly impressed by their lack of sanity. Interventions that embrace rather than stigmatize are relievingly corrective and have a self-fulfilling effect. In educative conversations it is more important to convey a general expectation of eventual understanding than to be completely accurate. Since one never does understand perfectly, it is also important to modify one's authoritative tone with some qualifications about such explanations being a "best guess" or "provisional understanding."

This style of intervention was first developed for children whose primitive preoccupations coexisted with fears of regression (Bornstein, 1949) and has variously been called "reconstruction upward" (R. M. Loewenstein, 1951; Greenson, 1967), "interpreting upward" (Horner, 1990), and simply "interpreting up." These phrases imply a contrast with the kind of interpretation helpful to neurotic-level patients, by which one works "from surface to depth" (Fenichel, 1941), addressing whatever defense is closest to conscious understanding. In interpreting up, one directly plumbs the depths, names their contents, and explains why that material would have been set off by the patient's life experiences. Oddly, this essential aspect of psychodynamic work with frightened patients is seldom spelled out in books on technique.

Supportive Technique: Relating Upset to Specific Stresses

This line of thought leads to a third principle of supportive therapy; namely, the *interpretation of feelings and life stresses rather than of defenses*. For example, therapists working with more disturbed people frequently have to sit through extended paranoid tirades when the patient is upset. It is tempting, in the face of an assault on the senses of a psychotic degree of fear and hatred, to try to interpret the projective defense or to contrast the client's distortions with the therapist's view of reality; but either of those strategies is likely to make the patient worry that the therapist is secretly in league with the persecutors. Yet just witnessing a disorganized psychotic outburst seems hardly therapeutic. So what is one to do?

First, one waits until the patient pauses for breath. It is better to wait too long than not long enough (this may mean sitting quietly and nodding sympathetically for most of the session), reminding oneself while one is waiting that at least the patient now trusts you enough to express uncensored feelings. Second, one makes a comment something like "You seem more upset than usual today," with no implication that the content of the upset is crazy. Finally, one tries to help the client find what it is that set off this intensity of feeling. Often, the real source of the patient's distress is only peripherally related to the topic of the rant; usually it is some life circumstance involving a separation (the patient's child is entering kindergarten, or a brother announced his engagement, or the therapist mentioned some vacation plans). Then one empathizes actively with how disconcerting separations are.

In this process, one must sometimes tolerate the odd role of seeming to endorse the person's distortions, and occasionally, as most strikingly dramatized in Robert Lindner's (1955) entertaining article "The Jet-Propelled Couch," one must even actively accept the patient's frame of reference. Sometimes only in being thus joined will the patient feel sufficiently understood to accept a subsequent interpretation (cf. Federn, 1952). The Spotnitz school of "Modern Psychoanalysis" (e.g., Spotnitz, 1976) has raised this style of therapy to a high art. Originally construed as "joining the resistance" or as practicing "paradigmatic psychoanalysis" (Coleman & Nelson, 1957), this approach has a lot in common with later "paradoxical intervention" techniques favored by some family systems therapists. Joining is not as cynical as it may seem, as there is always some truth in even the most paranoid constructions.

Examples of joining, in the service of eventual examination of misconstruals, include approaches like the following: A female patient storms into her therapist's office, accusing him of involvement in a plot to kill her. Rather than questioning the existence of the plot or suggesting that she is projecting her own murderous wishes, the therapist says, "I'm sorry! If I've been connected with such a plot, I wasn't aware of it. What's going on?" Another client falls into a miserable silence and when prodded confesses that he is responsible for the carnage in the Middle East. The therapist responds, "It must be terrible to carry that burden of guilt. In what way are you responsible?" Or a patient confides that the therapist's colleague and friend, the ward nurse, tried to poison him. The therapist says, "How awful. Why do you suppose she is mad enough at you to try to kill you?"

Note that in all these instances, the therapist does not express agreement with the patient's interpretations of events, but neither does he or she inflict the wound to the patient's pride of dismissing them. And most important, the therapist invites further discussion. Usually, once the client lets off enough steam, a more realistic understanding of what is going on will gradually replace the paranoid distortions. Sometimes the therapist can assist this process by gently asking about alternative explanations of the patient's perceptions, *but only after giving the client room to spill*. Often by the end of the session, the patient is reoriented to reality and leaves on an upbeat note.

By now the reader has probably assimilated how different psychoanalytic work with psychotic-level people is from therapy with neurotic individuals. Not everyone has the temperament to do this kind of work comfortably—it is facilitated by both counterphobia and omnipotence of a degree alien to the personalities of many therapists, and those without such qualities may be better off in other areas of mental health service. One of the most important things to learn in one's training is which kinds of people one enjoys and treats effectively, and which kinds one should refer.

Supportive therapy with psychotic and potentially psychotic people has different objectives and different satisfactions from therapy with healthier clients. Despite some prejudice against it in the name of cost containment (a position I regard as comparable to the argument that cancer patients should receive aspirin), psychotherapy with psychotic people is effective and is gratefully received (see, e.g., A Recovering Patient, 1986). Therapy with the severely disturbed can be lifesaving; expertise in it is much rarer than expertise treating healthier people; it is intellectually and emotionally stimulating; it nourishes one's creativity. At the same time, it can be emotionally depleting, confusing, and discouraging, and it inevitably confronts one with the limits on one's capacities to effect dramatic transformations.

PSYCHOANALYTIC THERAPY WITH BORDERLINE PATIENTS

The term *borderline* encompasses great diversity. Not only is a depressive person with borderline character structure quite different from a narcissistic or hysterical or paranoid borderline person, but there is a wide range of severity within the borderline category, extending from the border with the neuroses to the border with the psychoses

(Grinker et al., 1968)—somewhat arbitrary borders to begin with. Not surprisingly, the closer a person's psychology is to neurotic, the more positively he or she will respond to a more "uncovering" kind of treatment, whereas those clients who border on psychosis will react better to a more supportive style. People are not unidimensional; every neurotic-level person has some borderline tendencies, and vice versa. But in general, the treatment of choice for people with a borderline level of personality organization is *expressive psychotherapy*.

The aim of therapy for people with borderline structure is the development of an integrated, dependable, complex, and positively valued sense of self. Along with this process goes the evolution of a capacity to love other people fully despite their flaws and contradictions. A gradual movement from capricious reactivity to steady reliance on one's perceptions, feelings, and values is possible for borderline people, despite the difficulties they present to therapists, especially in the early phases of treatment.

Theorists with different beliefs about the origins of borderline personality structure have emphasized different aspects of treatment for it (e.g., Balint, 1968; Kernberg, 1975; Masterson, 1976; G. Adler & Buie, 1979; Giovacchini & Boyer, 1982; Pine, 1985; G. Blanck & R. Blanck, 1986; Searles, 1986; Stolorow, Brandchaft, & Atwood, 1987; Meissner, 1988), and often in books and articles on psychoanalytic therapy in general some mention is made of the special technical requirements for working with more troubled but not psychotic people (e.g., Eissler, 1953; Stone, 1954). There is sufficient controversy in the literature on technique with borderline clients that a few paragraphs cannot address all the divergences, but I shall mention a few generally accepted principles of treatment that will be comprehensible to people new to psychoanalysis.

Expressive Technique: Safeguarding Boundaries

Expressive therapy has many things in common with both supportive and uncovering treatments: The patient is encouraged to say everything that comes to mind; the therapist takes on the job of helping him or her make sense of it; and both parties expect that change and growth will occur through a combination of insightful learning and the provision of an ameliorative personal relationship. But the differences are significant. Most of them derive from the fact that the borderline person by definition does not have an integrated observing ego that sees things the same way the therapist does; instead, he or she is subject to shifting chaotically between different ego states, with no capacity yet for putting disparate attitudes together.

Although borderline patients have more capacity to trust than psychotically organized people do, and they thus do not require the therapist's continual demonstration that they are safe in the consulting room, they may take up to several years to develop the kind of therapeutic alliance that a neurotic client may feel within minutes of meeting the therapist. Whereas the psychotic person tends to fuse psychologically with the clinician and the neurotic one to keep a clear separate identity, the borderline person alternates—confusingly to self and others—between symbiotic attachment and hostile, isolated separateness. (Both states are upsetting: One raises the specter of engulfment, the other of desertion.)

Given this instability of ego state, a critical dimension of treatment with borderline patients is the *establishment of the consistent conditions of the therapy*—what Robert Langs (1973) has called the therapeutic frame. This includes not only arrangements as to time and fee but may also involve numerous other decisions about the boundaries of the relationship that rarely come up with other clients. Common concerns include, "Can I call you at home?" "What if I'm suicidal?" "Will you break confidentiality for any reason?" "How late can I cancel a session without being charged?" "Can I sleep on the floor in your waiting room?" "Will you write my professor and say I was too stressed out to take the exam?"

Some of these issues are articulated as questions; others come up in enacted form (e.g., one finds the client sleeping on the waiting room floor) as the limits of the relationship are tested. The possibilities for boundary issues are limitless with people in the borderline range, and the important thing for the therapist to know is not so much *what* conditions should be set (these may vary according to the patient's personality and the therapist's preferences) but how critical it is *that* they be set, consistently observed, and enforced by specific sanctions if the patient fails to respect them.*

Borderline-level clients will often react with anger to the practitioner's boundaries, but two therapeutic messages will be received nonetheless: (1) the therapist regards the patient as a grown-up and has confidence in his or her ability to tolerate frustration, and (2) the therapist refuses to be exploited and is therefore a model of self-respect. Usually the histories of people in the borderline range give evidence of their having had ample exposure to the opposite messages; they have

*Lest this sound harsh, let me stress that no matter how skilled the therapist is, most borderline clients will act in ways that provoke limits. It is disturbing to someone with separation–individuation issues to be indulged in every whim, much as it is to any adolescent whose parents do not insist on responsible behavior.

been indulged when regressed (and usually ignored when age appropriate), and they have been expected to be exploitable and allowed to exploit.

Therapists new to the treatment of borderline patients often wonder when all the preconditions of therapy will finally be worked out, a working alliance created, and the actual therapy begun. The experienced practitioner's response is that all the work with the conditions of treatment *is* the therapy. Once a neurotic-type alliance is achieved, the patient by definition will have taken a giant step developmentally. It is disconcerting to spend so much time on boundary issues with people who are often bright, talented, and articulate, and with whom one naturally wants to get on to other things. Niggling over limits is scarcely what we envisioned as constituting psychoanalytic treatment when we signed on for training. Thus, people working with their first borderline clients may suffer periodic fits of doubt about their competence.

Another aspect of the conditions of the therapy with borderline-level patients that I should mention in passing is that except for some people closer to the border of neurosis, it is generally better for the therapist and the client to work face to face. Although not as subject to overwhelming transferences as psychotically vulnerable people, borderline patients have more than enough transference without the therapist's creating more ambiguity by being out of the patient's line of vision. Also, again because intensity is hardly something needing encouragement in borderline clients, only an unusual set of circumstances (such as temporary suicidality or the need for increased support during withdrawal from an addiction) would warrant their coming more than three times a week, as in classical analysis.

Expressive Technique: Voicing Contrasting Feeling States

A second thing to attend to with borderline clients is the phrasing of interpretations. First, a contrast. With neurotic patients, one's comments should be infrequent enough to get the patient's attention ("less is more"), and one should interpret in a pithy, emotionally impactful way (Fenichel, 1941; Colby, 1951; Hammer, 1968). Often one interprets the underside of some conflict in which the patient is aware of only one area of feeling. For example, a woman in the neurotic range may be gushing about a friend with whom she is in a somewhat competitive situation in a way that suggests she is not in touch with any negative affects. The therapist may say something along the lines of, "But you'd also like to kill her." Or a man may be associating on and on about how independent and free spirited he is; the therapist may comment, "And yet you are always worried about what I think of you."

In these cases, the respective neurotic clients will know that the therapist has revealed a part of their subjective experience that they had been keeping out of consciousness. Because they can appreciate that the clinician is not being reductionistic, is not claiming that the disowned attitude is their *real* feeling and that their prior conscious ideas were illusory, they feel expanded in their awareness as a result of the interpretation. They feel understood, even if slightly wounded. But borderline clients to whom one talks this way will feel criticized and diminished, because unless the interpretation is phrased differently, the main message that will be received is, "You're utterly wrong about what you *really* feel." This misunderstanding derives from their tendency to be in one or another ego state rather than in a condition of complex identity in which ambivalence and ambiguity are tolerated.

For the above reasons, it is common for beginning therapists to think they are expressing solicitous understanding and to find that the borderline person reacts as if attacked. One way around this problem is to remind oneself that there is no observing ego in the borderline person that processes an interpretation as *additional* information about the self, and that consequently one must provide that function within the interpretation. So with a borderline client, one would have a better chance of being heard as empathic if one said, "I can see how much Mary means to you. Is it possible, though, that there is also a part of you—a part that you would not act upon of course—that would like to get rid of her because she's in some ways in competition with you?" Or, "You certainly have established that you have a very independent, self-reliant streak. It's interesting that it seems to coexist with some opposite tendencies, like a sensitivity to what I think of you." Such interventions lack the punch and beauty of an economy of words, but given the particular psychological problems of borderline people, they are much more likely than more trenchant formulations to be taken in as intended.

Expressive Technique: Interpreting Primitive Defenses

A third distinctive feature of effective therapy with patients in the borderline category is the *interpretation of primitive defenses as they appear in the relationship*. This work is not different in principle from ego psychological work with neurotic-level people, in that one analyzes defensive processes as they appear in the transference. But because the defenses of a borderline patient are so totalistic, and because he or she feels and comes across as entirely different in different ego states, the analysis of defense requires a special approach.

With borderline clients, it is generally not helpful for the therapist to make what psychoanalysts call genetic interpretations, in which a transference reaction is linked up to feelings that more appropriately belonged to a figure from the patient's past. In the neurotic range, one gets a lot of mileage out of an interpretation like, "Perhaps you are feeling so angry at me because you are experiencing me as like your mother." The neurotic patient often agrees, notices the differences between the therapist and the mother, and gets interested in other instances in which this distortion might have been operating. With borderline patients, reactions can vary from "So what?" (meaning, "You're a lot like my mother, so why wouldn't I react that way?") to "How's that supposed to be useful?" (meaning, "You're just talking party-line shrink talk now. When are you going to get down to helping me?") to "Right!" (meaning, "Finally you're getting the picture. The problem is my mother, and I want you to change her!"). These kinds of reactions can leave a beginning therapist completely bewildered, disarmed, and deskilled, especially if genetic interpretations were the most helpful aspect of his or her own personal therapy.

What *can* be interpreted with borderline clients is the nature of the here-and-now emotional situation with the therapist. For example, in an instance of anger, it is likely that in a borderline person the defense at work is not displacement or straightforward projection, as it would be in the above example of the neurotic person with the mother transference; instead, the patient is using projective identification. He or she is trying to unload the feeling of "bad me" (Sullivan, 1953) and the associated affect of rage by putting them on the therapist, but the transfer of image and affect is not "clean"; the patient maintains some feeling of both badness and anger despite the projection. This is the painful price paid by the borderline person, and inevitably shared by the therapist, for inadequate psychological separation.

Here is an essential and ultimately interpretable difference between borderline clients and both psychotic and neurotic ones. It will be covered in the next chapter in more detail, but in brief: The psychotic person when projecting is sufficiently out of touch with reality not to care whether or not a projection "fits." The neurotic person when projecting maintains an observing ego that is capable of noticing that he or she is projecting. Borderline patients when projecting cannot quite succeed in getting rid of the feeling being projected. They cannot take an attitude of indifference about how realistic the projected material is because reality testing in borderline people, unlike in psychotics, is intact. And they cannot relegate it to the unconscious part of the ego because, unlike neurotics, they have no observing-versus-experiencing ego differentiation in their personality makeup. So they keep feeling whatever is projected, along with the need to *make it fit* so that they will not feel crazy. As a result, the therapist receives the client's anger (or other strong affect) and also feels a rising countertransference anger as the client tries to make the projection fit by insisting that the *reason* he or she is angry is that the therapist is hostile. Soon, the therapist *is* hostile, on the basis of feeling worked over.* Such transactions account for the bad reputation borderline clients have among mental health professionals, even though they are not always unpleasant people and are usually responsive to enlightened treatment.

The kind of interpretation that may reach a borderline person in the above predicament is something like, "You seem to have a conviction that you are bad. You're angry about that, and you're handling that anger by saying that I am the one who is bad, and that it's my anger that causes yours. Could you imagine that both you and I could be some combination of good and bad and that that wouldn't have to be such a big deal?" This is an example of a here-and-now confrontation of a primitive defense. It represents an effort by the therapist, one that will have to be repeated in different forms for months at best, to move the patient from a psychology in which everything is black or white and all or nothing to one in which diverse good and bad aspects of the self, and a range of emotions, are all consolidated within an overall identity. This kind of interpreting does not come easily to most people, but fortunately, it improves with practice.

Expressive Technique: Getting Supervision from the Patient

A fourth technical dimension of work with borderline clients that I have found of great value is *asking the patient's help* in resolving the either/or dilemmas into which the therapist is typically put. This

*Borderline clients are renowned for exerting unconscious emotional pressures that seduce therapists out of role, invite inappropriate gratifications, and provoke hostile enactments. Consequently, they are often referred to as "manipulative." I prefer not to give that label to this subtle but powerful phenomenon, since we then have no word for the *conscious* manipulations characteristic of psychopathic people—a very different phenomenon in which the patient gets self-esteem from getting the better of someone. Someone with borderline organization has simply learned that competence gets ignored and incompetence gets attention. That the therapist *feels* manipulated does not equate to the client's deliberate exploitation.

technique, by which one in effect gets the patient to be one's supervisor, relates to the all-or-nothing way in which borderline people construe things. They tend to evoke in a therapist the sense that there are two mutually exclusive options for responding to a given situation, and that both would be wrong, for different reasons. Usually there is a test involved, in which if the therapist acts one way, he or she will fail according to one polarity of the patient's conflict, and if the other alternative is chosen, there will be an equal failure of the opposite sort.

For example, I once treated a 22-year-old man with an alcoholic father, who seemed not to notice his existence, and an overinvolved, anxious, intrusive mother, who took over her son's life to the extent of picking out his clothes each day. (I had met the parents and was thus in a position to know more about the real people who had influenced this man than one often knows with borderline clients.) As the therapy progressed, this patient would stop speaking for increasing amounts of time during our sessions. At first, it seemed as if he simply needed the space to get his thoughts together, but as the silences stretched out to 15 and then 20 minutes at a time, I felt that something less benign was going on and that I would be remiss in not addressing it.

If this patient had been in the neurotic range, I would have reminded him of his agreement to keep talking about whatever was on his mind and explored with him what was getting in the way of his willingness to do that; in other words, I would have done simple resistance analysis. But with this young man I could feel that something more primitive was going on, involving counterpoised terrors of engulfment and abandonment, and I knew we did not have enough of a working alliance for me to approach his silence as I would with a healthier person. If I remained quiet, I was fairly sure he would feel hurtfully neglected, as by his father; yet if I spoke, I suspected he would experience me as taking over, like his mother. My quandary at this juncture probably mirrored his sense that he would be damned if he did talk and damned if he didn't.

After trying for a while to figure out which intervention would be the lesser evil, it occurred to me to ask *him* to help me solve the problem. At least that way, whatever came out of our interaction would have an element of his autonomy in it. So I asked him how he wanted me to respond when he went into a long silence. He answered that he guessed he wanted me to ask him questions and to draw him out. I then commented that I would be glad to do that, but that he should know that I might be way off base in my pursuit of what he was thinking about since when he was quiet, I had no idea what was on his mind. (There had been evidence in the dreams and fantasies he had reported, while still talking, that he believed that others, like the fantasied omniscient mother of early infancy, could read his mind. I wanted to send a contrary and more realistic message.)

He brightened up and on that basis changed his mind, deciding that I should wait until he felt ready to talk. He then came for three sessions in a row in which he greeted me cheerfully, sat down, said nothing for 45 minutes, then departed politely when I said our time was up. Interestingly, whereas I had been in a miserable internal state before I got him to supervise me in this way, I was at peace with his silence afterward. A couple of years later, he was able to tell me that my willingness to take his direction in that matter marked the beginning of his ability to feel like a separate person in the presence of someone else. This technique thus reduces the therapist's immediate uneasiness; more important, it models an acceptance of uncertainty, affirms the patient's dignity and creativity, and reminds both parties nonjudgmentally of the cooperative nature of the work.

Expressive Technique: Promoting Individuation and Discouraging Regression

People with borderline levels of character organization need empathy as much as anyone else, but their mood changes and ego state fluctuations make it hard for clinicians to know how and when to convey it. Because they evoke loving countertransferences when they are depressed or frightened, and hateful ones when they act antagonistically, one may find oneself inadvertently rewarding them for regression and punishing them for individuation. Therapists trained to work with neurotic-level patients by fostering a contained regression may, out of habit, encourage some of the most unhealthy responses of borderline clients. An appreciation of their psychology, however, gives the therapist grounds for acting counterintuitively, that is, being relatively nonresponsive to states of subjective helplessness and showing appreciation for assertiveness—even when it takes the form of angry opposition.

The work of Masterson and his colleagues discussed in the previous chapter suggests a therapeutic approach based on attention to issues of closeness and distance. Masterson believes that the mothers of people diagnosed as borderline were deeply attached and responsive to their children in early infancy, but they discouraged the individuation that normally happens between 18 months and 3 years or so. The outcome of such parenting is that later on, whenever such people are in a regressed, dependent relationship, they feel safe; when alone, they suffer an anguished desperation that Masterson has evocatively called "abandonment depression." Closeness is thus comforting, yet with it comes a sense of being engulfed, controlled, and infantilized. Separateness, despite being abjectly painful, is eventually empowering.

Masterson's recommended technique with borderline clients stresses the need for the therapist to act in the opposite way the mother purportedly did, actively confronting regressive and self-destructive behaviors (e.g., "Why would you want to pick up men at bars?") and empathically endorsing all efforts toward autonomy and competence (e.g., "I'm glad to see you can tell me off when I make you angry"). His model emphasizes discouraging the clinging dependency that gives borderline patients no basis for self-esteem and taking pains to see the forward-moving, adaptive elements in even their most aggravating manifestations of self-assertion. Because one's natural countertransferences go in the converse directions, these attitudes are not always easy to take.

Expressive Technique: Interpreting during Quiescence

Pine (1985) contributed an important dictum to our literature on technique with clients who are struggling over separation and individuation: "Strike when the iron is cold." It has long been accepted that with neurotic-level people, the best time to make interpretations is when the patient is in a state of emotional arousal, so that the content of the therapist's observation is not intellectualized and the affective power of the issues being addressed is unmistakable. With borderline clients, an opposite rule applies, because when they are in a state of heightened emotionality, they are too upset to take anything in. One can comment on what happened in their rage or panic or desperate regression, but only after that state is over and they are internally reassured of having recovered from such a disturbing intensity of feeling.

Thus one might say to a borderline patient, "I was thinking. What you're talking about now, your tendency to feel murderous envy and to attack people when you're in that state . . . was something like that part of your outburst at me last week? It felt as if whatever I offered you, you had to destroy it." In a condition of emotional repose, a borderline client may be willing—even relieved —to hear that the therapist has named such a dynamic and tried to understand it. But in a state of intense feeling, he or she will usually receive interpretation not only as condemnation but also as an effort to dismiss passionately held attitudes as if they were contemptible. Telling someone in the throes of an envious rage that he or she is trying to destroy the therapist will only increase the person's helpless fury and shame over having such raw impulses. Talking about it later may be very fruitful.

Expressive Technique: Respecting Countertransference Data

A final aspect of the implications of a borderline diagnosis for psychotherapy concerns the *central role of the therapist's understanding of countertransference.* Much more than with either psychotic- or neurotic-level people, borderline clients communicate through powerful and unverbalized affect transmission. By this I mean that even though they may talk freely in therapy, the most important communications they send are often not in the content of their words but in the "background music" of their emotional state. The intuitive, affective, and imaginal responses of therapists when sitting with a borderline patient can often provide better data about the essence of what is going on between the two people than either cognitive reflection on the content of the patient's communication or recourse to ideas on theory and technique.

When one suddenly feels bored, or in a rage, or panicky, or overwhelmed with the wish to rescue, or diverted by sexual images, something is probably going on that is unconsciously instigated by the patient and that says something important about that person's internal state. For example, consider a paranoid man in treatment with a young woman. He is in a state of self-righteous indignation about mistreatment by some authority, and she notices that she feels weak, small, fearful of the patient's criticism, and distracted by fantasies of being attacked. She should consider the possibility that what she is feeling is a split-off, disowned part of the patient that is being projected into her in an almost physical way. If that idea seems reasonable after some reflection, it may be therapeutic (to both parties!) for her to say something like, "I know that you are in touch with feeling angry and energized, but I think there may also be a part of you that feels weak, anxious, and fearful of being attacked."

This area of the informational value of countertransference is a tricky one and must be addressed with discipline. Not every passing thought and emotion felt with a borderline patient is one that the patient put there. At their worst, therapists can do harm in the name of concepts like projective identification and induced countertransference; I have even heard of people getting into hassles with borderline patients over whose "fault" it is that the therapist is having strong reactions. I do not want to feed anyone's rationalizations in this direction. Decades of clinical evidence suggests that countertransference, like transference, is always a mixture of internally generated and externally stimulated material, sometimes weighted more in one direction, sometimes more in the other (Sandler, 1976, 1987; Roland, 1981; Gill, 1983; Tansey & Burke, 1989; Jacobs, 1991). Therapists should be insightful about their own dynamics and take emotional responsibility for their reactions, even when it is their patient who is obviously stirring them up. And even interpretations that the therapist is convinced are valid should be offered in a way that invites the client to take issue if the explanation feels wrong to him or her.

Having said all that, I want to add that the extreme contrary attitude, that one should regard countertransference as solely one's "own stuff," can also be inimical to clinical progress. Some psychoanalytic supervisors put so much stress on their students' understanding of their own dynamics that they foster a distracting degree of self-consciousness. No emotional energy is left over for reflecting on what can be learned about the patient from one's responses. A kind of navel gazing comes to substitute for therapeutic relatedness, and people of talent and compassion become reluctant to trust what are often excellent natural instincts because they fear they are acting something out.

If in the above example, for instance, the therapist had handled her countertransference with self-examination alone, reflecting on how she has a vulnerability to feeling small and frightened in the presence of angry men who remind her of her critical father, there would be little to do therapeutically with such an insight. It might help her to contain defensive reactions, an achievement not to be disdained, but it would not guide her toward what she could actively do for the patient. The worst thing that can happen if one mistakes one's own feelings for the client's is that one will be wrong, and if interpretations are made in a tone of hypothesis rather than pronouncement, the patient will be glad to point out the therapist's errors.

This concludes what I can say in a primer about some of the implications of developmental level of personality structure for treatment. The experienced clinician will understand that I have only scratched the surface. If this were a treatise on technique per se, each category would merit at least a chapter, or better yet, each would be the subject of its own book. And as if the above issues were not complex enough, let me now introduce the topic of the interaction of developmental and typological categories of personality structure and their complex relationship.

INTERACTION OF MATURATIONAL AND TYPOLOGICAL DIMENSIONS OF CHARACTER

Figure 4.1 sets out visually the ways in which many analytic diagnosticians implicitly map out their patients' personality structures. The developmental axis, though divided into the three main categories of

	Typological Dimension									
Developmental Dimension	Psychopathic	Narcissistic	Schizoid	Paranoid	Depressive	Masochistic	Obsessive compulsive	Hysterical	Dissociative	Other
Neurotic-to-healthy level Identity integration and object constancy Freudian oedipal Eriksonian initiative versus guilt										
Borderline level Separation–individuation Freudian anal Eriksonian autonomy versus shame and doubt										
Psychotic level Symbiosis Freudian oral Eriksonian basic trust versus mistrust										

FIGURE 4.1. Developmental and typological dimensions of personality.

organization discussed above, is actually a continuum, with differences of degree that gradually become great enough to warrant conceptualization as differences of kind. Individual people fluctuate somewhat maturationally; under enough stress an optimally healthy person can have a temporary psychotic reaction; and even the most delusional schizophrenic has moments of utter lucidity.

The maturational categories should by now make sense to the reader as constructs. Many of the typological ones should be familiar, even though they will not be discussed systematically until later in this book. Chapters 5 and 6 will cover in detail the psychoanalytic concept of defense, since the personality configurations on the typological axis represent the habitual use of one defense or one cluster of defenses.

At this juncture, I want to state an observation that may help the reader to interpret this grid. I think there is evidence that in every category on the horizontal axis, there is a range of character pathology from the psychotic to the neurotic–healthy areas. Yet people are not evenly distributed along all points of each continuum. Those categories that represent the habitual use of a primary defense will "load" more toward the psychotic end of the continuum; paranoid people, for example, who by definition depend on projective defenses, will be more common at the lower rather than at the upper end of the developmental axis. Those typological categories representing reliance on more mature defenses will load more toward the neurotic pole; a greater proportion of obsessional people, for example, will be at the neurotic end of the obsessive dimension than at the psychotic one.

Anyone's life experience with a diversity of human beings gives evidence that it is possible for someone to have a high degree of ego development and identity integration and still handle most anxieties with a primitive defense. Again taking the case of paranoid characters, most of us can think of people we have known whose personalities are distinctly paranoid but who have good ego strength, a clarity about their existence as individuated human beings, an elaborated and consolidated identity, and enduring relationships. They often find a home in professions like private detective work or law enforcement or covert operations, in which their paranoid tendencies work to advantage. The fact that healthier paranoid people do not usually seek psychotherapy (a fact intrinsically related to their paranoia) does not mean that they are not out there. The frequency with which people seek therapy and thereby get into mental health statistics is not the same across different types of personality structure because the categories reflect important differences in areas like one's disposition to trust, inclination to hope, willingness to part with money for nonmaterial benefits, and so forth.

Correspondingly, ordinary life experience also suggests that it is possible for people to rely centrally on a "mature" defense like intellectualization and nevertheless have poor reality testing, inadequate separateness, limited identity integration, and unsatisfying object relationships. Thus, while healthier obsessive people may be easier to find than those with psychotic leanings, any intake worker in an inpatient facility has seen people whose penchant for intellectualizing has crossed the line into delusion.

It is often more important clinically to have a sense of a client's overall developmental level than it is to identify his or her most appropriate typological descriptor. In the higher ranges especially, people rarely exemplify one pure personality type, since flexibility of defense is one aspect of psychological health or ego strength. But both types of assessment are important, as will be exemplified in certain instances of differential diagnosis that will be covered in Chapters 7 through 15.

SUMMARY

The subject of this chapter has been the implications for therapeutic technique of whether a given client is mainly neurotic, psychotic, or borderline in character structure. Neurotic-level people are usually excellent candidates for either psychoanalysis or traditional psychoanalytically oriented "uncovering" therapies; their ego strength also makes them responsive to many other kinds of intervention.

Patients at a symbiotic–psychotic level usually need supportive therapy, described as containing, among other things, an emphasis on safety, education, and attention to the effects of particular stresses.

Patients at a borderline level are most helped by expressive therapy, a mode of working in which boundaries are critical, contrasting ego states should be named, and primitive defenses should be interpreted. The patient's help may be solicited to resolve impasses. Interventions that are useful to borderline patients discourage regression and support individuation. The therapist builds understanding during periods of quiescence and respects information contained in countertransference.

Finally, character structure was diagrammed on two axes in order to illustrate graphically the principle of appreciating both developmental and typological dimensions of personality.

SUGGESTIONS FOR FURTHER READING

The standard text on classical psychoanalysis with people at a neurotic level of organization is still Greenson's (1967) *The Technique and Practice of Psychoanalysis*. My nominations for the most readable primers on conventional analytic therapy, of which there many, are the ones by Colby (1951) and Chessick (1969). Schafer's (1983) *The Analytic Attitude* articulates all the aspects of therapy that conventional books leave out. Among the texts on therapy that try to be generic across levels of character organization, I recommend those by Fromm-Reichmann (1950), Paolino (1981), Hedges (1983), and Pine (1985). The most readable book on therapy across developmental levels from an object relations perspective is probably Horner's (1991)

Psychoanalytic Object Relations Therapy. A particularly valuable self psychology perspective on treatment is Wolf's (1988) *Treating the Self*.

The best writing I know of about working with psychotic-level patients—and good sources in this area are much scarcer—includes work by Arieti (1955), Searles (1965), Lidz (1973), Giovacchini (1979), and Karon and VandenBos (1981). The longstanding need for a comprehensive book on supportive therapy has finally been filled by Rockland's (1992) excellent text.

The literature on the expressive therapies is confusing because of the diversity of approaches to people with borderline organization. A valuable recent primer by Kernberg and his colleagues (1989) translates his formulations into concrete clinical recommendations. Masterson's theory of technique, which has the virtue of being gracefully written, is perhaps best summarized in his 1976 book on treating the borderline adult. Gerald Adler's (1985) book is a readable description of yet another way of understanding and treating people in this group.

5
Primary (Primitive) Defensive Processes

Familiarity with the concept of defense and with the variety of defense mechanisms available to human beings is critical to the understanding of psychoanalytic character diagnosis. The major diagnostic categories used by analytic therapists to denote personality types refer implicitly to the persistent operation in an individual of a specific defense or constellation of defenses. Thus, a diagnostic label is a kind of shorthand for a person's habitual defensive pattern.

The term "defense" in psychoanalytic theory is in many ways unfortunate. What we end up calling defenses in mature adults begin as more global, inevitable, healthy, adaptive ways of experiencing the world. Freud is responsible for originally observing and naming some of these processes; his choice of the term "defense" reflects at least two aspects of his thinking. First, Freud was fond of military metaphors. When he was trying to make psychoanalysis palatable to a skeptical public, he frequently made analogies, for pedagogical purposes, comparing psychological operations to army tactical maneuvers, or compromises over military objectives, or battles with complex outcomes. Second, when he first encountered the most dramatic and memorable examples of what we now call defenses, most notably repression and conversion, he saw these processes operating *in their defensive function*. The emotionally damaged, predominantly hysterical people he first became fascinated by were trying to avoid reexperiencing what they feared would be unbearable pain. They were doing so, Freud observed, at a high cost to their overall functioning.

Ultimately it would be better for them to feel fully the overwhelming emotions they were afraid of, thereby liberating their energies (as per drive theory) for the task of getting on with their lives. Thus, the earliest context in which the defenses were talked about was one in which the doctor's task was to diminish their power.

In that context, the therapeutic value of weakening or breaking down a person's maladaptive defenses was self-evident. Unfortunately, in the climate of excitement in which Freud's early observations were greeted, the idea that defenses are somehow *by nature* maladaptive spread among the lay public, to the degree that the word acquired an undeservedly negative cast. Calling someone "defensive" is universally understood to be a criticism. Analysts also use the word in that way in ordinary speech, but when they are discussing defense mechanisms in a scholarly, theoretical way, they do not necessarily assume that anything pathological is going on when a defense is operating. In fact, analytically influenced therapists have sometimes understood certain problems, notably psychotic and close-to-psychotic "decompensations," as evidence of *insufficient* defenses.

The phenomena that we refer to as defenses have many benign functions. They begin as healthy, creative adaptations, and they continue to work adaptively throughout life. When they are operating to defend the self against threat, they are discernible as "defenses," a label that seems under those circumstances to fit. The person whose behavior manifests defensiveness is generally trying unconsciously to accomplish one or both of the following ends: (1) the avoidance or management of some powerful, threatening feeling, usually anxiety but sometimes overwhelming grief and other disorganizing emotional experiences; and (2) the maintenance of self-esteem. The ego psychologists emphasized the function of defenses in dealing with anxiety; object relations theorists, who emphasize attachment and separation, introduced the understanding that defenses operate against grief as well; and self psychologists have stressed the role of defenses in the effort to maintain a strong, consistent, positively valued sense of self.

Psychoanalytic thinkers assume, although it is not explicitly set down this way in our literature on diagnosis, that we all have preferred defenses that have become integral to our individual styles of coping. This preferential and automatic reliance on a particular defense or set of defenses is the result of a complex interaction among at least four factors: (1) one's constitutional temperament; (2) the nature of the stresses that one suffered in early childhood; (3) the defenses modeled—and sometimes deliberately taught—by parents and other significant figures; and (4) the experienced consequences of using particular defenses (in the language of learning theory, reinforcement effects). In psychodynamic parlance, the unconscious choice of one's favorite modes of coping is "overdetermined," expressing the cardinal analytic principle of "multiple function" (Waelder, 1960).

In this chapter and the next, I will cover the major defenses as they are currently understood by most analytic practitioners. Although there is no evidence that defenses emerge one after the other in a predictable, orderly sequence as a child develops, there is a fair degree of agreement among psychodynamic clinicians that some defenses represent a more "primitive" process than others. In general, the defenses that are referred to as primary or immature or primitive or "lower order" (Laughlin, 1970) are those that involve the boundary between the self and the outer world. Those that are conceived as secondary or more mature or advanced or "higher order" deal with internal boundaries, such as those between the ego or superego and the id, or between the observing and experiencing parts of the ego.

Primitive defenses operate in a global, undifferentiated way in a person's total sensorium, fusing cognitive, affective, and behavioral dimensions, while more advanced ones make specific transformations of either thought, feeling, sensation, behavior, or some combination of these. The conceptual division between more archaic and higher-order defenses is somewhat arbitrary, since some theoretically more mature defenses—somatization or acting out or erotization, for example—can be automatic and unmodified by secondary process thought. However, especially since Kernberg's calling attention to the operation of archaic forms of projection and introjection in borderline patients (e.g., 1976), it has become conventional in psychoanalytic writing to identify the following defenses as among those intrinsically "primitive": withdrawal, denial, omnipotent control, primitive idealization and devaluation, projective and introjective identification, and splitting of the ego. Except for the addition of dissociation to the list of primitive operations (for reasons that follow), I have chosen to adhere to this convention despite its ambiguities and conceptual limitations.

To qualify as primary, a defense has to show evidence of two qualities associated with the preverbal phase of development: a lack of attainment of the reality principle (see Chapter 2) and a lack of appreciation of the separateness and constancy of those outside the self. For example, the defense of denial is thought to be a manifestation of a more primitive process than the defense of repression. For something to be repressed, it has to have been known in some way and then consigned to unconsciousness. Denial is an instant, nonrational process. "This is not happening" is a more magical way of dealing with something unpleasant than "This happened, but I'll forget about it because it's too painful."

Similarly, the defense mechanism known as "splitting," in which a person segregates experiences into all-good and all-bad categories, with no room for ambiguity and ambivalence, is considered primitive because it is believed to derive from a time before the child has developed object constancy. The perception of mother when one feels gratified is thought to be an overall sense of "good mother," while the perception of the same person's presence when one is frustrated is experienced as "bad mother." Before the infant's maturation to the point when he or she can appreciate the reality that it is the same person in each situation, one whose presence sometimes feels good and sometimes feels bad, we assume each experience has a kind of total, discrete, defining quality. In contrast, a defense like rationalization is considered mature because it requires some sophisticated verbal and thinking skills and more attunement to reality for a person to make up reasonable explanations that justify a feeling.

To introduce one more level of complication to the evolving, contradictory, and variegated collection of observations that constitute contemporary psychoanalytic theory, it should also be noted that some defensive processes are implicitly seen in this theoretical approach as having both primitive and more mature forms. For example, "idealization" can denote an unquestioning, worshipful conviction that another person is perfect, or it can refer to a subtle, subdued sense that someone is special or superior, even though his or her limitations are acknowledged. "Withdrawal" can refer to the full renunciation of reality in favor of a psychotic state of mind, or it can refer to a mild tendency to deal with stress by daydreaming. Where it is the case that analysts tend to see a particular defense as having a continuum of development from earlier and more archaic to later and more discriminating forms, I will observe in what follows the convention of prefacing the relevant defense with the adjective "primitive."

The observant reader will notice that the so-called primitive defenses are simply ways that we believe the infant naturally perceives the world. These ways of experiencing are assumed by analytic thinkers to live on in all of us, whether or not we have significant pathology. Preverbal, pre-reality-principle, pre-object-constancy processes are the foundations upon which everyone's psychology is constructed. They pose a problem only if one lacks more mature psychological skills or if these defenses are persistently used to the exclusion of possible others. We all deny, we all split, we all have omnipotent strivings. Most of us also supplement these reactions with more sophisticated means of processing anxiety and assimilating a complex and disturbing reality. It is the absence of mature defenses, not the presence of primitive ones, that defines borderline or psychotic structure.

It is much harder to describe the primitive defenses than the more advanced ones. The fact that they are preverbal, prelogical, comprehensive, imaginal, and magical make them extremely unsuited for representation by the written word. I shall do my best to capture them in formal language, but the reader should be mindful that the representation of preverbal processes in words is to some degree an oxymoron. The following summary will give an overview of those defenses that are conventionally understood as primary.

PRIMITIVE WITHDRAWAL

When an infant is overstimulated or distressed, it will often simply fall asleep. Psychological withdrawal into a different state of consciousness is an automatic, self-protective response that one sees in the tiniest of human beings. Adult versions of the same process can be observed in people who retreat from social or interpersonal situations, substituting the stimulation of their internal fantasy world for the stresses of relating to others. A propensity to use chemicals to alter one's consciousness can also be considered a kind of withdrawal. Some professionals, including contributors to recent editions of the DSM, prefer the term "autistic fantasy" to withdrawal; this label refers to a specific version of the general tendency to shrink from personal contact.

Some babies are temperamentally much more inclined toward this way of responding to stress than are others; observers of infants have sometimes noted that it is the babies who are especially sensitive who are most likely to withdraw. Such constitutionally impressionable persons may generate a rich internal fantasy life and regard the external world as problematic or affectively impoverished. Experiences of emotional intrusion or impingement by caregivers and other early objects can reinforce withdrawal. When a person withdraws habitually and to the exclusion of other ways of responding to anxiety, analysts describe him or her as *schizoid*.

The obvious disadvantage of the defense of withdrawal is that it removes the person from active participation in interpersonal problem solving. People with schizoid partners are frequently at a loss as to how to get them to show some kind of emotional responsiveness. "He just fiddles with the TV remote control and refuses to answer me" is a typical complaint. People who chronically withdraw into their own minds try the patience of those who love them by their resistance to engaging on a feeling level. Those with serious emotional disturbance are hard to help because of their apparent indifference to the mental health workers who try to win their attention and attachment.

The main advantage of withdrawal as a defensive strategy is that while it involves a psychological *escape* from reality, it requires little *distortion* of it. People who depend on withdrawal console themselves not by misunderstanding the world but by retreating from it. Consequently, they may be unusually sensitive, often to the great surprise of those who write them off as dull nonparticipants. And despite their lack of a disposition to express their own feelings, they may be highly perceptive of feelings in others. On the healthier end of the schizoid scale, one finds people of remarkable creativity: artists, writers, theoretical scientists, philosophers, religious mystics, and other highly talented onlookers whose capacity to stand aside from ordinary convention gives them a unique capacity for original commentary.

DENIAL

Another early way in which unpleasant experiences can be handled by the infant is for him or her to refuse to accept that they are happening. Denial lives on automatically in all of us as our first reaction to any catastrophe; people who are informed of the death of someone important to them will inevitably utter "Oh, no!" as their initial response. This reaction is the shadow of an archaic process rooted in the child's egocentrism, in which a prelogical conviction that "If I don't acknowledge it, it isn't happening" governs experience. It was processes like this one that prompted Selma Fraiberg (1959) to title her classic popular book on early childhood *The Magic Years*.

Examples of people for whom denial is a bedrock defense are the Pollyana-like individuals who insist that everything is always fine and for the best. The parents of one of my patients continued to have one child after another even after three of their offspring had died from what any parents not in a state of denial would have realized was a genetically implicated affliction. They refused to mourn for the dead children, ignored the suffering of their two healthy sons, resisted advice to get genetic counseling, and insisted that their condition represented the will of God, who knew what was best for them. Experiences of rapture and overwhelming exhilaration, especially when they occur in situations in which most people would perceive some negative aspects to their circumstances, are similarly assumed to reflect the operation of denial.

Most of us use denial to some extent, with the worthy aim of making life less unpleasant, and many people have specific areas in which that defense predominates. Someone whose feelings get hurt in a situation in which it is inappropriate or unwise to cry is more likely to deny the hurt feelings than to acknowledge them fully and inhibit the crying response consciously. In crises or emergencies, a capacity to deny emotionally that one's survival is at risk can be lifesaving: One can take the most realistically effective and even heroic actions using denial. Every war brings tales of people who "kept their heads" in terrifying, life-threatening conditions, and saved themselves and their fellows.

Less benignly, denial can contribute to the contrary outcome. An acquaintance of mine refuses to get annual Pap smears, as if by ignoring the possibility of uterine and cervical cancer she can magically avoid it. Spouses who deny that their abusive partner is dangerous, alcoholics who insist that they have no drinking problem, mothers who ignore the evidence of sexual molestation of their daughters, elderly people who will not consider giving up a driver's license despite obvious impairment—all are familiar examples of denial at its worst. This psychoanalytic concept has made its way more or less undistorted into everyday language, partly because the word denial is, like withdrawal, not jargonized and partly because it is a concept of singular significance to 12-step programs and other enterprises that attempt to confront people on their use of this defense and thereby help them out of whatever hell it has created for them.

A component of denial can be found in the operation of most of the more mature defenses. Take, for instance, the consoling belief that the person who rejected you *really* desired you but wasn't ready for a full commitment. Such a conclusion includes denial that one was rejected as well as the more sophisticated excuse-making activity that we refer to as rationalization. Similarly, the defense of reaction formation, in which an emotion is turned into its opposite (e.g., hatred into love), constitutes a specific and more complex type of denial of the feeling being defended against than a simple refusal to feel that emotion.

The most obvious example of psychopathology that is defined by the use of denial is *mania*. In a manic state, people may deny to an astonishing degree their physical limitations, their need for sleep, their financial exigencies, their personal weaknesses, even their mortality. Where depression makes the painful facts of life supremely unignorable in the mind of the depressed person, mania makes them psychologically insignificant. People who use denial as their main defense are characterologically manic and are referred to as *hypomanic* by analytically oriented clinicians. (The "hypo" prefix, meaning "a little" or "somewhat," differentiates them from individuals who suffer full manic episodes.) "Cyclothymic" (meaning alternating emotion) has also been used for this category of people because of their observed tendency to cycle between manic and depressed moods, usually short of clinically diagnosable bipolar illness. Analysts understand this oscillation as the repetitive use of denial followed by its inevitable collapse as the person becomes exhausted in the manic condition.

As with most primitive defenses, unmodified denial in adults is usually cause for concern. Nonetheless, mildly hypomanic people can be delightful. Many comedians and entertainers show the quick wit, the elevated energy, the playfulness with words, and the infectious high spirits that characterize those who successfully screen out and transform painful affects for long periods of time. Yet the depressive underside of such people is often visible to their closer friends, and the psychological price exacted by their manic charm is often not hard to see.

OMNIPOTENT CONTROL

We assume that for the newborn, the world and the self are felt as one. Piaget recognized this (e.g., 1937) in his concept of "primary egocentrism" (a cognitive phase roughly equivalent to Freud's [1914b] "primary narcissism," during which primary process thought prevails). It follows that the source of all events is understood by the newborn as internal in some way; that is, if the infant is cold, for instance, and a caregiver perceives this and provides warmth, the baby has some preverbal experience of its having magically elicited the warmth. The awareness that there is a locus of control in separate others, outside the self, has not yet developed.

A sense that one can influence the world, that one has agency, is of course a critical dimension of self-esteem, one that begins with infantile and unrealistic but developmentally normal fantasies of omnipotence. It was Sandor Ferenczi (1913) who originally called attention to the "stages in the development of a sense of reality." He pointed out that at the infantile state of primary omnipotence or grandiosity, the fantasy that one is in control of the world is normal, that this naturally shifts, as the child matures, to a phase of secondary or derived omnipotence in which one or more primary caregivers are believed to be all-powerful, and that eventually, as the child matures further, he or she comes to terms with the unattractive fact that no one person's potency is unlimited. Most analysts suspect that a precondition for the mature adult attitude that one's power is not boundless is, paradoxically, the opposite emotional experience in infancy: a secure enough early life that one can freely enjoy the developmentally appropriate illusions of, first, one's own omnipotence, and second, that of the people on whom one depends.

Some healthy residues of the sense of infantile omnipotence remain in all of us and contribute to feelings of competence and effectiveness in life. There is a natural kind of "high" that we feel when we effectively exert our will. Anyone who has ever "had a feeling" of impending luck and then won some kind of gamble knows how delicious is the sense of omnipotent control. The conviction reported by former Vice President Quayle, who attributed it to his grandmother, that one can do anything he or she sets his mind to, is a piece of conventional American ideology that flies in the face of common sense and most human experience, but it nonetheless can be a powerfully positive and self-fulfilling fiction.

For some people, the need to feel a sense of omnipotent control, and to interpret experiences as resulting from their own unfettered power, is utterly compelling. If one's personality is organized around seeking and enjoying the sense that one has effectively exercised one's omnipotence, with all other practical and ethical concerns relegated to secondary importance, one can reasonably be construed as *psychopathic* ("sociopathic" and "antisocial" are synonyms of later origin). Ben Bursten (1973a), in a classic study of *The Manipulator*, has stressed that sociopathy and criminality are overlapping but not identical categories. This is another area in which ordinary understanding of a concept and more sophisticated psychoanalytic conceptualization are at odds; in lay speech, it has become common to assume that most criminals are psychopaths and vice versa. Yet many people who rarely break the law have personalities driven by the defense of omnipotent control. Bursten's study focuses on their use of conscious manipulation as a primary way of avoiding anxiety and maintaining self-esteem.

"Getting over on" other people is a central preoccupation and pleasure of individuals whose personalities are dominated by omnipotent control. Such people are common in enterprises that require guile, a love of stimulation or danger, and a willingness to subordinate other concerns to the central objective of making one's influence felt. They are found, for example, in leadership roles in businesses that require risk taking, in politics, in the military, in the CIA and other covert operations organizations, in sales professions, among cult leaders and evangelists, in the advertising and entertainment industries, and in most walks of life where the potential to wield raw power is high.

PRIMITIVE IDEALIZATION (AND DEVALUATION)

Ferenczi's formulation about how primitive fantasies of the omnipotence of the self are gradually replaced by primitive fantasies of the omnipotence of one's caregiver(s) continues to be valuable to psychoanalytic clinical theory. One can see how fervently a young child would need to believe that Mommy or Daddy can protect him or her from all the dangers of life. As we get older, we forget how frightening it is to children to confront for the first time the realities of hostility, vulnerability to illness and misfortune, mortality, and other terrors (see Brenner, 1982). One way that youngsters cushion themselves against these overwhelming fears is to believe that *someone*, some benevolent, all-powerful authority, is in charge. (In fact, this wish to believe that the people who are running the world are somehow more inherently wise and powerful than ordinary, fallible human beings lives on in most of us and can be inferred by our degree of upset whenever events remind us that such a construction is only a wish.)

The conviction of young children that their mother or father is perfectly capable of superhuman acts is the great blessing and curse of parenthood. It is an undisputed advantage in the boo-boo curing department, and there is nothing more touching than a child's total and loving trust, but in other ways it creates in parents a barely controllable exasperation. I remember one of my daughters, then about $2^1/_2$, throwing a full-scale tantrum when I tried to explain to her that I could not make it stop raining so that she could go swimming.

All of us idealize. We carry remnants of the need to impute special value and power to people on whom we depend emotionally. Normal idealization is an essential component of mature love (Bergmann, 1987). And the developing tendency over time to deidealize or devalue those to whom we have childhood attachments seems to be a normal and important part of the separation–individuation process. No 18-year-old voluntarily leaves home feeling it is a much better place than the one he or she is going to. In some people, however, the need to idealize seems relatively unmodified from infancy. Their behavior shows evidence of the survival of archaic and rather desperate efforts to counteract internal terror by the conviction that someone to whom they can attach is omnipotent, omniscient, and omnibenevolent, and that through psychological merger with this wonderful Other, they are safe. They also hope to be free of shame: A by-product of idealization and the associated belief in perfection is that imperfections in the self are harder to bear; fusion with an idealized object is a natural remedy.

Longings for the omnipotent caregiver naturally appear in people's religious convictions; more problematically, they are evident in phenomena like the insistence that one's lover is perfect, one's personal guru is infallible, one's school is the best, one's taste is unassailable, one's government is incapable of error, and similar illusions. In Guyana in 1978, more than 900 people willingly drank cyanide rather than face the fact that their leader, Jim Jones, had blundered. In general, the more dependent one is or feels, the greater the temptation to idealize. Numerous female friends have announced to me during pregnancy, a time of awesome confrontation with personal vulnerability, that their obstetrician is "wonderful" or "the best in the field."

When a person seems to live his or her life seeking to rank all aspects of the human condition according to how comparatively valuable they are in contrast to flawed alternatives, and seems to be motivated by a search for perfection both through merger with idealized objects and with efforts to perfect the self, we consider him or her *narcissistic*. While other aspects of a narcissistic personality organization have been emphasized in much of the psychoanalytic literature, a structural way of construing the psychology of such people is in terms of their dependence on the defense of primitive idealization. The other familiar aspects of narcissistic people can be understood as following from the use of that defense: Their need for constant reassurance of their attractiveness, power, fame, and importance to others (i.e., perfection) results from the condition of dependence on this defense, since self-esteem strivings in people who are organized around idealizing become contaminated by the idea that one must perfect the self rather than accept it in order to love it.

Primitive devaluation is only the inevitable downside of the need to idealize. Since nothing in human life is perfect, archaic modes of idealization are doomed to disappointment. The more an object is idealized, the more radical the devaluation to which it will eventually be subject; the bigger one's illusions are, the harder they fall. Therapists working with narcissistic people can ruefully attest to the damages that ensue when the patient who has thought that his or her therapist can walk on water decides instead that he or she cannot walk and chew gum at the same time. Treatment relationships with narcissistic clients are notoriously subject to sudden rupture when the patient becomes disenchanted with the therapist. However sweet it can feel in the countertransference to be the object of total idealization, it is nevertheless onerous, both because of the irritating aspects of an idealized role in which someone in effect believes you can stop the rain and because most therapists have learned the hard way that being put on a pedestal is only the precursor to being knocked off. A colleague of mine (J. Walkup, personal communication, May 1992) adds that it is also a straitjacket, tempting the therapist to deny his or her own ignorance, to find intolerable the modest goals of help and assistance, and to think that only one's best performance is "typical."

In ordinary life, one can see analogues of this process in the degree of hate and rage that can be aimed at those who seemed to promise much and then failed to deliver. The man who believed that his wife's oncologist was the only cancer specialist who could cure her is the one most likely to initiate a lawsuit if death eventually defeats the doctor. Some people spend their lives running from one intimate relationship to the next, in recurrent cycles of idealization and disillusionment, trading the current partner in for a new model every time he or she turns out to be a human being. The modification of primitive idealization is a legitimate goal of all long-term psychoanalytic therapy, but that enterprise has particular relevance in work with narcissistic clients because of the degree of unhappiness in their lives and in those of the people who try to love them.

PROJECTION, INTROJECTION, AND PROJECTIVE IDENTIFICATION

I am combining the discussion of two of the most primitive defensive processes, projection and introjection, because they represent opposite sides of the same psychological coin. In both projection and introjection, there is a lack of psychological boundary between the self and the world. As mentioned earlier, in normal infancy, before the child has developed a sense of which experiences come from inside and which ones have their sources outside the self, we assume that there is a generalized sense of "I" being equivalent to "the world." A baby with colic probably has the subjective experience of "Hurt!" rather than "Something inside me hurts." It cannot yet distinguish between an internally located pain like colic and an externally caused discomfort like pressure from diapers that are too tight. From this era of undifferentiation come the processes that later, in their defensive function, we refer to as projection and introjection. When these processes work together, they are considered one defense, called *projective identification*. Some writers (e.g., Scharff, 1992) distinguish between projective and introjective identification, but similar processes are at work in each kind of operation.

Projection is the process whereby what is inside is misunderstood as coming from outside. In its benign and mature forms, it is the basis for empathy. Since no one is ever able to get inside the mind of another person, we must use our capacity to project our own experience in order to understand someone else's subjective world. Intuition, leaps of nonverbal synchronicity, and peak experiences of mystical union with another person or group involve a projection of the self into the other, with powerful emotional rewards to both parties. People in love are well known for reading one another's minds in ways that they themselves cannot account for logically.

In its malignant forms, projection breeds dangerous misunderstanding and untold interpersonal damage. When the projected attitudes seriously distort the object on whom they are projected, or when what is projected consists of disowned and highly negative parts of the self, all kinds of difficulties predictably ensue. Others resent being misperceived and may retaliate when treated, for example, as judgmental, envious, or persecutory (attitudes that are among the most common of those that tend to be ignored in the self and ascribed to others). When a person uses projection as his or her main way of understanding the world and coping with life, he or she can be said to have a character that is *paranoid.**

Introjection is the process whereby what is outside is misunderstood as coming from inside. In its benign forms, it amounts to a primitive identification with important others. Young children take in all kinds of attitudes, affects, and behaviors of significant people in their lives. The process is so subtle as to be mysterious; yet when one sees it, it is unmistakable. Long before a child can make a subjectively voluntary decision to be like Mommy or Daddy, he or she seems to have "swallowed" them in some primal way.

In its problematic forms, introjection is, like projection, a very destructive process. The most notorious and striking examples of pathological introjection involve the process that has been labeled,

*Note that by the psychoanalytic definition, paranoia has nothing inherently to do with suspiciousness (which may be based on realistic, unprojected observation and experience), nor with whether or not an attribution is accurate. The fact that a projection "fits" does not make it any less a projection; and although it is easier to spot a projection when the attribution does *not* fit, it is also possible that there is some other, nondefensive reason for a misunderstanding of someone else's motives. Popular misuse of the word "paranoid" has wrongly equated it with "fearful" or "distrustful," much to the detriment of precision in language, even though it is true that what people project is usually unpleasant stuff to which they then react with fear and distrust.

somewhat inappropriately in view of its primitivity, "identification with the aggressor" (A. Freud, 1936).* It is well known, from both naturalistic observations (e.g., Bettelheim, 1960) and empirical research (e.g., Milgram, 1963), that under conditions of fear or abuse, people will try to master their fright and pain by taking on qualities of their abusers. "I'm not the helpless victim; I'm the powerful inflictor" seems to be the unconscious attraction to this defense. An understanding of this mechanism has critical importance to the process of psychotherapy. It crosses all diagnostic boundaries but is particularly evident in characterological dispositions toward *sadism*, *explosivity*, and what is often misleadingly called *impulsivity* (see "Acting Out" in Chapter 6).

A different way in which introjection can result in psychopathology involves mourning and its relation to depression (Freud, 1917a). When we love people or are deeply attached to them, we introject them, and their representations inside ourselves become a part of our identity ("I am Tom's son, Mary's husband, Sue's father, Dan's friend," etc.). If we lose any of the people whose image we have internalized, whether by death, separation, or rejection, not only do we feel that our *environment* is poorer for their absence in our lives but we also feel that we are somehow diminished, that a part of our *self* has died. An emptiness or sense of void comes to dominate our inner world. We may also, if we are focused on restoring the presence of lost objects rather than on giving them up, become preoccupied with the question of what failure or sin of ours drove them away. The appeal of this usually unconscious process is the implicit wish that if we can figure out what we did wrong, we can bring them back (another manifestation of infantile omnipotence). When mourning is avoided, unconscious self-criticism thus takes its place.

Freud (1917a) beautifully described the process of mourning as a slow coming to terms with this condition of loss, in which "the shadow of the object fell upon the ego" (p. 249). When a person is unable over time to separate internally from a loved one whose image has been introjected, and consequently fails to invest emotionally in other people (the function of the grieving process), he or she will continue to feel diminished, unworthy, depleted, and bereft. If one regularly uses

*Technically, the term identification has been reserved by most analysts for those internalizations that are experienced as subjectively voluntary (Schafer, 1968). The 3-year-old who wants to be "like Mommy" is identifying in a much less primitive way than the 2-year-old who simply takes on Mommy's qualities. "Identification" with the aggressor, because it is automatic, unconscious, and lacking in any subjective sense of option, is more properly understood as introjection, but at this point, after decades of use of the less precise term, we are stuck with it.

introjection to reduce anxiety and maintain continuity in the self, keeping psychological ties to unrewarding objects of one's earlier life, one can reasonably be considered characterologically *depressive*.

Melanie Klein (1946) was the first analyst to write about a defensive process that she found to be ubiquitous in more disturbed patients, which she called "projective identification." This fusion of projective and introjective mechanisms has been compactly described by Ogden (1982):

> In projective identification, not only does the patient view the therapist in a distorted way that is determined by the patient's past object relations; in addition, pressure is exerted on the therapist to experience himself in a way that is congruent with the patient's unconscious fantasy. (pp. 2–3)

In other words, the patient both projects internal objects and gets the person on whom they are projected to behave like those objects, as if the target person had those same introjects. Projective identification is a difficult abstraction, one that has inspired much controversy in the analytic literature (see Finell, 1986). Some have insisted that it is not qualitatively discriminable from projection per se, while others regard the introduction of the concept as having major clinical and theoretical significance (Kernberg, 1975). My own understanding of the term involves the ideas implied in the previous paragraph; that is, projection and introjection each have a continuum of forms, running from very primitive to very advanced (cf. Kernberg, 1976), and at the primitive end, those processes are fused because of their similar confusion of inside and outside. This fusion is what we call projective identification. In Chapter 4, I discussed briefly its operation in psychotic and borderline states.

To illustrate how that process differs from mature projection, consider the contrast between the following hypothetical statements from two young men who have come for an intake interview:

PATIENT A: (*Somewhat apologetically*) I know I have no reason to believe you're critical of me, but I can't help thinking that you are.

PATIENT B: (*In an accusatory tone*) You shrinks all love to sit back and judge people, and I don't give a shit *what* you think!

Let us assume that in reality, the therapist began the session with a genuinely friendly, interested, nonjudgmental attitude toward each client. The *content* of what is bothering each man is similar; both are worried that the therapist is taking a harsh, evaluative stance. Both are projecting an internalized critical object on to the therapist. Three aspects of their respective communications, however, make them very different from each other.

First, Patient A shows evidence of an observing ego, a part of the self that can see that his fantasy may not necessarily conform to reality; the projection in this case is ego alien. Patient B, on the other hand, experiences what is projected as an accurate depiction of the therapist's state of mind; his projection is ego syntonic. In fact, he believes in the reality of his attribution so absolutely that he is already launching a counterattack against the assault that he is certain the therapist is planning. The fusion of cognitive, affective, and behavioral dimensions of experience typical of primitive processes is discernible here.

Second, these patients differ in the extent to which their projective process has successfully done the job for which the defense was called upon, namely, to get rid of a troublesome feeling. Patient A has ejected the critical attitude and feels some relief in reporting it, while Patient B both projects it and keeps it. He ascribes a critical attitude to the other person, yet that does not relieve him of feeling censorious himself. Kernberg has described this aspect of projective identification as "maintaining empathy" with what has been projected.

Finally, these patients' respective communications will have very different emotional effects. The therapist will find it easy to like Patient A and will form a working alliance expeditiously. With Patient B, however, the therapist will rapidly begin feeling like exactly the sort of person that the patient is already convinced he is sitting with: uncaring, ready to judge, and reluctant to exert the amount of energy it will take to try to care about this man. In other words, the countertransference of the therapist toward the first man will be both positive and mild, while toward the second it will be both negative and intense.

The "self-fulfilling prophecy" quality of projective identification was once explained to me (B. Cohen, personal communication, February 1987) as a natural consequence of a person's being disturbed enough to have very primitive ways of perceiving reality, *short of psychosis*. A woman who is invested in staying anchored in reality will feel less crazy if she can induce in someone else the feelings she is convinced the other person already has. A frankly psychotic woman will not care whether her projection "fits," and will therefore spare others the pressure to confirm its appropriateness and hence her sanity.

Projective identification is a particularly powerful and challenging operation, as the reader can see, one that strains the therapist's capacities to help. While all the defenses in this section are considered primitive, this one, along with splitting, which I will discuss next, has a special reputation for causing headaches to clinicians. When one is caught in the patient's certainty about how the therapist "really" feels, along with the patient's unrelenting struggle to induce just those feelings, it takes a clear head and iron discipline to withstand the emotional barrage. Moreover, since all of us share in the predicament of being human, and hence contain already within ourselves all the different emotions, defenses, and attitudes that get projected on to us, there is always some truth in the projective identifier's belief. It can be very confusing to figure out in the heat of the clinical moment where the patient's defense ends and the therapist's psychology begins. Perhaps the capacity of this defense to threaten the therapist's confidence in his or her own mental health accounts for the fact that projective identification, along with splitting, is implicated in *borderline personality organization*. In particular, because the projective piece of it is so powerful, it is associated with borderline levels of paranoid personality.

Contrary to professional popular opinion, however, projective identification is not used exclusively by people whose character is essentially borderline. There are numerous subtle and benign ways that the process operates in everyday life irrespective of psychopathology. For example, when what is projected and identified with involves the loving, joyful affects, a contagion of good feeling can occur in a group. Even when what is projected and identified with is negative, as long as the process is not relentless, intense, and unmodulated by other interpersonal processes of a more mature sort, it is not unduly harmful.

SPLITTING OF THE EGO

Splitting of the ego,* usually referred to simply as "splitting," is the other interpersonally powerful process that is understood as deriving from a preverbal time, before the infant can appreciate that its caregivers have good and bad qualities and are associated with good and bad experiences. We can observe in 2-year-olds a need to organize their perceptions by assigning good and bad valences to everything in their world. That tendency, along with a sense of the difference

*Our terminology may be unfortunate here: One cannot have a split in the ego before an integrated ego has developed. And while we can aptly refer to splitting as a defense in a person whose ego has attained some kind of wholeness and then splits under stress, we should perhaps call it something else when a person is fixated on a pre-object-constancy, pre-integrated-ego state. Stolorow and Lachmann (1979) have made such a distinction in an important article on the "developmental prestages of defense."

between big and little (adult and child), is one of the primary ways in which young human beings organize experience. Before one has object constancy, one cannot have ambivalence, since ambivalence implies opposite feelings toward a constant object. Instead, one can be in either a good or a bad ego state toward an object in one's world.

In everyday adult life, splitting remains a powerful and appealing way to make sense of complex experiences, especially when they are confusing or threatening. Political scientists can attest to how attractive it is for any unhappy group to develop a sense of a clearly evil enemy, against which the good insiders must struggle. Manichean visions of good versus evil, God versus the devil, democracy versus communism, cowboys versus Indians, the lone whistle-blower against the hateful bureaucracy, and so on have pervaded the mythology of our culture. Comparably split images can be found in the folklore and organizing beliefs of any society.

The mechanism of splitting can be very effective in its defensive functions of reducing anxiety and maintaining self-esteem. Of course, splitting always involves distortion, and therein lies its danger. Scholarly studies of the "authoritarian personality" (Adorno, Frenkl-Brunswick, Levinson, & Sanford, 1950) in the post-World War II era explored the far-reaching social consequences of the use of splitting (not by that name) to make sense of the world and one's place in it. The authors of the original study on authoritarianism believed that certain right-wing beliefs were particularly likely to be associated with this kind of inflexibility, but later commentators established that left-wing and liberal forms of authoritarianism also exist (see Brown, 1965).

Clinically, splitting is evident when a patient expresses one nonambivalent attitude and regards its opposite (the other side of what most of us would feel as ambivalence) as completely disconnected. For example, a borderline woman experiences her therapist as all good, in contrast to the allegedly uncaring, hostile, stupid bureaucrats who work in the same setting. Or the therapist may suddenly become the target of unmodified rage, as the patient regards him or her as the personification of evil, neglect, or incompetence, when last week the therapist could do no wrong. If confronted with inconsistencies in his or her attributions, the client who splits will not find it arresting or worth pondering that someone who seemed so good has become so bad.

It is well known that in institutions like psychiatric hospitals and mental health centers, borderline patients not only split internally, they create (via projective identification) splits in the staff of the agency (Stanton & Schwartz, 1954; Main, 1957; G. Adler, 1972; Kernberg, 1981; Gunderson, 1984). Those mental health workers associated with a borderline client's care find themselves in repeated arguments in which some of them feel a powerful sympathy toward the patient and want to rescue and nurture, while the others feel an equally powerful antipathy and want to confront and set limits. This is one reason that splitting as a defense has a less than glowing reputation. Patients who use it as their customary way of organizing their experience tend to wear out their caregivers.

DISSOCIATION

I have, with considerable ambivalence, put *dissociation* with the primary defenses, both because it works so globally and strikingly on the total personality and because many dissociated states are essentially psychotic. It is, however, quite different from the above processes in that the others represent normal modes of operating that become problematic only if a person hangs on to them too long or to the exclusion of other ways of dealing with reality. Dissociation is different in that while any of us may be *capable* of dissociating under certain conditions (and this is disputable; much research indicates that only people with a high capacity to be hypnotized can use this defense), most of us are fortunate enough not to run into such conditions.

Dissociation is a "normal" reaction to trauma, but trauma cannot be said to be developmentally normal. Any of us, if confronted with a catastrophe that overwhelmed our capacity to cope, especially if it involved unbearable pain and/or terror, might dissociate. Out-of-the-body experiences during war, life-threatening disasters, and major surgery have been reported so often that only the most skeptical person can completely disregard the evidence for dissociative phenomena. People who undergo unbearable calamities at any age may dissociate; those who are repeatedly subject to horrific abuse as young children may learn to dissociate as their habitual reaction to stress. Where this is true, the adult survivor is legitimately conceptualized as suffering from a characterological dissociative disorder, or *multiple personality*.

There has been an explosion of research and clinical reporting on multiple personality and dissociation in the last two decades, all of which has underscored the fact that dissociative people exist in far greater numbers than anyone ever suspected. Perhaps there has been an increase in the kind of horrific child abuse that creates dissociation, or perhaps some threshold of public awareness has been crossed, mainly since the publication of *Sybil* (Schreiber, 1973), that has encouraged people who suspect that they may be regularly dissociating to show themselves sooner and in greater numbers to mental health professionals.*

The advantages of dissociating under unbearable conditions are obvious: The dissociator cuts off pain, terror, horror, and conviction of imminent death. Anyone who has had an out-of-the-body experience when he or she was in mortal danger, and even those of us without such a dramatic basis for empathy, can readily understand a preference for being outside rather than inside the sense of impending obliteration. Occasional or mild dissociation may facilitate acts of singular courage. The great drawback of the defense, of course, is its tendency to operate automatically under conditions in which one's survival is *not* realistically at risk, and when more discriminating adaptations to threat would extract far less from one's overall functioning.

Traumatized people may confuse ordinary stress with life threatening circumstances, becoming immediately amnestic or totally different, much to their own confusion and that of others. Outsiders, unless they also have a traumatic history, never suspect dissociation when a friend suddenly forgets some major incident or appears inexplicably changed. Rather, they conclude that their acquaintance is moody, or unstable, or a liar. There is thus a high interpersonal price paid by the habitual user of this defense.

SUMMARY

In this chapter I have described those defenses that analysts conventionally consider primitive or primary: withdrawal, denial, omnipotent control, primitive idealization and devaluation, primitive forms of projection and introjection, and splitting. I have also included dissociation because, in its most extreme form, it transforms the entire identity of the person using it. I have reviewed the normal origins of each defense (except dissociation, which is trauma induced) and mentioned adaptive and maladaptive functions of each. I have also identified the personality types associated with heavy reliance on each primary defense.

*The rapidly expanding literature on multiple personality and dissociation has not yet been integrated into mainstream psychoanalytic theory, but I have made an attempt to integrate it here (see Chapter 15), as an increased appreciation of dissociative conditions seems to be developing in analytic circles (cf. Herman, 1992; Lichtenberg, 1992).

SUGGESTIONS FOR FURTHER READING

Primitive forms of projection and introjection have inspired a few worthy books (Ogden, 1982; Sandler, 1987; Scharff, 1992); other primary defenses tend to be discussed in different writers' speculations about psychic development. Klein's "Love, Guilt, and Reparation" (1937) and "Envy and Gratitude" (1957) are highly illuminative of primitive processes and, unlike some of her work, not incomprehensible to beginning therapists. Balint (1968) was gifted in describing archaic dynamics in individuals; Bion (1959) was brilliant at discerning their operation in groups.

❖6❖

Secondary (Higher-Order) Defensive Processes

No summary of the defenses can be complete since virtually any psychological process can be used defensively. For the same reason, any selection of defensive operations from the range of existing possibilities must be arbitrary.* I have chosed the "mature," or "higher-order," defenses to be covered according to two criteria: (1) the frequency with which they are mentioned in psychoanalytic clinical literature and by practicing therapists and (2) their relevance to particular character patterns. The reader should understand that anyone else's list would be different, would emphasize other aspects of defense, and would reflect another writer's distinctive experience of psychoanalytic theory and practice.

*Anna Freud's (1936) *The Ego and the Mechanisms of Defense* covers denial, repression, reaction formation, displacement, rationalization, intellectualization, regression, reversal, turning against the self, identification with the aggressor, and sublimation. A more recent compendium by H. P. Laughlin (1970, 1979) delineates 22 major and 26 minor defense mechanisms, as well as numerous other "special" defensive reactions. The DSM-III-R enumerates 18. I have opted to describe a selection of operations that is more extensive, and more incorporative of later psychoanalytic models, than is A. Freud's modest listing. Yet because this is a text on diagnosis rather than on psychological processes per se, I shall cover only a portion of those enumerated in Laughlin's encyclopedic discussion.

REPRESSION

The most basic of the so-called higher-order defenses is repression. It was also one of the first to fascinate Freud, and it has enjoyed a long history of psychoanalytic clinical and empirical investigation. The essence of repression is *motivated forgetting or ignoring.* Its implicit metaphor recalls the early drive model with its idea that impulses and affects press for release and have to be held in check by a dynamic force. Freud (1915b) wrote that "the essence of repression lies simply in turning something away, and keeping it at a distance, from the conscious" (p. 146). If either an internal disposition or an external circumstance is sufficiently upsetting or confusing, it may be deliberately consigned to unconsciousness. This process may apply to a total experience, to the affect connected with an experience, or to one's fantasies and wishes associated with it.

Not all difficulty in paying attention or remembering constitutes repression. Only when there is evidence that an idea or emotion or perception has become consciously inaccessible *because of its power to upset* are there grounds for assuming the operation of this defense. Other attentional and memory deficits may result from toxic or organic conditions, or simply from the ordinary mental sifting of the important from the trivial. An example of the operation of repression in a global, massive way would be an experience of rape or torture that the victim later could not recall. Instances of what were once called the "war neuroses," now known as posttraumatic stress reactions, have been psychoanalytically explained by reference to the concept of repression.* In such cases, a person is unable to remember at will certain horrifying, life-threatening events but may be troubled by intrusive flashbacks of them, a phenomenon that Freud would have put under the colorful label "the return of the repressed." Early psychoanalytic observation made much of such phenomena.

Later analytic theory applied the term repression more to internally generated ideas than to trauma. Repression was seen as the means by which children deal with developmentally normal but unrealizable and frightening strivings, such as the wish to destroy one parent and solely possess the other: They slowly learn to relegate them to unconsciousness. Contemporary analysts assume that one must have attained

*In Chapter 15 I shall present a contemporary argument that this kind of forgetting should be understood as dissociation rather than repression, and further, that repression proper represents a subset of dissociative processes (the BASK model of dissociation [Braun, 1988]). Since this formulation has not yet received attention and acceptance by the general psychoanalytic community, I have chosen in this chapter to present repression more classically, as the prototypic neurotic-level defense and component of other more advanced defensive processes.

a sense of the wholeness and continuity of the self before one is capable of handling disturbing impulses by repression. For people whose early experiences did not permit their attainment of this constancy of identity, troublesome feelings tend to be handled with more primitive defenses like denial, projection, and splitting (Myerson, 1991).

A clinically inconsequential example of repression, the kind that Freud (1901) regarded as part of the "psychopathology of everyday life," would be a speaker's momentarily forgetting the name of a person he or she was introducing, in a context in which there was evidence for some unconscious negative feeling by the speaker toward that person. In all three of these variants of repression—the severe, profound instances of unremembered trauma, the developmentally normal processes that allow children to reject infantile strivings and seek love objects outside the family, and the trivial and often entertaining instances of its operation—one can see the basically adaptive nature of the process. If one were constantly aware of the whole panoply of one's impulses, feelings, memories, images, and conflicts, one would be chronically overwhelmed. Like other unconscious defenses, repression becomes problematic only when it (1) fails to do its job (i.e., dependably keeping disturbing ideas out of consciousness so that the person can go about the business of accommodating to reality), or (2) gets in the way of certain positive aspects of living, or (3) operates to the exclusion of other more successful ways of coping. Overreliance upon repression, along with certain other defensive processes that often coexist with it, has generally been considered the hallmark of the *hysterical personality*.

Freud's early efforts to get hysterical patients to bring into consciousness both the traumatic events of their histories and the urges and feelings they had been raised to consider unacceptable yielded fascinating information. From working with this population he originally concluded, as mentioned in Chapter 2, that repression caused anxiety. According to his original mechanistic model, the anxiety that was such a frequent concomitant of hysteria was caused by a repressive bottling up of drives and affects. These feelings pressed for discharge and hence caused a chronic state of tension.* Later, as he revised his theory in light of accumulating clinical observations, he reversed his version of cause and effect, regarding repression and other defense mechanisms as the *result* rather than the cause of anxiety. In other words, preexisting irrational fear created the need to forget.

This later formulation of repression as the elemental defense of the ego, the automatic suppressor of countless anxieties that are simply inherent in living one's life, has become an accepted psychoanalytic

*Some irreverent commentators have dubbed this the "coitus-interruptus" theory of the relationship of repression to anxiety.

premise. Nevertheless, Freud's original postulation of repression as the instigator of anxiety is not without some intuitive appeal, in that excessive repression may ultimately cause as many problems as it solves. This process, labeled by Mowrer (1950) the "neurotic paradox," whereby attempts to quell one anxiety only generate others, is the core characteristic of what was once (in a much more comprehensive use of the term than is typical now) called neurosis. Along these lines, Theodor Reik used to contrast the emotionally healthy person, who can stand in front of the window at Tiffany's admiring the jewelry and tolerating a passing fantasy of stealing it, with the neurotic person, who looks in the window and runs in the opposite direction. When psychoanalytic ideas first captured the imagination of the educated public, such popularized examples of the pathological operation of repressive defenses contributed to a widespread overvaluation of the goals of removing repression and shedding inhibitions, and also to the assumption that these processes were the essence of all psychoanalytic therapies.

An element of repression is present in the operation of most of the higher-order defenses (although it is arguable that denial rather than repression is operating in instances in which it is unclear whether or not the person originally acknowledged something before losing that knowledge). For example, in reaction formation, the turning of an attitude into its opposite, such as hate into love or idealization into contempt, the original emotion can be seen as repressed (or denied, depending on whether it was ever consciously felt). In isolation, the affect connected with an idea is repressed (or denied, as above). In reversal, there is a repression of the original scenario that is now being turned around. And so forth. Freud's original belief that repression was a sort of grandfather of all other defensive processes can be seen sympathetically in this light, despite the current consensus in the analytic community that the processes described in Chapter 5 predate repression in the child by at least a year and a half.

REGRESSION

Regression is a relatively uncomplicated defense mechanism, familiar to every parent who has watched a child slide backwards into the habits of a prior maturational stage when tired or hungry. Social and emotional development does not progress in a straight line; there is a fluctuation to personal growth that becomes less dramatic as we age, but never entirely goes away. Almost anyone, if tired enough, will begin to whine. The "rapprochement subphase" of the separation–individuation process that Mahler described as a universal feature of the last part of every child's second year, when the toddler who has just declared independence from the mother goes back and hides under her skirt, is only one example of the tendency of human beings to cling to the familiar right after having achieved some new level of competence.

In long-term psychotherapy and psychoanalysis, this tendency is easy to observe. The patient who has finally summoned up the courage to try out a new way of behaving, especially if it involves new behavior toward the therapist (e.g., expressing criticism or anger, confiding masturbation fantasies, or asking for a break on fees or scheduling with more self-assertion than was permitted in childhood), will frequently revert to old habits of thought, feeling, and behavior in subsequent sessions. The therapist who does not appreciate the ebb and flow inherent in developmental change may be dismayed by this phenomenon (the countertransference may resemble the normal exasperation of a parent who finally succeeds in getting a young child to sleep through the night, and then gets a week of bedroom visits at 3:00 A.M.) until it becomes clear that despite the regressive dimension of the client's struggle, the overall direction of change is forward.

Strictly speaking, it is not regression when a person is aware of needing some extra comfort and asks to be held or reassured, nor is it regression when one deliberately seeks out a means—through competitive sports, for instance—of discharging primordial levels of drive. To qualify as a defense mechanism, the process must be unconscious. Thus, the woman who lapses unwittingly into compliant, little-girlish ways of relating right after realizing some ambition or the man who thoughtlessly lashes out at his wife just after attaining some new level of intimacy with her are regressing in the psychoanalytic meaning of the term, since their respective actions have not been consciously chosen and pursued.

Some people use the defense of regression more than others. For example, some of us react to the stress of growth and change by getting sick. Many who do not get diagnosably ill may nonetheless feel terrible physically and revert to their beds. This process is never conscious (if it is, it is properly called malingering), and it may cause anguish both to the regressed person and to those involved with him or her. This variant of regression, known as *somatization*,* is usually resistant to change and challenging to address therapeutically (see McDougall, 1989).

*I am using this term in accordance with psychoanalytic convention, in which somatization (physical impairment related to emotional stress) is distinguished from *conversion* (marked physical impairment like paralysis or blindness, that cannot be accounted for physiologically). Somatization in this context refers to a more general physical debility.

Some hypochondriacal people, the patients who drive physicians to distraction with a litany of vague and changing complaints that never to respond to treatment, use regression to the sick role as a primary means of coping with upsetting aspects of their lives. By the time they are persuaded to consult a therapist, they have usually built up an additional and virtually impenetrable wall of defensiveness deriving from having repeatedly been treated like a spoiled child or willful attention seeker. They expect clinicians to try to expose them as malingerers. Consequently, the therapist whose client uses regression to the sick role as a favored defense must have almost superhuman reserves of tact and patience—all the more so if the patient's pattern of taking to the sickbed has been reinforced by other rewards of that position ("secondary gain"; see Chapter 14).

The conclusion that a person complaining of physical pain or exhaustion is using the defense of regression as a primary reaction to emotional stress must not be reached hastily or unreflectively, since the stress of disease itself will cause a regressive reaction in an afflicted person. People can get sick because they are unconsciously depressed; they can also get depressed because they are medically ill. It has been widely noted, however, that somatization and hypochondria, as well as other kinds of regression into relatively helpless and childlike modes of dealing with life, can be a kind of cornerstone of a person's character. Where regression constitutes someone's core strategy for dealing with the challenges of living, he or she may be legitimately characterized as an *infantile personality*.*

ISOLATION

One way in which people may deal with anxieties and other painful states of mind is by isolating feeling from knowing. More technically, the affective aspect of an experience or idea can be sequestered from its cognitive dimension. Isolation of affect can be of great value: Surgeons could not work effectively if they were constantly attuned to the physical agony of patients or to their own revulsion, distress, or sadism when cutting into someone's flesh; generals could not plan battle strategy if they were in continual touch with the graphic horrors of war;

*This category did not survive officially after the second edition of the DSM, though many analytic diagnosticians have not abandoned it. Kernberg (1984) has argued that the description of the histrionic personality in the DSM-III and subsequent manuals has subsumed aspects of the older concept of infantile personality organization. The Dependent Personality Disorder diagnosis in the later editions of the DSM implies a reliance on regression.

police officers could not investigate violent crimes without becoming unglued.

The "psychic numbing" that Lifton (1968) has described as a consequence of catastrophe exemplifies the operation of isolation of affect on a social level. Therapists who have worked with survivors of the Holocaust have been struck by their wooden descriptions of atrocities that defy the ordinary imagination. The political scientist Herman Kahn (1962) wrote an influential book on the probable outcome of a nuclear conflagration, in which the most horrific consequences of atomic disaster were detailed in an almost jovial tone of detachment. With respect to its adaptive utility in extreme situations, isolation is a degree more discriminative than dissociation: The experience is not totally obliterated from conscious experience, but its emotional meaning is cut off.

Isolation can also become, by means of a certain style of child rearing mixing with a child of a certain temperament, a core defense in the absence of trauma. We all know people who claim that they have no emotional responses to things about which the rest of us have powerful feelings; such people sometimes make a virtue out of the defense of isolation and idealize the condition of expressing only rational concerns. Our cultural tendency to admire the capacity to isolate affect from intellect is discernible in the widespread devotion of old "Star Trek" fans to the character of Mr. Spock, the Vulcan. The fact that isolation is appreciated as a defensive rather than a natural position is betrayed by the decision of the writers of that series to give Spock a latent emotional side, the contribution of his Earthling mother.

Isolation is considered by psychoanalytic thinkers to be the most primitive of the "intellectual defenses" and the basic unit of psychological operation in mechanisms like intellectualization, rationalization, and moralization. These defenses will be considered separately in the following sections, but they have in common the relegation to unconsciousness of the personal, gut-level implications of any situation or idea or occurrence. When one's primary defense is isolation, and the pattern of one's life reflects the overvaluation of thinking and the underappreciation of feeling, one's character structure is considered *obsessive*.

INTELLECTUALIZATION

Intellectualization is the name given to a higher-order version of the isolation of affect from intellect. The person using isolation typically reports that he or she has no feelings, while the one who intellectualizes talks *about* feelings in a way that strikes the listener as emotionless. For example, the comment, "Well, naturally I have some anger about that," delivered in a casual, detached tone, suggests that while the idea of feeling anger is theoretically acceptable to the person, the actual expression of it is still inhibited. When patients in psychoanalysis are intellectualizing their treatment, they tend to summarize their experiences on the couch in a tone that sounds more like a weather report on their psyche than a disclosure of something that has moved them. In the 1988 presidential campaign, when Michael Dukakis responded with intellectualization to a question about his reaction to the hypothetical rape of his wife, the public scorned him for his obvious defensiveness.

Intellectualization handles ordinary emotional overload in the same way that isolation handles traumatic overstimulation. It shows considerable ego strength for a person to be able to think rationally in a situation fraught with emotional meaning, and as long as the affective aspects of that circumstance are eventually processed with more emotional acknowledgment, the defense is operating effectively. Many people feel that they have made a maturational leap when they can intellectualize under stress rather than giving an impulsive, knee-jerk response. When someone seems unable to leave a defensively cognitive, antiemotional position, however, even when provoked as in the Dukakis example above, others tend intuitively to consider him or her emotionally dishonest. Sex, banter, artistic expression, and other gratifying adult forms of play may be unnecessarily truncated in the person who has learned to depend on intellectualization to cope with life.

RATIONALIZATION

The defense of rationalization is so familiar that it hardly needs explication here. Not only has this term seeped into common usage with a connotation similar to the one used in psychoanalytic writing, it is also a phenomenon that most of us find naturally entertaining—at least in others. "So convenient a thing it is to be a *reasonable Creature*," Benjamin Franklin remarked, "since it enables one to find or make a Reason for everything one has in mind to do" (quoted in K. Silverman, 1986, p. 39). Rationalization may come into play either when we fail to get something we had wanted, and we conclude in retrospect that it was actually not so desirable (sometimes called "sour grapes rationalization" after the Aesop fable of the fox and the grapes), or when something bad happens, and we decide that it was not so bad after all ("sweet lemon rationalization"). An example of the first kind would be the conclusion that the house we could not afford was too big for us anyway; an example of the second would be the universally popular rationalization of those who value education: "Well, it was a learning experience."

The more intelligent and creative a person is, the more likely it is that he or she is a good rationalizer. The defense operates benignly when it allows someone to make the best of a difficult situation with minimal resentment, but its drawback as a defensive strategy is that virtually anything can be—and has been—rationalized. People rarely admit to doing something just because it feels good; they prefer to surround their decisions with good reasons. Thus, the parent who hits a child rationalizes aggression by allegedly doing it for the youngster's "own good"; the therapist who insensitively raises a patient's fee rationalizes greed by deciding that paying more will benefit the person's self-esteem; the serial dieter rationalizes vanity with an appeal to health.

MORALIZATION

Moralization is a close relative of rationalization. When one is rationalizing, one unconsciously seeks cognitively acceptable grounds for one's direction; when one is moralizing, one seeks ways to feel it is one's *duty* to pursue that course. Rationalization converts what the person already wants into reasonable language; moralization puts it into the realm of the justified or morally obligatory. Where the rationalizer talks about the "learning experience" that some disappointment provided, the moralizer will insist that it "builds character."

The self-righteous quality of this particular transformation of impulse makes others regard it as either amusing or vaguely unpleasant, although in certain social and political situations, leaders who exploit their constituents' wish to feel morally superior can produce mass moralization so effortlessly that the public that has been thus seduced hardly blinks. The belief of the colonialists that they were bringing higher standards of civilization to the people whose resources they were plundering is a good example of moralization. Hitler was able to indulge his own murderous fantasies by persuading an astounding number of followers that the obliteration of Jews, homosexuals, and gypsies was necessary for the ethical and spiritual improvement of the human race. The Spanish Inquisition was another social movement now notorious for the moralization of aggression, greed, and strivings for omnipotence.

At a less catastrophic level, most of us have witnessed someone who defended having savagely criticized a subordinate on the grounds that it is a supervisor's duty to be frank about an employee's failings. In doctoral oral defenses, hostile examiners have been known to make comments like, "Would we be doing this student any favors by withholding the critique that this study deserves?" One of my friends, an interior decorator, moralized the vanity behind her decision to have an expensive facelift by explaining that alas, it was her obligation to present an appealing appearance to her customers. Bette Davis reported having been in conflict over her wish to continue her acting career during World War II, but she resolved her discomfort by noting, "But then I felt that's what the enemy wanted—to destroy and paralyze America. So I decided to keep on working" (quoted in Sorel, 1991).

Moralization may be usefully regarded as a developmentally advanced version of splitting. Although I have not seen it presented that way in the psychoanalytic literature, it makes sense that an inclination to moralize would be the natural later stage of the primitive tendency to make gross good–bad distinctions. While splitting occurs naturally in the child before there is an integrated self capable of ambivalence, moralization resolves, by recourse to principle, mixed feelings that the evolving self has become able to suffer. From moralization one can infer the operation of a superego, albeit usually a rigid and punitive one.

Moralization is the preeminent defense in a characterological organization that analysts call *moral masochism* (Reik, 1941). Some obsessive and compulsive people are also wedded to this defense. In psychotherapy, moralizers can create vexing dilemmas for clinicians, who find that when they confront certain self-defeating attitudes or behaviors, their patients regard them as deficient in virtue for not seeing the issue the same way they do. One patient of mine, an obsessive compulsive man on the neurotic end of the borderline continuum, kept imploring me to make a moral judgment about his compulsive masturbation, with the hope that that would resolve his conflict about it. "How would you feel if I said I thought it was getting in the way of your going out and developing relationships with women?" I asked. "I'd feel criticized, deeply ashamed—I'd want to crawl in a hole," he responded. "How about if I said that given your repressive background, it was an achievement to have found any kind of sexual satisfaction, and your masturbation represents a forward-moving tendency in your sexual development?" I offered. "I'd think you were depraved."

Moralization thus illustrates the caveat that even though a given defense may be considered a "mature" mechanism, it can still be maddeningly impervious to therapeutic influence. Working with someone in the neurotic range whose character is defined by the chronic, inflexible use of a particular defensive strategy can be as arduous as working with overtly psychotic patients.

COMPARTMENTALIZATION

Compartmentalization is another of the intellectual defenses, probably more closely related to dissociative processes than to rationalization and moralization, although rationalization is often called on to support it. Like isolation of affect, it is on the more primitive side; its function is to permit two conflicting conditions to exist without conscious confusion, guilt, shame, or anxiety. Whereas isolation involves a rift between cognition and emotion, in compartmentalization, there is a rift between incompatible cognitive sets. When someone compartmentalizes, he or she holds two or more ideas, attitudes, or behaviors that are essentially and definitionally in conflict, without appreciating the contradiction. To an unpsychologically minded observer, compartmentalization is indistinguishable from hypocrisy.

Examples of everyday compartmentalization of which most of us are occasionally guilty include such simultaneous attitudes as a professed belief in the Golden Rule and also in the principle of looking out for Number One, espousing the importance of open communication while defending the position of not speaking to somebody, deploring prejudice yet savoring ethnic jokes. On the more pathological end of the compartmentalization continuum, we find people who are great humanitarians in the public sphere yet defend the abuse of their children in the privacy of their homes. In recent times, the public has been reminded of the phenomenon of the preacher who rails against sin while enthusiastically committing more than his share of it. More than one crusader against pornography has been found to have an extensive collection of erotica. Sin that is committed with a clear sense of guilt, or in a dissociated state at the time of commission, is not properly regarded as revealing the defense of compartmentalization; the term applies only if the discrepant activities or ideas are both accessible to consciousness. Upon confrontation, the person using compartmentalization will rationalize the contradictions away.

UNDOING

Just as moralization can be considered a more grown-up version of splitting, *undoing* can be regarded as the natural successor to omnipotent control. There is a magical quality about the defense that betrays its archaic origins, even though the person engaging in defensive undoing can often be induced, via an appeal to his or her observing ego, to see the meaning of what amounts to superstitious behavior. Undoing is a term that means exactly what one would think: the unconscious effort to counterbalance some affect—usually guilt or shame—with an attitude or behavior that will magically erase it. An everyday example would be a spouse's arriving home with a gift that is intended to compensate for last night's temper outburst. If that motive is conscious, we cannot technically call it undoing, but when undoers are not aware of their shame or guilt, and therefore cannot consciously own their wish to expiate it, the label applies.

Many religious rituals have an aspect of undoing. The effort to atone for sins, even those committed only in thought, may be a universal human impulse. Around the age when children can cognitively grasp the fact of death, one sees numerous magical rituals that have a component of undoing. The childhood game of avoiding cracks in the sidewalk lest one break mother's back is psychoanalytically comprehensible as the undoing of unconscious death wishes for the mother, which create more fear than they did before the concept of death had taken on a more mature meaning. Omnipotent fantasies are discernible in the implicit belief expressed in this behavior that one's hostile feelings are dangerous: The thought is tantamount to the deed.

One of my patients used to give me flowers occasionally. As she was quite disturbed and would have experienced my rejecting such gifts, or even analyzing her disposition to give them, as a profound repudiation of her generous impulses, for a long time I did not attempt to explore with her the meaning of this behavior. Eventually, however, she was able to figure out herself that she tended to bring me bouquets when she had been unusually angry at me the previous session. "I guess they were really for your grave," she explained, grinning.

People who have a high degree of remorse for their past sins, mistakes, and failures, whether real, exaggerated, or committed only in thought, may make a lifetime project out of undoing. Adlai Stevenson, for example, who accidentally killed his young cousin when he was a boy, devoted the rest of his life to public service. A 79-year-old, middle-class Caucasian woman whom I studied in connection with research on the psychology of characterological altruists (McWilliams, 1984) had for decades dedicated herself to the cause of equal justice for nonwhite people; her background included her having inadvertently insulted a woman of color, whom she had deeply loved, when she was about 9. Tomkins's (1964) study of committed abolitionists suggested a similar organization of personality around the defense of undoing.

When undoing is a central defense in a person's repertoire, and when acts that have the unconscious significance of expiating past crimes comprise the main support to the individual's self-esteem, we consider his or her personality to be *compulsive*. I want to stress here, since the terms "compulsion" and "compulsive" are so often associated with undesirable behaviors, that the concept of compulsivity is neutral as to moral content. In other words, one can be a compulsive drinker, but one can also be a compulsive humanitarian.*

TURNING AGAINST THE SELF

Anna Freud tended to use simple, everyday language, and her use of the term "turning against the self" is no exception. The concept means what a lay person would assume, that is, the redirecting of some negative affect or attitude from an external object toward the self. If one is critical of an authority whose goodwill seems essential to one's security, and if one thinks that person cannot tolerate criticism, one feels safer aiming the critical ideas inward. For children, who have no choice about where they live and who may pay a high price for offending a touchy caregiver, the defense of turning against the self can distract them from the much more upsetting fact that their well-being depends on an undependable adult. However unpleasant it is to feel self-critical, it is emotionally preferable to acknowledging a realistic threat to one's survival under conditions in which one has no power to change things.

One of my patients spent her formative years living in the care of a suicidal mother and an on-again-off-again, self-centered father. Her family's security was so precarious that even at the subsistence level they were in trouble: Some of this woman's earliest memories concern her parents' being thrown out of their apartments for nonpayment of rent. Rather than feel chronic terror that her mother would kill herself and her father would disappear on some self-indulgent project—both of which were serious possibilities—she became adept at believing that if only she were a better person, her parents would give her their love and protection. This conviction, which had been adaptive in

*"Obsessive" and "compulsive" are not necessarily pejorative terms when applied to personality structure, even though these labels derive from attempts to understand pathological states of obsession and compulsion. The sufferer of ego-alien, persistent, unwanted thoughts (obsessions) or persistent, unwanted acts (compulsions) may be desperate for help. In contrast, a person happily obsessed with writing a novel or pleasurably engaged in compulsive gardening is hardly to be regarded as "sick." In describing character, which may be highly adaptive and healthy, "obsessive" applies to thinking styles, "compulsive" to acting modes of adaptation.

childhood, caused her continual suffering as an adult when she reacted to any unhappy circumstance with self-attack rather than with creative efforts to improve her situation. It took years of therapy for her to realize at an emotional level that she was no longer a powerless child in a dysfunctional family, whose only hope for a sense of efficacy lay in the project of improving herself internally.

Most of us retain some tendency to turn negative affects, attitudes, and perceptions against the self because of the illusion that the process gives of our being more in control of upsetting situations than we may be. Turning against the self is a popular defense among healthier people, who are aware of and resistant to temptations to deny or project unpleasant qualities; they prefer to err in the direction of considering that a problem is their fault rather than someone else's. Automatic and compulsive use of this defense is common in people with depressive personalities and in some kinds of characterological masochism.

DISPLACEMENT

Displacement is another defense that is popularly appreciated without much distortion of its technical psychoanalytic meaning. At the age of 11 one of my daughters, observing our dog attack its pull toy right after being scolded for misbehavior, commented, "Look at that! She's taking her anger out on the toy—just like people!" The term displacement refers to the redirection of a drive, emotion, preoccupation, or behavior from its initial or natural object to another because its original direction is for some reason anxiety ridden.

The classic cartoon about the man bawled out by his boss, who goes home and yells at his wife, who in turn scolds the kids, who kick the dog is a study in displacement. The "triangulation" emphasized by family therapists in the tradition of Murray Bowen is a displacement phenomenon. I have noticed that in couples in which one partner is unfaithful, the other partner directs most of his or her reactive hatred not to the mate who has strayed but to the "other" woman or man. Tirades about "that home wrecker," implying that the partner was an innocent victim of a cynical seduction, seem to protect an already anguished person from risking any further threat to the relationship that might be created if the betrayed party's rage were aimed directly at the adulterous mate.

Lust can also be displaced; sexual fetishes seem explicable as the reorientation of erotic interest from a human being's genitals to some unconsciously related area, like feet or even shoes. If events in a man's history have made vaginas seem dangerous, some other female-associated object may be substituted. Anxiety may itself be displaced; Freud's famous patient the "Wolf Man" was treated in his later years by Ruth Mack Brunswick for a morbid preoccupation with his nose that came to be understood as the displacement of frightening, mutilatory fantasies about his penis (Gardiner, 1971). When a person uses displacement of anxiety from some other area to a specific object that symbolizes the dreaded phenomenon (e.g., a terror of spiders, which have the unconscious significance of maternal engulfment, or a horror of knives, which unconsciously equate with phallic penetration), he or she has a phobia (Nemiah, 1973). If a person has a pattern of displaced, fearful preoccupations in many aspects of his or her life, we consider the person's character to be *phobic*.

Certain lamentable cultural trends such as racism, sexism, heterosexism, and the general blaming of societal problems on disenfranchised groups who have little power to fight back contain a large element of displacement. So does the tendency toward scapegoating that one finds in most organizations and subcultures. Transference, in clinical as well as extraclinical manifestations of transference that Sullivan called "parataxic distortions," contains displacement (of feelings toward important early objects) as well as projection (of internal features of the self). Benign forms of displacement include the diverting of aggressive energy into creative activity—a great deal of housework gets done when people are in a snit about something—and the redirecting of erotic impulses from impossible or forbidden sexual objects toward an appropriate partner.

REACTION FORMATION

The defense of *reaction formation* is an intriguing phenomenon. Evidently, the human organism is capable of turning something into its polar opposite in order to render it less threatening. The traditional definition of reaction formation involves this conversion of a negative into a positive affect or vice versa. The transformation of hatred into love, or longing into contempt, or envy into attraction, for example, can be inferred from many common transactions.

Perhaps the earliest age at which the process is discernible to the onlooker is in a child's third or fourth year; by this time, if a new baby arrives, the displaced older sibling is likely to have enough ego strength to handle its anger and jealousy by converting them into a conscious feeling of love toward the newborn. It is typical of reaction formation that some of the disowned affect "leaks through" the defense, such that observers can sense there is something a bit excessive or false in the conscious emotional disposition. With a preschool sister who has been displaced by a younger brother, for instance, there may be a distinct flavor of her "loving the baby to death": hugging him too hard, singing to him too loudly, bouncing him too aggressively, and so on. Most adult older siblings remember a story about themselves pinching the new baby's cheeks until it screamed, or offering it some delicacy that was actually poisonous, or committing some similar transgression that was allegedly motivated by love.

A more accurate way to depict reaction formation than as the turning of an emotion into its opposite might be to note that it functions to deny ambivalence. It is a basic psychoanalytic assumption that no disposition is totally unmixed. We can hate the person we love or resent the person to whom we feel grateful; our emotional situation does not simply reduce to one or the other position.* It is a common misunderstanding of psychoanalytic interpretation that the analyst delights in exposing the fact that one *seems* to feel "x" but *really* feels "y"; in fact, it is psychoanalytically correct only to say that while one may feel "x," one *also* (unconsciously, perhaps) feels "y." In reaction formation, one persuades the self that all that is felt is one polarity of a complex emotional response.

One can see from the example of the displaced sibling who finds a way to avoid feeling negative affects and to experience only positive ones, at an age when finer discriminations between shades of feeling and (more important) between feelings and actions are not yet maturationally possible, how valuable such a defense can be. Other situations in which its operation is mostly benevolent include circumstances in which competitive feelings, which include both murderous and admiring components, lead a child to emulate a competent friend rather than to reject him or her. In adults one sees reaction formation, but ordinarily we assume that grown people would be better off acknowledging all aspects of their emotional reactions to any given situation and applying their inhibition to the domain of behavior rather than that of feeling.

Reaction formation is a favored defense in those psychopathologies in which hostile feelings and aggressive strivings are of paramount concern and are experienced as in danger of getting out of hand. Paranoid people, for instance, often feel only hatred and suspicion

*Freud made the charmingly dubious argument, evidently out of his personal wish to believe that his mother had not entertained any negative feelings toward him as a baby, that there is one exception to the otherwise sacrosanct psychoanalytic premise that no state of feeling is ever unambivalent: the love of a mother toward a male infant. Most psychoanalysts have not accepted his ideas on this topic (see Stolorow & Atwood, 1979; Gay, 1988).

when the external observer suspects that they also feel longing and dependency; obsessive and compulsive people frequently believe that they have only respect and appreciation for the authorities that others suspect them of simultaneously resenting.

REVERSAL

Another way that one can cope with feelings that present a psychological threat to the self is by enacting a scenario that switches one's position from subject to object or vice versa. For example, if one feels that the yearning to be cared for by someone else is shameful or dangerous, one can vicariously satisfy one's own dependency needs by taking care of another person and unconsciously identifying with that person's gratification in being nurtured. This particular version of *reversal* is a time-honored device of therapists, who are often uncomfortable with their own dependency but happy to be depended upon.

As soon as children are old enough to play with dolls or "action figures" (as boys' dolls are currently marketed), they can be said to be using reversal. An advantage of reversal is that one can shift the power aspects of a transaction so that one is in the initiating rather than the responding role. Control–mastery theorists call this "passive-into-active transformation." The defense operates constructively when the scenario being reversed is a benign one and destructively when the reversed situation is intrinsically negative. In fraternity hazing and other abusive rites of passage, for instance, one's experience of persecution during one's own initiation is transformed later into a situation that is felt as positive by virtue of its being a switch from passive to active, from victim to victimizer.

Sometimes in clinical practice one encounters reversal being used in a way that challenges one's therapeutic resourcefulness. I worked for a long time with a man who had had a deeply depressed and alcoholic mother. Every morning as a boy, he would come into the kitchen to see her drooping over a cup of coffee, cigarette in hand, looking exhausted and miserable. His presenting problem was a vulnerability to depression that had originated in his unsatisfactory relationship with this miserable, potentially suicidal woman. When he would come in for a session, he would often scan my face and announce, "You sure look tired today" or "You certainly seem to be down in the dumps about something." Occasionally he was right, but more commonly I was in a good mood and struck by the inaccuracy of his observation. As time went on, I increasingly challenged his assumption about my fatigue or despondency, saying that I was not aware of feeling tired or depressed. Instead of finding this interesting, and using my comment as a springboard to understand what he was displacing or projecting, he would reverse roles with me psychologically, announcing that while I might *think* I was okay, I obviously was not; that he was an unusually sensitive observer of people, and he knew a depressed person when he saw one.

This man had essentially made himself the therapist and me the patient, thus reversing a situation that was very difficult for him. His childhood experience of unreliable maternal authority had not given him grounds for any emotional security in a role that invited him to depend, especially on a female object. In this case, although his use of reversal protected him from acknowledging some deeply disturbing feelings, it had had the unfortunate side effect of making it hard for him to be in relationships that were emotionally reciprocal. Part of the stimulus for his depressive symptoms was a series of failed friendships and love affairs in which his tendency to recreate the scenario of a needy child and empathically limited parent, with himself in the latter position, eventually rankled potential intimates.

Another subject in my research on altruism (McWilliams, 1984) was an attractive, successful man in his 40s whose greatest satisfactions in life lay in his activity as a volunteer for an international agency that arranged for the adoption of hard-to-place children (some were of stigmatized ethnic origin, some had physical handicaps or deformities, and some suffered congenital diseases). In his words, "I can't describe the high I get when I hand the baby to the adoptive mother and know that a new life is beginning for that kid." His personal history included the sudden, shattering death of his mother when he was two, followed by a short period of great distress, followed by his informal adoption by a housekeeper, who later married his father and became in every psychological sense his mother. Whenever he successfully arranged an adoption, he felt the elation of rescuing someone as he had been rescued (although until I worked with him, he had never made a conscious connection between his own background and his humanitarian concerns) and the relief that this time the situation was reversed: He was the rescuer, the one with the power, and it was the other party who was the helpless, dependent child.

The reader may be noticing that as these higher-order defensive processes are discussed, there are no single personality types that reflect an overdependence on them. Psychologically healthier people tend not only to use more mature defenses, such as reversal, they also handle anxiety and other difficult emotional states by recourse to varying defensive modes. Consequently, they are less readily typed by one label.

IDENTIFICATION

It may seem odd for *identification* to be included in a list of defense mechanisms, since most of us consider the capacity to identify with another person, or with some aspect of another person, as a benign and nondefensive tendency. That some kinds of identification have very few if any defensive components (e.g., the kind that psychologists with a social learning orientation have called "modeling") is well established, but psychoanalytic thinkers continue to regard many instances of identification as motivated by needs to avoid anxiety, grief, shame, or other painful affects; or to restore a threatened sense of self-cohesion and self-esteem. Like the other mature defensive processes, identification is a normal aspect of psychological development that becomes problematic only under certain circumstances.

Freud (1923) was the first to suggest a distinction between nondefensive and defensive identification by differentiating what he called "anaclitic" identification (from the Greek word meaning "to lean on") from "identification with the aggressor." The first type he considered to be motivated by an uncomplicated wish to be like a valued person ("Mommy is generous and comforting, and I want to be just like her"). The second he regarded as an equally automatic but defensively motivated solution to the problem of feeling threatened by the power of another person ("I'm afraid of Mommy's punishment for my hostile impulses; if I *become* her, her power will be inside rather than outside me"). Many acts of identification were assumed by Freud to contain elements of both a straightforward taking in of what is loved and a defensive becoming like what is feared.

Analysts use the word identification to connote a mature level of deliberately, yet at least partly unconsciously, becoming like another person. This capacity evolves in a natural developmental line from the earliest infantile forms of introjection, which have the quality of swallowing the other person whole, to more subtle, discriminating, and subjectively voluntary processes of selectively taking on another person's characteristics. Identificatory potential is assumed to evolve and modify throughout life and to be the emotional basis of psychological growth and change. In fact, the opportunity that close relationships provide for mutually enriching identifications accounts for the value that analysts have traditionally placed on emotional intimacy (e.g., see the argument to this effect in the Blancks' [R. Blanck & G. Blanck, 1968] book on marriage). In a way that parallels how primitive projection transforms itself over the life span of an emotionally healthy person into a greater and greater capacity for empathy, archaic forms of identification gradually transmute to more and more discerning and nuanced ways to enrich the self by accumulating the qualities of admired others.

Freud's most familiar paradigm of defensive identification was the oedipal situation. In this famous scenario, the young child reaches an age, usually around 3, in which his* wishes for exclusive possession of the mother run into the harsh fact of the father's claim on her love and physical availability. He fears that his father, whose superior power is obvious, will kill or maim him in retaliation for his own wishes to kill or maim his father, whom he views as a rival, and the child resolves the anxiety connected with such fantasies by identification ("Maybe I can't get rid of father—whom I love anyway and don't really want to dispose of—or get mother all to myself—which would also have its problems, but I could be *like* father and grow up to have someone *like* mother as my exclusive partner"). Freud felt that this fantasy, which he considered normal and universal, was the prototype for identification with the aggressor—in this case an imagined aggressor.†

Identification is inherently a neutral process; it can have positive or negative effects depending on who is the object of the identification. A major part of the process of psychotherapy is the rethinking of old and now problematic identifications that were entered into automatically, resolved a conflict for the child at the time, and are now causing conflict in adulthood. For example, a minister that I worked with had survived the ordeal of having an abusive, alcoholic father and an ineffectual, phobic mother by emulating his tough Uncle Harry, a man who solved all interpersonal problems with his fists. This resolution was highly adaptive for my patient throughout his adolescence in a chaotic family in a series of hostile urban neighborhoods; he could deck anybody that got in his way, and as a result, nobody messed with him. This was the way he attained relief of anxiety, discharge of troubling feelings that were unwelcome in his home, restoration of his self-esteem, and a guarantee of others' respect. In his later professional life, however, when he threatened to beat up several obnoxious church elders, he *lost* the respect of many in his congregation, who did not regard his behavior as consistent with a Christian sensibility. He

*I am deliberating using the masculine pronoun here since Freud's depiction of this process was based on his understanding of male children and was then extended to females in a way that most subsequent thinkers, especially female ones, have found somewhat contrived and unempathic to the situation of the little girl (e.g., see Horney, 1926; Thompson, 1964; Chasseguet-Smirgel, 1971; J. B. Miller, 1973; D. Silverman, 1986; Chodorow, 1989; Fast, 1990; D. Bernstein, 1993).

†Most contemporary analysts see identification with the aggressor as having much earlier roots, in fears and fantasies typical of the first year, as mentioned in Chapter 5 (see Segal, 1964).

presented himself for therapy knowing that he had to develop new ways of coping with stress, and as he came to understand the nature of his early identifications and the current price he paid for them, he did.

Because identification can seem to be a remedy for all the complexities of life, it may be used more frequently as a defense when a person is under emotional stress, especially of the sort that puts a strain on older subjective versions of who one is. Death or loss will predictably instigate identification, both with the absent love object and then with those who come to replace that person in the survivor's emotional world. The yearning of adolescents to find heroes whom they may emulate in their effort to address the complex demands of looming adulthood has been noted for centuries; in fact, the dissatisfaction of contemporary teenagers with the heroes now offered by Western culture has been connected by some psychoanalytic observers with the alarming increase in adolescent suicides over recent decades (e.g., Hendin, 1975).

Some people seem to identify more easily and reflexively than others, as if they are blotters for whatever psychological ink comes in their direction. Those who suffer from basic confusions of identity, of whatever severity, are obviously at risk here, as anyone who has studied cult behavior can attest. Conversion experiences contain a heavy component of defensive identification. Even quite healthy people with some area of identity disturbance, such as a hysterically organized woman with unconscious feelings that her gender is a problem, can be more than usually subject to identifying with someone in the environment who gives the impression of having a better handle on life's difficulties.

The capacity of human beings to identify with new love objects is probably the main vehicle through which people recover from emotional suffering, and the main means by which psychotherapy of any kind achieves change. Repeatedly, research on the treatment process finds the emotional quality of the relationship between patient and therapist to be more highly correlated with outcome than any other specifiable factors (Strupp, 1989). In some recent analytic writing on the therapy process, relationship is stressed to such an extent that interpretation, once seen as the mainstay of psychological healing, may hardly be mentioned at all (e.g., Loewald, 1957; Levenson, 1972; Greenberg & Mitchell, 1983; Meissner, 1991).

In psychoanalytic treatment, the patient's propensity to make identifications with the therapist is cherished for its reparative potential and is also safeguarded as far as possible from abuse. Practitioners try to avoid exploiting the patient's readiness to identify by exemplifying general qualities of human virtue (such as compassion, curiosity, tolerance of difference, and a sense of ultimate responsibility for one's behavior) while being reserved about showing specifics of their personal attributes, giving advice, or sharing particular opinions. Freud's repeated warning to analysts to avoid falling into the temptation to present themselves in a grandiose way as saviors, healers, or prophets to their patients remains a guiding maxim in the field; narcissistic misuse of a patient's wish to identify remains a professional taboo—albeit one that, like other taboos, is probably broken much more frequently than most of us would admit.

ACTING OUT

Another mechanism that merits discussion here is the general category of "acting out." I enclose the term in quotation marks to call attention to the frequency with which the label currently gets applied to all kinds of behavior that the labeler happens not to like, often in a tone quite at odds with the original nonpejorative meaning of the term. Most readers of this text have probably heard the term bandied about disapprovingly and will not be aware of the more professional, technical use of the concept.

To my knowledge, the earliest appearances of the phrase "acting out" occurred in psychoanalytic descriptions of patients' actions outside the office, when their behavior seemed to embody feelings toward the analyst that the patient was unaware of having or was too anxious to let into consciousness, especially in the analyst's presence (Freud, 1914a). Later on, "acting out" became used more generally to describe behavior that is driven by unconscious needs to master the anxiety associated with internally forbidden feelings and wishes, and with powerfully upsetting fears, fantasies, and memories (Aichhorn, 1936; Fenichel, 1945). By *enacting* frightening scenarios, the unconsciously anxious person turns passive into active, transforming a sense of helplessness and vulnerability into an experience of agency and power, no matter how negative the drama that is played out (cf. Weiss, Sampson, & the Mount Zion Psychotherapy Research Group, 1986).

A teacher I saw in treatment several years ago, whose relationship to her judgmental mother had left her both frightened of and deeply hungry for intimacy, began a sexual affair with a colleague named Nancy a few weeks after entering therapy. It seemed to me that she was beginning to feel some wish for closeness with me, was unconsciously assuming that I (like her mother) would be scornful of her longings, and was handling her unconscious and forbidden strivings by acting out aspects of what she wished and feared with someone who bore my name. This kind of enactment, assuming my interpretation of it is accurate, happens frequently in analysis, especially with patients who have a childhood basis for fearing an authority's rejection of their needs and feelings.

The term *acting out* thus properly refers to any behavior that is assumed to be an expression of transference attitudes that the patient does not yet feel safe enough to bring into treatment in words. It may also be used to label the process by which any attitude, in or out of treatment, may be discharged in action with the unconscious purpose of mastering fears that surround it. What is acted out may be predominantly self-destructive, or predominantly growth enhancing, or some of each; what makes it acting out is not its goodness or badness but the unconscious and fearsome nature of the impulses that propel the person into action and the compulsive, automatic way in which the acted-out behavior is undertaken. The current popularity of calling any unappreciated behavior—in obstreperous children, for example, or in rude acquaintances—"acting out" is psychoanalytically unjustified. The negative cast that the phrase has acquired may reflect the fact that beneficial kinds of acting out do not call attention to themselves in the way that destructive ones do.

A number of imposing labels created by analysts to depict classes of behaviors that are usually unconsciously motivated fall under the general heading of acting out. These include, for example, exhibitionism, voyeurism, sadism, masochism, perversion, and all the "counter" terms: counterphobia, counterdependency, counterhostility, and so on.* All tend, when applied to specific acts that are understood as defensive, to assume underlying fear or other disavowed negative feelings. Freud's early observation that we act out what we do not remember remains astute, especially if we assume that the reason we do not remember is that something very painful went along with the unremembered and now-enacted state.

To the extent that there is an identifiable population of persons who rely on acting out to deal with their psychological dilemmas, that group would fall into the category of *impulsive personalities*. This nomenclature is misleading, as it implies an uncomplicated readiness to do whatever one feels like doing at the moment. Psychotherapeutic

*As in other areas in which psychoanalytic terminology is attached to human inclinations, the assumption is *not* made that any of these processes are inherently negative or even inherently defensive. People are assumed to have normal voyeuristic and exhibitionistic needs, for example, that are ordinarily discharged in socially acceptable ways of looking and being looked at. Masochistic and sadistic strivings are likewise seen as normal aspects of human experience, which find positive expression in acts of personal sacrifice or dominance, respectively.

experience has led most thoughtful clinicians to believe that what may look like spontaneous, uncomplicated impulsiveness is often unconsciously and very complexly driven behavior, behavior that is anything but innocently expressive and random. Hysterically organized people are famous for acting out unconscious sexual scenarios; addicted people of all kinds can be conceptualized as repeatedly acting out their relation to their preferred substance (in such cases, of course, chemical dependency can complicate what was already a psychological addiction); people with compulsions are by definition acting out when they succumb to internal pressure to engage in their particular compulsive acts; sociopathic people may be reenacting a complicated pattern of manipulation. Thus, the defense may be seen in many contrasting clinical presentations.

SEXUALIZATION (INSTINCTUALIZATION)

Some writers on defensive processes might subsume sexualization under acting out since its operation usually takes an enacted form. I have chosen to present it separately, partly because it is possible to sexualize without acting out (a process that is more accurately referred to as *erotization*) and partly because it is a concept of such general and interesting significance that it deserves some special attention.

Freud originally assumed that basic sexual energy, a force he referred to as libido, underlay virtually all human activity. (Later in his theorizing, impressed with the prevalence of human destructiveness, he decided that aggressive strivings were equally fundamental and motivating, but most of the language of his clinical theory derives from a time before that shift in his thinking). One consequence of his biological, drive-based psychological theory was his tendency to regard sexual behaviors as expressing a *primary* motivation, not a derivative and defensive one. Obviously, sexuality is a powerful basic dynamism in human beings, and much human sexual behavior amounts to relatively direct expressions of the reproductive imperative of our species. Clinical experience and research findings (e.g., Stoller, 1968, 1975, 1980, 1985; Money, 1980, 1988) over the decades since Freud's work, however, have impressed most psychoanalytically sympathetic thinkers with the extent to which sexual activity and fantasy are used defensively: to master anxiety, to restore self-esteem, to offset shame, or to distract from a sense of inner deadness.

People may sexualize any experience with the unconscious intention of converting terror or pain or other overwhelming sensation into excitement. This process has also been referred to in the analytic literature as *instinctualization*. Sexual arousal is a reliable means of feeling alive; a child's fear of death—by abandonment, abuse, or other dreaded calamity—can be mastered psychologically by turning a traumatic situation into a life-affirming one. Studies of people with unusual sexual proclivities have often turned up infantile experiences that overwhelmed the child's capacity to cope and were consequently transformed into self-initiated sexualizations of the trauma. For example, Stoller's (e.g., 1975) work with sexually masochistic people, those who report needing to feel pain in order to achieve erotic gratification, revealed that a significant number of them had suffered invasive and painful medical treatments as young children.

In a more general way, most of us use sexualization to some degree in order to cope with and spice up troublesome aspects of life. There are some common differences between people of opposite gender in what they tend to sexualize: For example, women are more apt to sexualize dependency and men to sexualize aggression. Some people sexualize money, some sexualize dirt, some sexualize power, and so forth. Many of us sexualize the experience of learning; the erotic presence of talented teachers has been noted at least since the time of Socrates. The tendency of people to erotize their reaction to anyone with superior power may explain why political figures and other celebrities are typically deluged with sexually available admirers, and why the potential for sexual corruption and exploitiveness is so great among the influential and famous.

The susceptibility of those in a relatively weak position to converting their envy, hostility, and fear of mistreatment into a sexual scenario, one in which they compensate for a relative lack of official power with recourse to a very personal erotic power, is one of the reasons it is socially important to have laws and conventions protecting those who are structurally dependent on others (employees on employers, students on teachers, sergeants on lieutenants, etc.). We all need to be discouraged from the temptations created by our own defenses as well as from the possibility of crass exploitation by the authorities in our lives.

At the risk of belaboring a point that applies to all defensive processes, let me stress that sexualization is not inherently problematic or destructive. People's individual sexual fantasies, response patterns, and practices are probably more idiosyncratic than almost any other psychological aspect of their lives; what turns one person on erotically may leave another cold. If I happen to sexualize the experience of someone's handling my hair (even if the childhood genesis of my doing so was a defensive sexualizing of my mother's abusive hair yanking), and my sexual partner loves to run his or her fingers through it, I am not likely to go into psychotherapy. But if I sexualize the experience of being frightened by abusive males, and I have repeated affairs with men who beat me up, I might well seek help. As with every other defense, it is the context and consequences of its use in adulthood that determine whether it is reasonably to be regarded (by self and others) as a positive adaptation, an unremarkable habit, or a pathological affliction.

SUBLIMATION

At one time, the concept of *sublimation* was widely understood among the educated public and represented a trendy way of looking at many different individual proclivities. Contemporarily, with the receding centrality of drive theory in general psychoanalytic thinking, it is referred to less in psychoanalytic literature, and it is less appreciated popularly as a concept. The original idea was that sublimation was the "good" defense, the one that by definition represented a creative, healthful, socially acceptable or beneficial resolution of internal conflicts between primitive urges and inhibiting forces.

Sublimation was the label Freud originally gave to the expression of biologically based impulses (which to him included urges to suck, bite, mess, fight, copulate, look at others and be looked at by them, inflict injury, endure pain, protect the young, etc.) in a socially valuable form. For example, Freud would have said that a periodontist may be sublimating sadism; a performing artist, exhibitionism; a lawyer, the wish to kill one's enemies. Instinctual strivings, according to him, become influenced by the circumstances of one's individual childhood; certain drives or conflicts take on special salience and may be creatively directed into useful activities.

This defense was considered to be the healthiest means of resolving psychological predicaments for two reasons: First, it fostered behavior beneficial to the species; second, it *discharged* the relevant impulse instead of wasting a lot of emotional energy either transforming it into something different (e.g., as reaction formation would do) or counteracting it with an opposing force (e.g., denial, repression). Such energy discharge was assumed to be inherently beneficial: It kept the human organism in proper homeostasis (Fenichel, 1945).

Sublimation remains a concept to which one finds references in the analytic literature when a writer is referring to someone's finding a creative and useful way to express problematic impulses and conflicts. In contrast to a common misunderstanding that the object of psychotherapy is to rid oneself of infantile strivings, the psychoanalytic position about health and growth includes the assumption that the infantile parts of our natures remain alive throughout adulthood. We do not have the choice to divest ourselves of them; we can only handle them in better or worse ways.

The goals of analytic therapy include the understanding of all aspects of the self, even the most primitive and disturbing ones, the development of compassion for oneself (and others, as one's need to project and displace one's previously disowned qualities lessens), and the expansion of one's freedom to resolve old conflicts in new ways. They do not include purging the self of its loathed aspects or obliterating primitive desires. That sublimation is considered the apogee of ego development says a great deal about the basic psychoanalytic attitude toward the human organism and its inherent potentials and limits, and about the implicit values informing psychoanalytic diagnosis.

This concludes my review of defensive operations that are pertinent to an understanding of the organization of individual character. I should remind the reader here that this book is about personality *structure*, not just personality *disorders*. Even though its focus is on the clinical task of diagnosis, which presumes that the person coming for help is suffering in some way, one must remember that the problem for which help has been sought may not lie in the patient's basic character. It may, for example, be a response to some stress that would tax the reserves of anyone, with any kind of character structure.

But just *how* a person suffers will reflect his or her personality organization. And how someone else can help mitigate the suffering requires a sensitivity to personality differences. Cactus and ivy will both grow when given light and water, but the gardener who does not appreciate the differences between the two plants will not bring each to full flower. An understanding of variation among people in their basic character is essential to the conduct of effective psychotherapy whether or not the problem to be addressed is characterological. A therapeutic stance that is helpful to an obsessive person troubled by depression will differ from the one that helps another depressed client whose basic personality is more hysterically organized.

All of us have powerful childhood fears and yearnings, handle them with the best defensive strategies available at the time, and maintain these methods of coping as other demands replace the early scenarios of our lives. The object of a sensitive psychodiagnostic process is not to evaluate how "sick" someone is, or to determine which people are beyond the pale of what is socially defined as normal (McDougall, 1980), but to understand the *particularity* of a person's suffering and strength so that one can relieve the former and build on the latter.

In the following chapters, I shall describe the major psychodynamically significant personality organizations. Each category, as I have mentioned, constitutes a characterological reliance on a defense or group of defenses. Each comprises a developmental range from people who are frankly psychotic to those who are exemplars of psychological health. I shall describe subjective as well as objective aspects of working with someone with each personality type and, where possible, translate psychoanalytic generalities and abstractions into reportable clinical transactions.

SUMMARY

This chapter has covered the most common and clinically relevant of the secondary, or "higher-order," defenses: repression, regression, isolation, intellectualization, rationalization, moralization, compartmentalization, undoing, turning against the self, displacement, reaction formation, reversal, identification, acting out, sexualization, and sublimation. Adaptive and maladaptive examples of each have been given, along with commentary about related character types. Finally, some general comments about the relationship of defense to character were made in the service of transition to the topics of the next chapters.

SUGGESTIONS FOR FURTHER READING

As I mentioned at the end of Chapter 5, commentary on the defenses is usually embedded in other topics and is seldom the subject of a book. Anna Freud's (1936) and H. P. Laughlin's (1970, 1979) writings are the exceptions, and both are very readable. For the intrepid, Fenichel (1945) covered the topic with his usual thoroughness in Chapters 8 and 9 of *The Psychoanalytic Theory of Neurosis*.

II
TYPES OF CHARACTER ORGANIZATION

Each chapter of this section covers a major character type. Order of presentation is arbitrary but runs roughly from low to high levels of object-relatedness. I have organized the discussion along the following lines: (1) considerations of drive, affect, and temperament; (2) adaptive and defensive operations of the ego; (3) object relational patterns that contribute to development of the character type, become internalized, and repeat as "scripts"; (4) experiences of the self (conscious and unconscious ways one sees oneself and how one supports self-esteem); (5) transference and countertransference outcomes of having internal representations of self and others and their recurrent relations; (6) implications for treatment; and (7) considerations of differential diagnosis.

RATIONALE FOR CHAPTER ORGANIZATION

The first four categories I have taken directly, although with some additional elaboration, from Pine (1990), who has summarized drive, ego, object relational, and self aspects of individual psychology as follows:

> Broadly speaking, under these four terms I am referring, respectively, to the domains of (a) drives, urges, wishes; (b) defense, adaptation, reality testing, and defects in the development of each;

> (c) relationships to significant others *as experienced* and as carried in memory, with whatever attendant distortions such experiences and memories may entail; and (d) subjective experience of self in relation to such phenomena as boundaries, esteem, authenticity, and agency. (p. 13)

Like Pine, I see these four perspectives as implicit in the psychoanalytic tradition and as useful for sorting out different aspects of psychological complexity.

I have added the category of affect to Pine's first domain (cf. Tomkins, 1962, 1963, 1991, 1992; Kernberg, 1976; Isaacs, 1990; Spezzano, 1993). Much of what is implied in the concept of drive in psychodynamic writing is actually affective in nature. In spite of the emphasis on emotion that has characterized psychoanalytic description ever since Breuer and Freud (1893–1895) saw abreaction as a necessary condition of recovery from hysterical afflictions, and in spite of the value that therapists continue to place on emotional as opposed to intellectual insight, the role of affect in organizing and defining personality structure is still understated in most formal psychoanalytic theories.

I have also included temperament here. The significance Freud attached to innate individual differences in areas like direction and strength of drive looks quite reasonable in retrospect. Since therapy deals only with those aspects of self that are modifiable, clinicians do not think much about inborn leanings. Yet knowing someone's constitutional endowment contributes to reasonable goals. And commenting on such factors to one's clients helps them to accept their basic temperamental dispositions and to come to terms realistically with certain facts of their nature.

The next two topics under each personality type are intended to illuminate the interpersonal style characteristic of someone with that diagnosis and the requirements for effective therapy with such a person. Countertransference details are given for both diagnostic and therapeutic reasons. One's emotional reactions contain important diagnostic information, often the only clues (especially in more disturbed patients) for differentiating between two character types with contrasting therapeutic requirements. In addition, countertransference information may prepare therapists for what they are going to feel working with any client; they can then improve their chances of handling their feelings effectively. I have included here ideas about how to pass what control–mastery theorists would regard as characteristic "tests" of patients with different types of personality (Weiss, Sampson, & the Mount Zion Psychotherapy Research Group, 1986).

Finally, the differential diagnosis sections are included to alert the practitioner to possible alternatives to a given diagnosis, especially when any of the alternatives have important therapeutic consequences. It can be disastrous, for example, to misunderstand a hysterical woman as a fundamentally narcissistic one, or a narcissistic man as characterologically obsessive, or a person with multiple personality disorder as schizophrenic. And yet all these mistakes are made all the time because the manifest appearance and symptomatology of patients in each pair above can be virtually identical. For all the assets of the DSM, its checklist approach to diagnosis lends itself to these kinds of errors.

CHARACTER, CHARACTER PATHOLOGY, AND SITUATIONAL FACTORS

The following descriptions include both disturbed and healthy versions of each character type. Everyone has character. In most of us, it is not "disordered." We all have features of several personality styles no matter which tendencies are paramount in us. Many people who do not fit neatly into one category are adequately described as a combination of two types of organization (paranoid–schizoid, depressive–masochistic, etc.). Assessment of someone's character structure, even in the absence of a personality disorder, gives the therapist an idea of what kinds of interventions will be assimilable by the client and what style of relatedness will make him or her most receptive to efforts to help. Even though no one corresponds point for point to a textbook description, most people can be located in a general area that gives a clinician some orientation toward how to be therapeutic.

Dynamics are not pathology. It is appropriate to consider someone as having a pathological character, or a personality disorder, only when his or her defenses are so stereotypical that they prevent psychological growth and adaptation. An obsessive man organizes his life around thinking, achieving self-esteem in creative acts of thought such as scholarship, logical analysis, detailed planning, and judicious decision making. A pathologically obsessive one ruminates unproductively, accomplishing no objective, realizing no ambition, hating himself for going in circles. A depressive woman finds satisfaction in taking care of others; a pathologically depressive one cannot take care of herself.

It is also important to distinguish between character and responsivity. Certain situations elicit aspects of anyone's personality that may be latent under other circumstances: Losses bring out one's depressive side; threats to security arouse paranoia; battles for control breed obsessive rumination; sexual exploitation evokes hysteria. In making a diagnosis the therapist should be careful to weigh the relative impact of situational factors and characterological ones. It is a common mistake to assume, regardless of context, that if a patient reacts in accordance with the description of a particular character type, he or she has that kind of personality.

A Chinese graduate student who is in treatment with one of my supervisees has numerous preoccupations that are basically narcissistic: She is acutely sensitive to how she is perceived, spends most of her emotional energy on maintaining her self-esteem, suffers envy of American students to whom everything seems to come easily, and worries constantly about whether she "fits in." The genuine warmth with which she relates to her therapist, however, and the affection that colors my supervisee's countertransference, belie a conclusion that she has an essentially narcissistic personality. The stresses of adapting to a new community have simply exacerbated the latent concerns about acceptability, identity, and self-esteem with which anyone would struggle if culturally displaced. In addition to illustrating a caveat about confusing personality with reactivity, this example points to the critical importance of transference and countertransference data in assessment.

LIMITS ON PERSONALITY CHANGE

Analytic experience suggests that while personality can be substantially *modified* by therapy, it cannot be *transformed* (the drive-theory homily for this observation was "You can change the economics but not the dynamics"). That is, a therapist can help a depressive client to be less destructively and intransigently depressive but cannot change him or her into a hysterical or schizoid character. People maintain their core internal scripts, conflicts, expectations, and defenses, yet they may vastly expand their autonomy and realistic self-esteem if they appreciate the components of their basic personality. The increased freedom comes from mastery and choice in behavior that previously was automatic; the self-acceptance comes from understanding how they got their particular combination of tendencies. Whether or not a therapy contract includes an agreement to modify character, an appreciation of its nature by both parties will facilitate their work.

This section gives in-depth descriptions of psychopathic, narcissistic, schizoid, paranoid, depressive, manic, masochistic, obsessive, compulsive, hysterical, and dissociative personalities. A more comprehensive text would contain chapters on several other well-documented character prototypes, including passive aggressive, sadistic, explosive, impulsive, infantile, hypochondriacal, psychosomatic, and phobic organizations. My decision to omit these other types had several determinants, primary among which was my effort to write a book that would give therapists a general overview of psychoanalytic character diagnosis, not a treatise on every type of character. I wanted its scope to be adequately broad but not to weigh down the reader's book bag, expense account, or fortitude.

Secondarily, I lack enough direct, personal clinical experience with some character types to write about them confidently. For example, although I have supervised a few therapies of clients with agoraphobia and other phobic reactions, I have never myself worked intensively with someone with a phobic personality. Even when I know the pertinent literature on certain kinds of people, I cannot bring them to life without a strong experiential level of understanding. In the case of patients who are characterologically phobic, the reader may be consoled that the chapter on this topic in MacKinnon and Michels (1971) remains very illuminating.

Finally, it is my impression that most of the personality types I have omitted operate more commonly as melodic variations than as symphonic themes. For example, while people whose personalities are best described as sadistic are not unknown, sadism is more often an ingredient in psychopathy or dissociation than an organizing principle in someone's character. Impulsivity tends to be a feature of borderline personality organization in general, and sometimes of psychopathic or hysterical structure. Infantile personality is probably best seen as a subset of hysteria. Hypochondria is usually symptomatic of characterological narcissism. Passive aggressive patterns may, for different reasons, characterize someone of almost any kind of personality organization. While it behooves readers to know that all kinds of idiosyncratic character structures exist, and that an ability to conceptualize them sensitively has significant clinical implications, no text can cover every important variety of personality organization.

7
Psychopathic (Antisocial) Personalities

I will begin discussing the typological categories of personality organization with what are probably the most unpopular and intimidating patients encountered in mental health practice, those who are essentially psychopathic. I am following Meloy (1988) in using the older term for this personality type because of its established place in psychoanalytic history. I will be using "sociopathic" and "antisocial" as synonyms, unlike some earlier analytic writers who saved these terms for people in criminal subcultures who were not necessarily characterologically psychopathic.

People whose personalities are structured along psychopathic lines range from extremely psychotic, disorganized, impulsive, sadistic people like Richard Chase (Biondi & Hecox, 1992; Ressler & Schactman, 1992), who randomly murdered, dismembered, and drank the blood of his victims (in the delusion that his own blood was poisoned, and he needed it to survive), to urbane, polished charmers like some of the characters depicted by Stewart (1991) in his disturbing report on malfeasance at the highest levels of American corporate management.

The psychopathic continuum loads heavily in the borderline-to-psychotic direction, because by definition the diagnosis refers to a basic failure of human attachment and a reliance on very primitive defenses. With Bursten (1973a), however, I would argue that there do exist people in the higher ranges of functioning whose personalities show more sociopathy than any other features and who warrant a diagnosis as high-level psychopaths. Such people have enough identity integration, reality testing, and capacity to use more mature defenses to be considered as in the neurotic range, but their core ways of thinking and acting nevertheless show an antisocial sensibility. An example would be a successful and socially prominent forger. Bursten's criterion for diagnosing psychopathy, that the organizing preoccupation of the person is "getting over on" or consciously manipulating others, captures the essence of psychopathic psychology. Conceived this way, the diagnosis of characterological sociopathy has nothing to do with overt criminality and everything to do with internal motivation.

DRIVE, AFFECT, AND TEMPERAMENT IN PSYCHOPATHY

There is some evidence that people who become antisocial have more basic aggression than others. The fact that infants differ in temperament from birth (something any parent with more than two children always knew) has now been established scientifically (Thomas, Chess, & Birch, 1968). Some of the areas in which infants have demonstrated innate variability include activity level, aggressivity, reactivity, consolability, and similar factors that might influence development in a psychopathic direction. Adoption research and twin studies (Schulsinger, 1977; Mednick, Gabrielli, & Hutchings, 1984) have suggested the operation of some genetic factor in sociopathy that, though not determinative, lays the groundwork for it if other disposing factors exist (Vandenberg, Singer, & Pauls, 1986). Neurochemical and hormonal research (Wolman, 1986; Meloy, 1988) points to the probability of a biological substrate for the higher levels of affective and predatory aggression found in antisocial people.

Reactivity of the autonomic nervous system consistently tests lower in diagnosed psychopaths (Lykken, 1957; Hare, 1970; Loeb & Mednick, 1977), a fact that has been regarded as explanatory of the increased sensation seeking of such people and of their apparent "inability to learn from experience" (Cleckley, 1941). In short, people who become antisocial seem to have inborn tendencies toward aggressivity and a higher-than-average threshold for pleasurable excitement. Whereas most of us can get emotional satisfaction from good music, loving sex, natural beauty, a clever joke, or a job well done, the psychopath may need a sharper, more jolting experience to feel alive and well. Appreciating this fact about an antisocial patient may foster a tolerant attitude in the therapist, who will need lots of cognitive support for remaining committed to a person who is extremely difficult to love.

As for the main feelings with which sociopathic people are concerned, it is hard to specify them because of the inability of antisocial people to articulate emotion. They act instead of talking. They seem to have a sense of basic arousal without the sense of having specific affects. When they do feel, what they are likely to experience is either blind rage or manic exhilaration. In the section below on object relations, some reasons for this "massive affect block" (Modell, 1975) will be suggested. Meanwhile the reader should note that one way in which the effective treatment of psychopaths is markedly different from therapy with people of other character types is that the clinician cannot expect to connect with the patient by reflecting his or her feelings.

DEFENSIVE AND ADAPTIVE PROCESSES IN PSYCHOPATHY

The primary defensive operation in psychopathic people is omnipotent control. They also use projective identification, many subtle dissociative processes, and acting out. The need to exert power takes precedence over all other aims. It defends against shame and, especially in brutal psychopaths, distracts others from seeing the sexual perversions that often underlie criminality (Ressler & Schactman, 1992). The sociopath's famous absence of conscience (Cleckley, 1941) evidences not only a defective superego (Johnson, 1949) but also a lack of primary reciprocal attachments to other people. To the antisocial person, the value of others reduces to their utility in allowing one to demonstrate clout.

Psychopathic people will brag outright about their con jobs, conquests, and scams if they think the listener can be thereby impressed with their power. There is nothing unconscious about this process; it is literally shameless. Law enforcement agents are repeatedly astounded at how readily criminals will confess to homicide yet will hide lesser offenses (sexual compulsions, taking a few dollars from a murder victim's handbag), evidently because these are seen as signs of weakness (N. Susalis, personal communication, May 7, 1993). Kernberg (1984) refers to the psychopath's "malignant grandiosity," a phrase that rings true to anyone who has experienced a sociopathic person's effort to triumph sadistically by sabotaging therapy. It is important to distinguish between psychopathic manipulation and what is frequently labeled manipulation in hysterical and borderline patients.* The former is a deliberate, syntonic attempt to use others; the latter makes others *feel* used, while the patient is relatively unaware of a specific manipulative intent.

Experienced clinicians have long noted how psychopaths—those who have escaped self-destruction and incarceration—tend to "burn out" in middle age, often becoming surprisingly upright citizens. They also become more amenable to psychotherapy and may profit from it more than younger people with their diagnosis. This change is partially explicable by hormonal decreases that may reduce internal pressures toward action, but it is also likely that it results from the loss of physical power that occurs at mid-life. As long as omnipotent defenses are unthwarted by limits, a person will have no reason to develop more mature adaptations. Older adolescents and young adults of all personality types, especially healthy young men,† typically have omnipotent feelings: Death is far away, and the prerogatives of adulthood are at hand. Infantile grandiosity is reinforced. But reality has a way of catching up with most of us. By the age of forty or so, death is no longer an abstraction, one's physical strength has declined, one's reaction time is down, one's health cannot be taken for granted, and the long-term costs of hard living have begun to appear. These facts of life can have a very maturing effect.

As for projective identification, in sociopathic people a reliance on this process may reflect not only a developmental arrest and a general reliance on primitive defenses but also the consequences of their inarticulateness. Their inability and/or disinclination to express emotions verbally means that the only way they can get other people to understand what they are feeling is to evoke that feeling in them. In the section on transference and countertransference I shall say more about this. The dissociative defenses of psychopaths are commonly noted but hard to evaluate in specific instances. Dissociative phenomena range

*As noted in Chapter 4, I recommend reserving the term "manipulation" for the sociopathic variety, since it is conscious and deliberate, with very different origins from those that motivate people of other character types. Hysterical and borderline patients try to get their needs met by indirect means that exasperate others and provoke attributions of manipulation. The application of the term "manipulative" to the psychopath is simply descriptive, whereas with other clinical populations it tends to be both judgmental and preemptive of more useful ways of understanding what is going on with the patient.

†One reason that psychopathy is more common in males may be that females confront realistic limitation earlier. Women are not as physically strong as men; they must cope from early adolescence with the nuisance of menstruation and the threat of pregnancy; they are at greater risk of rape and physical abuse; and as primary caregivers, they are humbled by the discrepancy between their images of ideal maternal effectiveness and the emotional realities of trying to rear civilized children.

from trivial instances of the minimizing of one's role in some blunder to total amnesia for a violent crime. Dissociation of personal responsibility is a critical diagnostic indicator of psychopathy; the batterer who explains that he and his lover had a "tiff" and he "guesses he lost his temper" or the seemingly contrite cheater who claims to have "used bad judgment in this instance" is showing characteristic sociopathic minimization. When an interviewer picks this up, he or she should ask for specifics: "What exactly did you do when you lost your temper?" or "What exactly did you judge wrong?" (usually the answer to the latter shows regret about getting caught, not about cheating).

When a psychopathic person claims to have been emotionally dissociated or amnestic during some experience, especially during the perpetration of an offense, it is hard to tell whether the experience was in fact dissociated or whether words to this effect are a manipulative evasion of responsibility. Given the frequency of severe abuse in the histories of people diagnosed as antisocial, and given the causal relationship between abuse and dissociation, it would be unimaginable for dissociation not to be a frequent concomitant of a psychopathic personality; still, the unreliability of accounts by antisocial people makes the topic a vexing one. I will say more on this in the comments below on differential diagnosis and in Chapter 15.

Acting out is virtually definitional of psychopathy. Not only do sociopathic people have an internal goad toward action when aroused or upset, they have no experience of the increase in self-esteem that comes from control of impulse. Psychopaths are often seen as lacking anxiety (e.g., Ellis, 1961), but I suspect that Greenwald (1974) is right that the immediacy of their acting out, combined with their refusal to admit "weak" feelings, account for this (see also Deutsch, 1955). In other words, they do feel anxiety but act out so fast to relieve themselves of such a toxic feeling that the observer has no chance to see it. Moreover, they would never admit to it if asked. Greenwald stresses the pleasure that antisocial people in therapy attain as they develop a capacity to acknowledge anxiety and control their responses to it.

OBJECT RELATIONS IN PSYCHOPATHY

The childhood backgrounds of antisocial people are often rife with insecurity and chaos. Confusing amalgams of harsh discipline and overindulgence have been noted in the literature (Abraham, 1935; Aichhorn, 1936; Redl & Wineman, 1951; Greenacre, 1958; Akhtar, 1992). Especially in the histories of more destructive, criminal psychopaths, one can find virtually no consistent, loving, adequately protective family influences. Weak, depressed, or masochistic mothers and explosive, inconsistent, or sadistic fathers have been linked with psychopathy, as have alcoholism and other substance abuse in the family of origin. Patterns of moves, losses, and family break-ups are also common. Under unstable and frightening circumstances like these, the normal confidence in one's early omnipotent feelings and later in the power of others to protect the young self could not possibly develop in a natural way. The absence of a sense of power at developmentally appropriate times may impel children in this predicament to spend the rest of their lives seeking confirmations of their omnipotence.

Psychopathic people cannot acknowledge ordinary emotions because they associate them with weakness and vulnerability. It may also be common in their individual histories for no one to have helped them put words to emotional experiences. Because of the affect block in the psychopathic individual, they have no concept of using language to articulate feelings; whereas most of us use words to express ourselves, psychopathic people use them to manipulate. They have no internalized basis for understanding another role for speech. Clinical observations suggest that in their families of origin there was little emphasis on the expressive and communicative functions of language; instead, words were used mostly to control others.

The deficits of their caregivers in articulating and responding to emotional needs is related to another piece of clinical lore: Children who become sociopathic have been indulged materially and deprived emotionally. The parents of an antisocial patient of mine used to get her extravagant gifts (a stereo, a car) when she seemed upset. It did not occur to them to draw her out and listen to her concerns. This kind of "generosity" is particularly destructive; in the case of my patient, it left her no way to formulate her lingering sense that there was something missing in her life.

The most penetrating recent psychoanalytic thinking about psychopathy (e.g., Kernberg, 1984; Meloy, 1988) emphasizes the failure, from whatever accidents of temperament and rearing, of internalization. The antisocial person simply never (to any normal degree) attached psychologically, incorporated good objects, or identified with caregivers. He or she did not take love in and never loved. Instead, identification may have been with a "stranger selfobject" (Grotstein, 1982) experienced as predatory. Meloy (1988) writes of "a paucity of deep and unconscious identifications with, initially, the primary parent figure and ultimately the archetypal and guiding identifications with the society and culture and humankind in general" (p. 44).

An alternative origin of a character organized around omnipotent fantasies and antisocial behavior is a personal history in which parents or other important figures were deeply invested in the child's demonstration of power and sent repeated messages that life should pose no limits on the prerogatives of a person so inherently entitled to exert dominance. Such parents tend to react with outrage when teachers, counselors, or law-enforcement agents try to set limits on their youngster, identifying with the child's defiance and acting out their own hatred of authority. Like all character types, psychopathy can be "inherited" in that the child imitates the defensive solutions of the parents.

When the main source of someone's characterological psychopathy is parental modeling and reinforcement of manipulative and entitled behavior, the prognosis is probably better than when the condition is rooted in the chaotic, dramatically abusive situations previously mentioned. At least the child of indulgent, corrupting parents has succeeded in identifying with someone and is not completely devoid of a capacity to connect. It may be that this kind of family breeds healthier psychopaths and that harsher, turbulent backgrounds produce more deeply disturbed ones, but good research on this question remains to be done.

THE PSYCHOPATHIC SELF

As stated above, one of the constitutional aspects of a predisposition toward psychopathy is a degree of aggression that would make one under any circumstances a difficult child to calm down, to comfort, and to mirror lovingly. A child who is innately hyperactive, demanding, distractible, and headstrong needs much more active, energetic parenting than a placid, easily consoled youngster. He or she also arguably needs much more direct involvement by a father figure than most preschoolers in Western societies get (see Herzog, 1980; Cath, 1986; McWilliams, 1991; Diamond, 1993). I have personally known highly aggressive children who were observably too much for one parent but who had a capacity to attach if given enough stimulation and loving discipline. Given our cultural tendencies to assume that one caregiver, usually the mother, is enough, we are probably raising many more psychopaths than we would otherwise see.

But sociological conjectures aside, the condition of being viewed from day one as a problem child would make it very hard for a potential psychopath to find self-esteem via the normal route of feeling the caregivers' love and pride. Since outside objects fail, the only object to cathect is the self and its privately driven power. Self-representations, then, may be polarized between the desired condition of personal omnipotence and the feared condition of desperate weakness. Aggressive and sadistic acts may stabilize the sense of self in a sociopathic person by both reducing unpleasant states of arousal and restoring self-esteem.

David Berkowitz, the famous "Son of Sam" serial killer, began his murders of young women after learning that his biological mother was something of a slattern rather than the elevated figure of his imagination (Abrahamsen, 1985). An adoptee, he had attached his self-esteem to the fantasy of having a superior "real" mother, and when this illusion was shattered by the truth, he went on a compensatory rampage. Similar connections between some blow to a persons's grandiosity and his or her subsequent criminality have been noted in many sensational cases, but observation of manipulative people in ordinary life suggests that this pattern in its essentials is not limited to psychopathic killers. Anyone whose fondest images of self reflect unrealistic notions of superiority, and who runs into evidence that he or she is only human, will attempt to restore self-esteem by exerting power.

In addition, the more chaotic the environment of a child, and the more exhausted or inadequate the caregivers, the more likely it is that the youngster will not run into effective limits and not have to take seriously the consequences of impulsive actions. From a social learning theory point of view, grandiosity in a child would be the expectable result of an upbringing that lacked consistent discipline. The condition of having much more energy than one's caregiver would teach the lesson that one can ignore the needs of others, do whatever feels compelling at the time, and handle any adverse consequences by escaping, dissimulating, and seducing or bullying others.

One other feature of self-experience in the psychopathic patient that deserves mention is *primitive envy*, the wish to destroy that which one most desires (Klein, 1957). Although antisocial people rarely articulate envy, many of their behaviors demonstrate it. One probably cannot grow up unable to love without knowing that there is something out there that other people enjoy that one lacks. Active devaluation and depreciation of anything in the tenderer realms of human life are characteristic of sociopaths of all levels of severity; antisocial people in the psychotic range have been known to kill what attracts them. Ted Bundy, for example, described his need to destroy pretty young women (who, others noted, resembled his mother) as a kind of "owning" them (Michaud & Aynesworth, 1983). The killers portrayed in Truman Capote's (1965) *In Cold Blood* exterminated a happy family "for no reason" except presumably that they *were* a happy family toward whom the exterminators could not bear to feel their consuming envy.

TRANSFERENCE AND COUNTERTRANSFERENCE WITH PSYCHOPATHIC PATIENTS

The psychopath's basic transference to a therapist is a projection of his or her internal predation, the assumption that the clinician intends to use the patient for selfish purposes. Not having had any emotional experience with love and empathy, the antisocial patient has no way to understand the generous aspects of the therapist's interest and will try to figure out the practitioner's "angle." If the patient has reason to believe that the therapist can be used to promote some personal agenda (such as giving a good report to the judge or probation officer), he or she may be uncannily charming, so much so that an inexperienced clinician may be taken in.

The usual countertransference to the patient's preoccupation with using the therapist or outsmarting the therapist's exploitive agenda is shock and resistance to the sense that one's essential identity as a helper is being eradicated. The naive practitioner may succumb to the temptation to try to prove helpful intent. When that fails, hostility, contempt, and moralistic outrage toward the psychopathic person are common reactions. These "unempathic" feelings in ordinarily compassionate people should be understood, paradoxically, as a kind of empathy with psychopathic psychology: The client is unable to care about the therapist, and the therapist finds it almost as hard to care about the client. Outright hatred of the patient is not uncommon, and is no cause for worry, since the capacity to hate is a kind of attachment (Bollas, 1987). If one can tolerate the experience of internal coldness and even hatred, one will get an unpleasant but useful glimpse of what it is like to be a psychopathically organized person.

Other common countertransference reactions are complementary rather than concordant (Racker, 1968; see Chapter 2) and chiefly involve fear of a peculiarly ominous kind. People who work with psychopaths frequently comment on their cold, remorseless eyes and worry that such patients have them "under their thumb" (Meloy, 1988). Eerie forebodings are common. Again, it is important that the clinician tolerate these upsetting reactions rather than try to deny or compensate for them, since minimizing the threat posed by a true sociopath is unwise (both realistically and because it may prompt the client to demonstrate his or her destructive power).

Finally, the experience of being actively, even sadistically depreciated can provoke intense hostility or hopeless resignation in the clinician. Awareness that devaluing messages constitute a defense against envy is cold intellectual comfort in the face of a psychopath's unmitigated scorn, but it helps.

THERAPEUTIC IMPLICATIONS OF THE DIAGNOSIS OF PSYCHOPATHY

In light of the bad reputation of antisocial patients, I should say at the outset that I have known of many psychopathic people who were helped very much by enlightened psychotherapy. The therapist cannot be grandiose, however, about how much can be accomplished, and more than with patients in other diagnostic categories, it is critical that a careful assessment be done to see whether or not any individual sociopathic patient is treatable. Some are so damaged, so dangerous, or so determined to destroy the therapist's objectives that psychotherapy would be an exercise in futility and naivete. As the specific evaluation of treatability is beyond the scope of this text, I refer the reader to Meloy's (1988) excellent chapter on applying Kernberg's structural interview technique to assessing whether psychotherapy should be undertaken with any individual psychopathic person.

Meloy also makes a critical distinction between the roles of evaluator and therapist, a discrimination that is unnecessary with patients of most other character types (since they lack the psychopath's aim of defeating the clinician) yet is essential with this population. Meloy's explanation of the phenomenon of *therapeutic nihilism* (Lion, 1978) also fits my own experience:

> It is the stereotypical judgment that all psychopathically disturbed individuals, or antisocial personality disorders, *as a class*, are untreatable by virtue of their diagnosis. Such a judgment ignores both individual differences and the continuous nature of severity of psychopathology. I have most commonly observed this reaction in public mental health clinicians who are assigned patients on referral from probation, parole, or the court; and assume, because of the coercive nature of the treatment referral, that . . . any psychotherapeutic gain is impossible.
>
> Such reactions are often the product of attitudes that have been internalized as an "oral tradition" during training from senior, teaching clinicians. They are rarely the product of direct, individual experience. It is, in a sense, a mass retaliatory attitude where moral judgment impinges on professional assessment. The behavioral pathology of the psychopath, to devalue and dehumanize others,

> becomes the concordant identification of the clinician doing to the psychopath what the clinician perceives the psychopath doing to others. (Meloy, 1988, p. 325)

These attitudes may also reflect the fact that in most training programs—even those that send graduate students into internship and practicum placements at jails and drug treatment centers full of psychopathic people—very little if any attention is paid to the development of the technical skills appropriate for this group. When novice therapists apply techniques that are effective with other populations and fail, they may blame the patient rather than the limitations of their training.*

Once one has decided to work with a sociopathic person—or realized that a patient one had been seeing some other way is basically sociopathic—the most important feature of treatment is *incorruptibility*: of the therapist, the frame, and the conditions that make therapy possible. It is much better to err on the side of inflexibility than to show, in the hope that it will be seen as empathy, what the patient will see as weakness. Antisocial people do not understand empathy. They understand using people, and they will feel a sadistic triumph over, not a grateful appreciation for, a therapist who wavers from the strict boundaries of the treatment contract. Anthony Hopkins gave a chilling demonstration of the psychopath's talent for finding someone's Achilles's heel in his character's manipulation of the detective played by Jodie Foster in *The Silence of the Lambs*. Any aspect of therapeutic technique that can be interpreted as weakness and vulnerability will be.

It is unrealistic to expect love from antisocial people, but one can earn their respect by coming across as tough-minded and exacting. When I work with sociopathic patients, I insist on payment at the beginning of each session and send the client away in its absence—no matter how reasonable the explanation offered. Like most therapists who were initially taught to bend over backwards to consider the special needs of each patient, I had to learn from experience that not bending at all is the right response to the special needs of the psychopath. In the early part of therapy I do not analyze patients' assumed motives for testing the solidity of the contract, I merely remind them that our deal was that they would pay up front and that

*Karon and VandenBos (1981) have made a comparable critique of the equally prevalent and inadequately supported belief that schizophrenia is not effectively treatable by psychodynamically informed therapy. Psychopathic patients at a psychotic level of personality organization thus may have two strikes against them.

I will hold up my end of the deal—the application of my expertise to help them understand themselves better—if they hold up theirs.

Related to incorruptibility is an *uncompromising honesty:* talking straight, keeping promises, making good on threats, and persistently addressing reality. Honesty includes the therapist's private admission of intense negative feelings toward the patient, both countertransferences and realistic perceptions of danger. If such reactions are denied, countertransferences may be acted out and legitimate fears may be minimized. Therapists must make peace with their own antisocial tendencies so that they have a basis for identifying with the patient's psychology. With respect to money discussions, for example, the therapist should nondefensively admit selfishness and greed when giving a rationale for the fee.

Except for admissions like the above that legitimately pertain to the therapeutic contract, honesty does not mean disclosure; self-revelation will only be interpreted as frailty. Nor does it mean moralizing. When analyzing the patient's destructive actions, it is futile to invite the expression of assumed feelings of badness since the patient lacks a normal superego and doubtless committed the sins in order to feel good (omnipotent) rather than bad (weak). One must restrict oneself to addressing the possible reality outcomes of amoral behavior. Probes into presumed struggles with conscience tend to evoke responses like the one attributed to Willie Sutton when he was asked why he robbed banks: "Because that's where the money is."

The therapist's unrelenting emphasis on the realistic risks of each grandiose design need not be humorless just because the matters at hand have serious consequences. One of my colleagues, a woman renowned for her talent with antisocial clients, reports the following banter with a court-remanded car thief:

> "The man was explaining to me how brilliant his scheme had been for the heist he had almost pulled off, how if only one little unforeseen thing hadn't happened, it would have been the perfect crime. As he talked, he was getting more and more excited and animated, and I agreed with some admiration that he had almost gotten away with the theft. It started to feel like we were co-conspirators. Eventually, he got so carried away that he asked, 'Would you do something like that?'
>
> " 'No,' I answered.
>
> " 'Why not?' he asked, a little deflated.
>
> " 'Two reasons,' I said. First, there's *always* some little thing that can go wrong, even with a brilliant plan. Life isn't that controllable. And then I'd be in jail, or in a mental hospital

involuntarily, like you are, talking to some shrink I didn't choose myself. And second, I wouldn't because I have something that you don't: a conscience.

" 'Yeah,' he said. 'You know how I could get one of those?' "

Of course, the first step in developing a conscience (more technically, a superego) is to care about someone to the degree that that person's opinion matters. Without moralizing, the therapist moves the patient along toward more responsible behavior simply by *being a consistent, nonpunitive, nonexploitable object.* Greenwald (1958, 1974), who worked with antisocial people in the Los Angeles underworld, describes how he connects with psychopaths in terms that they understand. He reasons that since power is the only quality antisocial people respect, power is the first thing the therapist must demonstrate. Greenwald (1974) gives the following instance:

> A pimp came to see me and started to discuss his way of life. He said, "You know I'm ashamed to show myself and so on, but after all, it's a pretty good way to live and most guys would want to live that way, you know, to live as a pimp. It's not bad—you get girls out hustling for you—why shouldn't you do it? Why shouldn't anybody do it?" I said, "You're a jerk." He asked why. I replied, "Look, I live off the earnings of call girls. I wrote a book about them; I got respect for it; I got famous from it; they made a movie out of it. I made much more money off call girls than you ever will, and you, you schmuck, you can get arrested any day and be sent to jail for ten years, whereas I get respect, honor, and admiration." This he could understand. He saw that somebody whom he considered similar to him had a superior way of accomplishing the same ends. (p. 371)

Greenwald has his own free-wheeling but still essentially incorruptible style with psychopathic patients. He is not the only therapist who has discovered the utility of "outpsyching the psychopath" or "conning the con" as a way of demonstrating that he deserves respect. Like my colleague previously quoted, he can own enough psychopathic impulses in himself that he does not feel fully alienated from the emotional world of his clients. Tellingly, he reports that in the second or third year of intensive treatment with him, sociopathic patients typically go into a serious and often psychotic depression. He understands this as evidence that they have started to care about him in a genuine way rather than as an object to manipulate and, realizing this, descend into a state of misery about their psychological dependency. This depression, which only slowly lifts, compares in its essentials to the feelings of the infant in the second 6 months of life as described by Klein (1935), when the mother's existence as a separate person outside the baby's control makes its painful impact on the child.

In contrast with appropriate therapy with people of other diagnoses, the therapist of a psychopathic client must adopt an attitude of *independent strength verging on indifference*. One cannot be emotionally invested in the patient's changing because as soon as an antisocial person sees that need, he or she will sabotage psychotherapy to demonstrate the clinician's impotence. It is better to invest in simply increasing one's understanding, setting the tone that one will do one's job competently, and communicate that it is up to the patient to take advantage of therapy or not. This principle is analogous to the lesson every police officer learns about investigating a crime: Never show the suspect that it is important to you to get a confession.

The most skilled interviewer of antisocial people I know is the chief of detectives in my town, a man with an exceptional record of evoking confessions—often movingly tearful ones—from rapists, child torturers, murderers, and serial killers. Listening to tapes of his interrogations, one is struck by his attitude of respect and his quiet conviction that even the most monstrous perpetrator has a need to tell someone the truth. The suspects' responsiveness to being treated with dignity is poignant—the more so in light of their knowledge that the interviewer's agenda is to prosecute. No one interrogated by him has ever complained of betrayal, even as he testifies against them in court on the basis of their confession. "He treated me fair," they report.

These phenomena raise the question of whether the fabled callousness of the psychopath is a response to environments that are either abusive (as was childhood, later replicated by a savage subculture) or incomprehensible (as is a therapist's wish to help). The fact that these killers and maimers are palpably relieved to confess to someone who wants to incarcerate them suggests that even the most incorrigible felon has a primitive sense of accountability and can gain something from a relationship.* The sadistic murderer Carl Panzram (Gaddis & Long, 1970) extended lifelong friendship to a prison guard who once showed him ordinary kindness. Rigorous tough-mindedness

*This observation does *not* equate to an argument for "leniency" toward dangerous criminals. Understanding that psychopathic people are human beings who may be helped in certain ways should not be confused with wishful thinking that psychotherapy can transform a compulsive killer into a model of citizenship. The public needs reliable protection from antisocial people whether or not their crimes are psychodynamically comprehensible and whether or not they can profit individually from a therapeutic relationship.

and rock-bottom respect seem to be a winning combination with antisocial people.

Over the course of treatment, as the psychopathic person's omnipotent control, projective identification, domination by envy, and self-destructive activities are doggedly analyzed in this atmosphere, the patient will in fact change. Any shift from using words to manipulate to using them for honest self-expression is a substantial achievement that may occur just through the antisocial person's repeated exposure to someone with integrity. Any instance where the client inhibits an impulse and learns something about pride in self-control should be seen as a milestone. Since even a small movement toward human relatedness in a psychopath may prevent an immense amount of human suffering, such progress is worth every drop of sweat the practitioner secretes in its service.

DIFFERENTIAL DIAGNOSIS

It is not usually hard to spot the antisocial features in any client whose personality has a psychopathic component. Whether those features are central enough to define the person as characterologically psychopathic is a more subtle question. Psychologies that can easily be misunderstood as essentially sociopathic include paranoid, dissociative, and narcissistic conditions. In addition, some people with hysteroid personalities become misdiagnosed as antisocial, a topic that will be discussed in Chapter 14.

Psychopathic versus Paranoid Personality

There is a great deal of overlap between predominantly psychopathic psychologies and those that are more paranoid in organization; many people have strong strains of both kinds of orientations. Both antisocial and paranoid people are highly concerned with issues of power, but from different perspectives. Unlike psychopaths, people with essentially paranoid character structure have profound guilt, the analysis of which is critical to their recovery from suffering. Thus, it is critical to assess with anyone who has both paranoid and sociopathic features which tendencies predominate.

Psychopathic versus Dissociative Personality

There is also considerable overlap between psychopathic and dissociative conditions. It is critical for an interviewer to evaluate whether a patient is a basically psychopathic person who uses some dissociative defenses or whether he or she is a multiple personality with one or more antisocial or persecutory alter personalities. The prognosis for the former kind of patient is guarded, whereas essentially dissociative people, when accurately diagnosed, respond much more quickly and favorably to therapy. Unfortunately, this evaluation can be exceedingly difficult, even when done by an expert. Both primarily dissociative and primarily psychopathic people have a deep distrust of others, and for different reasons (terror of abuse vs. omnipotent triumph), both will dissimulate, comply superficially, and subvert the therapist.

I do not recommend trying to make this differential diagnosis when some important consequence hinges on it—for instance, when a man who has committed homicide may plead not guilty by reason of insanity if he can convince a professional that he has multiple personality disorder. The differential diagnosis is hard enough without that complication, although regrettably, it is such a pivotal legal distinction that evaluators will have to develop some procedures to make it more reliable. Hypnosis holds some promise in this area. I shall say more on this differential in Chapter 15.

Psychopathic versus Narcissistic Personality

Finally, there is a very close connection between psychopathic and narcissistic conditions. Both character types reflect a subjectively empty internal world and a dependence on external events to provide self-esteem. Some theorists (Kernberg, 1975; Meloy, 1988) put psychopathy and narcissism on one dimension, characterized overall as narcissistic; the psychopath is considered as on the pathological end of the narcissistic continuum. I would argue that antisocial and narcissistic people are different enough to warrant a continuum for each. Most sociopathic people do not idealize repetitively, and most narcissistic ones do not depend on omnipotent control. But many people have aspects of both character types, and self-inflation can characterize either one.

Because treatment considerations are quite different for the two groups (e.g., sympathetic mirroring comforts most narcissistic people but antagonizes antisocial ones) despite the things they have in common and the number of people who have aspects of each orientation, it seems to me more useful to differentiate carefully between them.

SUMMARY

In this chapter the psychopathic personality has been portrayed as expressing an organizing need to feel one's effect on others, to manipulate them, to "get over on" them. Constitutional predispositions to antisocial behaviors were briefly summarized, along with attention to the rage and mania that may briefly interrupt the affect block characteristic of sociopathic persons. Psychopathy was discussed in terms of the defenses of omnipotent control, projective identification, dissociation, and acting out; of object relations marked by instability, pandering, emotional misunderstanding, exploitation, and sometimes brutality; and a self structure dominated by grandiose efforts to avoid a sense of weakness and envy. Unempathic transference and countertransference reactions were discussed, along with the treatment requirements of the therapist's incorruptibility, consistency, and independence of the need to be seen as helpful. Psychopathic character was distinguished from paranoid, dissociative, and narcissistic types.

SUGGESTIONS FOR FURTHER READING

Unfortunately, texts on psychotherapy as a general process rarely give psychopathic clients much attention, and there is a paucity of good analytic literature on this group. Readers who want more information on disciplined psychodynamic work with the antisocial population thus have limited resources. At this point, Bursten's (1973a) study *The Manipulator* and Meloy's (1988) book *The Psychopathic Mind* are the most comprehensive, readable explorations of the topic known to me. Akhtar (1992) also has a good chapter on the topic in *Broken Structures*.

8

Narcissistic Personalities

People whose personalities are organized around maintaining their self-esteem by getting affirmation from outside themselves are called narcissistic by psychoanalysts. All of us have vulnerabilities in our sense of who we are and how valuable we feel, and we try to run our lives so that we can feel good about ourselves. Our pride is enhanced by approval and injured by disapproval from significant others. In some of us, concerns with "narcissistic supplies," or supports to self-esteem, eclipse other issues to such an extent that we may be considered excessively self-preoccupied. Terms like "narcissistic personality" and "pathological narcissism" apply to this disproportionate degree of self-concern, not to ordinary responsiveness to approval and sensitivity to criticism.

Narcissism, normal as well as pathological, is a topic to which Freud (1914b) gave recurrent attention. He borrowed the term from the Greek myth of Narcissus, the youth who fell in love with his reflection in a pool of water and eventually died of a kind of longing that his image could never satisfy. Yet Freud had little to say about therapy for those in whom narcissistic concerns were central. Alfred Adler (e.g., 1927) and Otto Rank (e.g., 1929) both wrote on topics we would now include under narcissism, but their respective estrangements from Freud made their work unfamiliar to many therapists. Since the early psychoanalytic era, it has been noted that some people have problems with self-esteem that are hard to construe solely in terms of drives and unconscious conflicts, and are correspondingly hard to treat by reference to conflict-based models of therapy. A deficit model seems to fit their experience better: There is something *missing* from their inner lives.

Preoccupied with how they appear to others, narcissistically organized people may privately feel fraudulent and loveless. Ways of helping them to develop self-acceptance and to deepen their relationships awaited the expansion of dynamic psychology into areas that Freud had only begun to touch. Attention to concepts like basic security and identity (Sullivan, 1953; Erikson, 1950, 1968), the self as opposed to the more functionalist concept of the ego (Winnicott, 1960b; Jacobson, 1964); self-esteem regulation (A. Reich, 1960); attachment and separation (Spitz, 1965; Bowlby, 1969, 1973); developmental arrest and deficit (Kohut, 1971; Stolorow & Lachmann, 1978); and shame (Lynd, 1958; Lewis, 1971; Morrison, 1989) contributed to our understanding of narcissism.

As new theoretical areas were explored in the post-Freudian years, old areas were reworked in ways that led to improvements in treating narcissistic problems. Much clinical ferment followed challenges by object relations theorists (Horney, 1939; Fairbairn, 1954; Balint, 1960) to Freud's concept of "primary narcissism," the assumption that the infant cathects self before others. Thinkers who stressed primary *relatedness* understood narcissistic pathology not as fixation on normal infantile grandiosity but as compensatory for early disappointments in relationship. Around the same time, notions like containment (Bion, 1967), the holding environment (Winnicott, 1945, 1960a; Modell, 1976), and mirroring (Winnicott, 1967; Kohut, 1968) were redefining theories of therapy. These ideas were more applicable than earlier models of psychopathology and treatment to people for whom the continuity of a sense of self, and the esteem attached to it, were fundamentally problematic.

It is also likely that when Freud was writing, narcissistic problems of the kind that are epidemic today were less common. Psychoanalytically influenced social theorists (e.g., Fromm, 1947; Slater, 1970; Hendin, 1975; Lasch, 1978, 1984) have argued that the vicissitudes of contemporary life reinforce narcissistic concerns.* The world changes rapidly; we move frequently; the media exploit our insecurities and pander to our vanity and greed; secularization dilutes the internal norms that religious traditions once provided. In mass societies and in

*In the United States, a climate of narcissistic absorption may not be so recent a development as some contemporary social critics suggest. In the early 1800s, Alexis de Tocqueville noted that a society that touted equality of opportunity left citizens concerned with how to demonstrate their claim to special worth. Without a class system to provide visible levels of status, they would try to accumulate observable evidence of their proper "place"—which could not be an inferior station without reflecting on their personal failure. Compare E. M. Forster's (1921) description of Leonard Bast:

times of rapid change, the immediate impression one makes on others may be more compelling than one's integrity and sincerity, qualities that are prized in smaller and more stable communities where people know each other well enough to make judgments based on someone's history and reputation.

Many of Freud's patients suffered from too much internal commentary about their goodness or badness, a condition he came to describe as reflecting a "harsh superego." In contrast, contemporary clients often feel subjectively empty rather than full of critical internalizations; they worry that they "don't fit in" rather than that they are betraying their principles, and they may ruminate about observable assets such as beauty, fame, wealth, or the appearance of political correctness rather than more private aspects of their identity and integrity. Image replaces substance, and what Jung (1945) called the *persona* (the self one shows to the world) becomes more vivid and dependable than one's actual person.

In "The God Complex," Ernest Jones (1913) was the first analytic writer to depict the more overtly grandiose kind of narcissistic person. Jones described a type of man characterized by exhibitionism, aloofness, emotional inaccessibility, fantasies of omnipotence, overvaluation of his creativity, and a tendency to be judgmental. He portrayed such people as on a continuum of mental health from psychotic to normal, commenting that "when such men become insane they are apt to express openly the delusion that they actually are God, and instances of the kind are to be met within every asylum" (p. 245). Wilhelm Reich (1933) devoted a section of *Character Analysis* to consideration of the "phallic-narcissistic character," represented as "self-assured . . . arrogant . . . energetic, often impressive in his bearing . . . [who] will usually anticipate any impending attack with an attack of his own" (pp. 217–218). This familiar type appears in its essentials in the description of the narcissistic personality in recent editions of the DSM.

As psychoanalytic observations of personality continued, it became clear that the overtly grandiose personality was only one form

---

He knew that he was poor, and would admit it: he would have died sooner than confess any inferiority to the rich. . . . Had he lived some centuries ago, in the brightly coloured civilizations of the past, he would have had definite status, his rank and income would have corresponded. But in his day the angel of Democracy had arisen, enshadowing the classes with leathern wings, and proclaiming: "All men are equal—all men, that is to say, who possess umbrellas," and so he was obliged to assert gentility, lest he slipped into the abyss where nothing counts and the statements of Democracy are inaudible. (1921, pp. 45–46) of what we would today construe as a narcissistic problem or "disorder of the self" (Kohut & Wolf, 1978). Current analytic conceptualization recognizes many different external manifestations of a core difficulty with identity and self-esteem. Bursten (1973b) has suggested a typology of narcissistic personalities that includes craving, paranoid, manipulative, and phallic narcissistic subvarieties. Further, many writers have observed that in every vain and grandiose narcissist hides a self-conscious, shame-faced child, and in every depressed and self-critical narcissist lurks a grandiose vision of what that person should or could be (A. Miller, 1975; Meissner, 1979; Morrison, 1983). What narcissistic people of all appearances have in common is an inner sense of, and/or terror of, insufficiency, shame, weakness, and inferiority. Their compensatory behaviors might diverge greatly yet still reveal similar preoccupations. Hence, individuals as different as Judy Garland and Socrate's problematic student Alcibiades might be reasonably regarded as narcissistically organized.

DRIVE, AFFECT, AND TEMPERAMENT IN NARCISSISM

Very little controlled research has been done on the topic of constitutional and temperamental contributions to narcissistic personality organization in adulthood. Unlike antisocial people, who pose obvious and costly problems to society and therefore inspire funding for scientific investigation into psychopathy, narcissistic individuals are quite diverse, often subtle in their pathology, and not so patently damaging. Successful narcissistic people (monetarily, socially, politically, militarily, or however their success is manifested) may be admired and emulated. The internal costs of narcissistic hunger for recognition are rarely visible to onlookers, and injuries done to others in the pursuit of narcissistically driven projects may be rationalized as trivial or necessary side effects of competence ("You can't make an omelet without breaking eggs"). Also, recognition of more subtle kinds of narcissism as treatable character problems is an achievement of only the past two or three decades.

Consequently, most of the ideas we have on predispositions to narcissistic personality structure come from clinical observation. The most recurrent theme in the literature on this topic seems to be that people at risk for developing a narcissistic character may be constitutionally more sensitive than others to unverbalized emotional messages. Specifically, narcissism has been associated with the kind of infant who seems preternaturally attuned to the unstated affects, attitudes, and expectations of others. Alice Miller (1975) believes, for example, that many families contain one child whose natural intuitive talents are unconsciously exploited by its caregivers for the maintenance of *their* self-esteem and that this child grows up confused about whose life he or she is supposed to lead. According to her, such gifted children are more likely than untalented youngsters to be treated as narcissistic extensions* and are hence more apt to become narcissistic adults.

On a different note, in discussing more entitled, grandiose narcissistic clients, Kernberg (1970) has suggested that they may have either an innately strong aggressive drive or a constitutionally determined lack of tolerance for anxiety about aggressive impulses. Such dispositions would partially explain the lengths to which narcissistic people may go to avoid acknowledging their own drives and appetites: They may be scared of their power. Beyond these speculations, we know little about temperamental propensities that may contribute to a narcissistic character structure.

As for the main emotions associated with narcissistic personality organization, shame and envy are recurrently stressed in the clinical literature. Feelings of shame and fears of being shamed pervade the subjective experience of narcissistic people. The early analysts underestimated the power of this emotional set, often mistaking it for guilt and making guilt-oriented interpretations that narcissistic patients found unempathic. Guilt is the conviction that one is sinful or has committed wrongdoings; it is easily conceptualized in terms of an internal critical parent or the superego. Shame is the sense of *being seen as* bad or wrong; the audience here is outside the self. Guilt carries with it a sense of an active potential for evil, whereas shame has connotations of helplessness, ugliness, and impotence.

The narcissistic person's vulnerability to envy is a related phenomenon. If I have an internal conviction that I am lacking in some way and that my inadequacies are always at risk of exposure, I will be envious toward those who seem content or who have assets that I believe would make up for what I lack. Envy may also be the root of the much-observed judgmental quality of narcissistically organized persons, toward themselves and toward others. If I feel deficient and I perceive you

*Analysts refer to people who are needed to prop up the self-esteem of others as "narcissistic extensions" of those who use them this way. The term carries an exploitive connotation when the extension is not appreciated as a separate person, but it can also indicate more benign forms of pride and reflected renown. In fantasies and dreams, physical images of narcissistic extensions are common, as when a man imagines his lover as his missing breast or a woman imagines a man as her penis. The narcissistic yearning to extend the self beyond the limit of gender is a universal aspect of heterosexual romantic love (Bergmann, 1987; Kernberg, 1991).

as having it all, I may try to destroy what you have by deploring, scorning, or criticizing it.

DEFENSIVE AND ADAPTIVE PROCESSES IN NARCISSISM

Narcissistically structured people may use a whole range of defenses, but the ones that they depend on most fundamentally are idealization and devaluation. These defenses are complementary, in that when the self is idealized, others are devalued, and vice versa. Kohut (1971) originally used the term "grandiose self" to capture the sense of self-aggrandizement and superiority that characterizes one polarity of the inner world of narcissistic people. This grandiosity may be felt internally, or it may be projected. There is a constant "ranking" process that narcissistic people use to address any issue that faces them: Who is the "best" doctor? What is the "finest" preschool? Where is the "most rigorous" training? Realistic advantages and disadvantages may be completely overridden by concerns about comparative prestige.

For example, a woman I know was determined that her son would go to the "best" college. She took him to see several exclusive schools, pulled strings where she had any, and even wrote thank-you notes to deans of admission with whom he had interviewed. By mid-April, he had been accepted by Amherst, Columbia, Princeton, the University of Chicago, and Williams, and he was on the waiting list at Yale. Her response was a sense of devastation that he had been rejected by Harvard. The young man elected to attend Princeton. Throughout his freshman year, his mother badgered Harvard to take him as a transfer student. Although he thrived at Princeton, when Harvard finally capitulated to his mother's relentless entreaties, there was no question about his destination.

The subordination of other concerns to issues of general valuation and devaluation is of note here. This mother knew that professors in her son's chosen field considered Harvard inferior to Princeton in that area; she also knew that Harvard undergraduates received less attention than those at Princeton; and she was aware that her son would suffer socially at Harvard for missing his freshman year there. Nevertheless, she persisted. Although not a narcissistic character, this woman used her son as a narcissistic extension in this instance because she had a defensive belief system that included the conviction that her own life would have been dramatically transformed had she gone to Radcliffe, the "best" school for women at the time she was applying to college.

In an instance where a parent's valuation and devaluation were characterological, a patient of mine, a college student with artistic and literary sensibilities, was told by his grandiose father that he would support his becoming a doctor (preferably) or a lawyer (if he proved untalented in the natural sciences), but nothing else. Medicine and law commanded money and respect; any other career would reflect badly on the family. Because this young man had been treated like a narcissistic extension his whole life, he saw nothing unusual in his father's position.

A related defensive position in which narcissistically motivated people are trapped concerns perfectionism. They hold themselves up to unrealistic ideals and either convince themselves that they have attained them (the grandiose outcome) or respond to their falling short by feeling inherently flawed rather than forgivably human (the depressive outcome). In therapy, they may have the ego-syntonic expectation that the point of undergoing treatment is to perfect the self rather than to understand it and to find more effective ways of handling its needs. The demand for perfection is expressed in chronic criticism of self or others (depending on whether or not the devalued self is projected) and in an inability to find joy amid the ambiguities of human existence.

Sometimes narcissistic people handle their self-esteem problem by regarding someone else—a lover, a mentor, a hero—as perfect and then feeling inflated by identification with that person ("I am an appendage of So and So, who can do no wrong"). Some have lifelong patterns of idealizing someone and then sweeping him or her off the pedestal when an imperfection appears. Perfectionistic solutions to narcissistic dilemmas are inherently self-defeating: One creates exaggerated ideals to compensate for defects in the sense of self that are felt as so contemptible that nothing short of perfection will make up for them, yet since no one is perfect, the strategy is doomed, and the depreciated self emerges again.

OBJECT RELATIONS IN NARCISSISM

From the above description of some of their ego processes and essential predicaments, the reader has probably already concluded that relationships between narcissistic people and others are overly burdened with the self-esteem issues of the narcissistic party. Although it is rare for a person with a narcissistic personality disorder to come to therapy with the explicit agenda of becoming a better friend or family member or lover, it is not uncommon for such a person, especially if he or she is at least middle-aged, to be aware that something is wrong in interactions with others. One problem in helping such patients is conveying to them what it would be like to accept a person nonjudgmentally and nonexploitively, to love without idealizing, and to express genuine feelings without shame. Narcissistic people may have no concept of such possibilities; the therapist's acceptance of them will be the prototype for their emotional understanding of intimacy.

Self psychologists have coined the term "selfobjects" for the people in our lives who nourish a sense of identity and self-regard by their affirmation, admiration, and approval. The term reflects the fact that individuals in that role function as objects outside the self and also as part of one's self-definition. By helping to modulate self-esteem, they augment or replace what most of us also do internally. We all have selfobjects, and we need them. If we lose them we feel diminished, as if some vital piece of us has died. Yet reality and morality require that others be more than selfobjects, that we see them in terms of who they are and what they need, not just in terms of what they do for us.

The narcissistic person needs selfobjects so greatly that other aspects of relationship pale, and may even be unimaginable, as they were to my client whose father would not support his being anything but a doctor or lawyer. Thus, the most grievous cost of a narcissistic orientation is a stunted capacity to love. Despite the importance of other people to the equilibrium of a narcissistic person, his or her consuming need for reassurance about self-worth leaves no energy for others except in their function as selfobjects and narcissistic extensions. Hence, narcissistic people send confusing messages to their friends and families: Their need for others is deep, but their love for them is shallow.

Most analysts believe that people get this way by having been used as narcissistic appendages themselves. I have mentioned Alice Miller's theories in this vein. Narcissistic patients may have been critically important to parents or other caregivers, *not because of who they really were but because of what function they fulfilled.* The confusing message that one is highly valued, but only for a particular role that one plays, makes a child feel that if his or her real feelings, especially hostile or selfish ones, are found out, rejection or humiliation will follow. It fosters the development of what Winnicott (1960a) called the "false self," the presentation of what one has learned is acceptable.*

Most parents regard their children with a combination of

*A crucial difference between the etiologies of psychopathy and narcissism may be that whereas the antisocial person emerges from a background of essential neglect, the narcissistically organized person emerges from a particular kind of attention or even doting, in which support is given on the implicit condition that the child cooperate with a parent's narcissistic agenda.

narcissistic needs and true empathy. Every child is treated to some degree as a narcissistic extension, and in moderation, children enjoy being treated this way. Making parents feel proud, as if they also had been admired when their son or daughter is esteemed, is one of the sweeter pleasures of childhood. As usual, the issue is one of degree and balance: Does the child also get attention unrelated to whether the parent's aims are furthered?

A markedly nonnarcissistic attitude toward offspring informs the remarks of an 85-year-old friend of mine who reared 12 children during the Depression, all of whom have turned out well despite borderline poverty and some painful losses:

> "Every time I'd get pregnant, I'd cry. I'd wonder where the money would come from, how I was going to nurse this child and take care of everything else. But around the fourth month I'd begin to feel life, and I'd get all excited, thinking, 'I can't wait till you come out and I find out who you are!' "

I quote this to contrast her sentiments with those of a prospective parent who "knows" who the child is going to be: Someone who realizes all the parent's failed ambitions and brings reflected glory to the family.

A related aspect of the upbringing of people who become narcissistic is an family atmosphere of constant evaluation. If one has an agenda for a child that is vital to one's own self-esteem, then every time that child disappoints, he or she will be criticized, either directly or covertly. No one has ever brought up a child without criticism, but the background message that one is not good enough in some vague way is altogether different from specific feedback on behaviors that offend. An evaluative atmosphere of perpetual praise and applause, which one finds in a minority of families with narcissistic children, is equally damaging to the development of realistic self-esteem. The child is always aware of being judged, even if the verdict is positive. He or she knows on some level that there is a false quality to the attitude of constant admiration, and despite the conscious sense of entitlement that may issue from such a background, it creates a nagging worry that one is a bit of a fraud, undeserving of this adulation that seems tangential to who one really is.

Thus we see again how certain character structures can be "inherited," though parents do not have to have narcissistic personalities themselves to rear a son or daughter who is disturbed narcissistically. Parents may have narcissistic needs toward a particular child (as in the case of the woman whose son had to go to Harvard) that set the stage for that child's not being able to discriminate between genuine feelings and efforts to please or impress others. What is a nonissue to one parent is a central one to another. We all want for our children the things we lacked, a harmless desire as long as we spare them any pressure to live their lives for our sakes.

An interesting twist on a narcissistic dynamic was Martha Wolfenstein's (1951) article on "The Emergence of Fun Morality," depicting how liberal intellectual parents in the 1950s, having grown up during hard times, gave their children the message that they should feel bad about themselves if they were not *having fun*. People whose options were drastically curtailed by some disaster such as war or persecution are particularly apt to send signals that their children should live the life they never had. Typically—the most dramatic case being the offspring of Holocaust survivors—the children of traumatized parents grow up with some identity confusion and feelings of vague shame and emptiness (see Fogelman & Savran, 1979; Bergmann, 1985; Fogelman, 1988). The communication that "unlike me, you can have it all" is particularly destructive, in that no one can have it all; every generation will face its own constraints. For self-esteem to be contingent on such an unrealistic goal is a crippling inheritance.

THE NARCISSISTIC SELF

I have already alluded to many of the self-experiences of people who are diagnosably narcissistic. They include a sense of vague falseness, shame, envy, emptiness or incompleteness, ugliness, and inferiority, or their compensatory counterparts: self-righteousness, pride, contempt, defensive self-sufficiency, vanity, and superiority. Kernberg (1975) describes such polarities as opposite ego states, grandiose (all-good) versus depleted (all-bad) definitions of self, which are the only options narcissistic persons have for organizing their inner experience. The sense of being "good enough" is not one of their internal categories.

Narcissistically structured people are aware at some level of their psychological fragility. They are afraid of falling apart, of precipitously losing their self-esteem or self-coherence (e.g., when criticized) and abruptly feeling like nobody rather than somebody (Goldberg, 1990a). They sense that their identity is too tenuous to hold together and weather some strain. Their fear of the fragmentation of their inner self is often displaced into a preoccupation with their physical health; thus, they are vulnerable to hypochondriacal preoccupations and morbid fears of death.

One subtle outcome of the perfectionism of narcissistic people is the avoidance of feelings and actions that express awareness of either personal fallibility or realistic dependence on others. In particular, remorse and gratitude are attitudes that narcissistic people tend to deny (McWilliams & Lependorf, 1990). Remorse about some personal error or injury includes an admission of defect, and gratitude for someone's help acknowledges one's need. Because the narcissistic person tries to build a positively valued sense of self on the illusion of not having failings and not being in need, he or she fears that the admission of guilt or dependency exposes something unacceptably shameful. Sincere apologies and heartfelt thanks, the behavioral expressions of remorse and gratitude, may thus be avoided or compromised in narcissistic people, to the great impoverishment of their relationships with others.

By definition, the assessment of narcissistic personality organization expresses the interviewer's observation that the patient needs external affirmation in order to feel internal validity. Theorists diverge rather strikingly in stressing either the grandiose or depleted aspects of narcissistic self-experience, a difference of emphasis most familiar in the disagreement between Kernberg and Kohut on how to understand and treat narcissistic characters, about which I shall say more later. Disputes on this question go back at least as far as differences of opinion between Freud (1914b), who stressed the individual's primary love of self, and A. Adler (1927), who emphasized how narcissistic defenses compensate for feelings of inferiority. Which came first in the evolution of pathological narcissism, the grandiose self-state or the depleted–shamed one, may be the psychoanalytic equivalent of a chicken–egg riddle. From a phenomenological standpoint, these contrasting ego states are intimately connected, much as depression and mania are opposite sides of the same psychological coin.

TRANSFERENCE AND COUNTERTRANSFERENCE WITH NARCISSISTIC PATIENTS

Transference in the treatment of narcissistic clients feels qualitatively different from what one is used to with most other kinds of people. Even in the highest-functioning, most cooperative person with this type of character, the ambiance in the therapeutic relationship contrasts with that created by other motivated and healthy patients. Typically, the therapist first notices the patient's lack of interest in transference explorations that would be taken in as illuminative and helpful by other kinds of people. Comments or questions about how the patient is feeling toward the therapist may be received as distracting, annoying, or irrelevant to the client's concerns. It is not unusual for the client to conclude that the therapist is raising this topic out of conceit or a need for mirroring. (Such silent hypotheses constitute projections, of course, even if they are true, but they tend to be unverbalized, and they can rarely be usefully interpreted, at least in the beginning phases of treatment.)*

Narcissistic patients do have strong reactions to the therapist. They may devalue or idealize in powerful ways. Yet they are curiously uninterested in the meaning of those reactions and are genuinely confused about why the clinician is attentive to them. Typically, their transferences are so ego syntonic as to be inaccessible to exploration; a narcissistic patient believes he or she is devaluing the therapist because the therapist is objectively second-rate or idealizing him or her because the therapist is objectively wonderful. Efforts to make such reactions ego alien will usually fail, at least initially: The devalued practitioner who points out the patient's critical attitude will be perceived as defensive, and the idealized one who comments on the patient's overvaluation will be further idealized as someone whose perfection includes an admirable humility.

Beginning therapists get a lot more devaluing transferences than idealizing ones. If it is any consolation for the misery one endures at being the object of subtle and relentless disparagement, being the recipient of a narcissistic idealizing transference is not much better. In both circumstances one has the feeling that one's reality as a human being with some expertise, who is sincerely trying to help, has been extinguished. In fact, this countertransference sense of having been obliterated, being ignored as a real person, is diagnostic of a narcissistic dynamic.

Related to these phenomena are countertransferences that include boredom, irritability, sleepiness, and a vague sense that nothing is happening in the treatment. A typical comment about a narcissistic client from a therapist in supervision: "She comes in every week, gives me the news of the week in review, critiques my clothing, dismisses all my interventions, and leaves. Why does she keep coming back? What is she getting out of this?" A strange sense that one does not quite exist in the room is also common. Extreme drowsiness is

*The early psychoanalysts noticed this and concluded that narcissistic patients did not have transferences because their libidinal energy was all directed toward the self; this was another basis for doubting their treatability. Contemporary analytic theory acknowledges that narcissistic clients do have transference reactions but of a different sort from those of other patients.

perhaps the most unpleasant of the countertransference reactions to narcissistic patients; every time I experience this, I find myself generating biological explanations (I didn't get enough sleep last night; I just ate a big lunch; I must be coming down with a cold), and then once that patient is out the door and another one is inside, I am wide awake and interested. Occasionally one's countertransference to an idealizing person is a sense of grandiose expansion, of joining the patient in a mutual admiration society. But unless the therapist is also characterologically narcissistic, such reactions are both unconvincing and short-lived.

The psychoanalytic explanation for these phenomena relates to the special kind of transference generated by narcissistic people. Rather than projecting a discrete internal object such as a parent on to the therapist, they externalize an aspect of their self. Specifically, instead of the patient's feeling that the therapist is like mother or father (although sometimes one can see aspects of such transferences), he or she projects either the grandiose or the devalued part of the *self*. The therapist thus becomes a container for the internal process of self-esteem maintenance. He or she is a selfobject, not a fully separate person who feels to the patient *like* a previously known, well-delineated figure from the past.

To be used for a self-esteem maintaining *function* rather than perceived as a separate *person* is disconcerting, even unnerving. The dehumanizing effect of the narcissistic person's attitude accounts for some of the negative countertransference reactions analytic practitioners have described in connection with the treatment of such clients. Yet most therapists also report that they easily tolerate, control, and derive empathy from such reactions once they understand them as comprehensible and expectable features of the treatment of this kind of psychology. The disposition to feel flawed as a therapist is a virtually inevitable mirror of the patient's core worries about self-worth; it is relieving to substitute a revised clinical formulation for ruminations about what one is doing wrong.

Heinz Kohut and other analysts of a self psychology bent (e.g., Bach, 1985; Stolorow et al., 1987; Wolf, 1988; Rowe & MacIsaac, 1989) think in terms of several subtypes of selfobject transferences that appear in narcissistic patients, including mirroring, twinship, and alter-ego patterns. Although an explication of such concepts is beyond the scope of this book, readers who find that the description of narcissistic character pathology fits a patient they have previously been construing some other way may find it helpful to explore the language of self psychologists for conceptualizing their clients' experience.

THERAPEUTIC IMPLICATIONS OF THE DIAGNOSIS OF NARCISSISM

A therapist who is able to help a narcissistic person to find self-acceptance without either inflating the self or disparaging others has done a truly good deed, and a difficult one. A primary requisite for treating narcissistic pathology is patience: No one with a track record for changing the psychology of narcissistic patients has done it very fast. Although modification of any kind of character structure is a long-term undertaking, the requirement of patience may be more keenly felt with narcissistic clients than with those of other character types because of one's having to endure countertransference reactions of boredom and demoralization.

Because currently there are competing theories of etiology and therapy, it is hard to summarize conventional psychodynamic wisdom about treating narcissistic patients. Most arguments are variants on a complex disagreement between Kohut and Kernberg that appeared in the 1970s and 1980s. The gist of their respective positions is that Kohut (1971, 1977, 1984) sees pathological narcissism *developmentally* (the patient's maturation was going along normally and ran into some difficulties in the resolution of normal needs to idealize and deidealize), while Kernberg (1975, 1976, 1984) views it *structurally* (something went awry very early, leaving the person with entrenched primitive defenses that differ in kind rather than in degree from normality). Kohut's conception of a narcissistic person can be imaged as a plant whose growth was stunted by too little water and sun at critical points; Kernberg's narcissist can be viewed as a plant that has mutated into a hybrid.*

A consequence of their differing theories is that some approaches to narcissism stress the need to give the plant plenty of water and sun so that it will finally thrive, and others propose that it must be pruned of its aberrant parts so that it can become what it should have been. Self psychology adherents thus recommend benign acceptance of idealization or devaluation and unwavering empathy for the patient's experience. Kernberg advocates the tactful but insistent confrontation of grandiosity, whether owned or projected, and the systematic interpretation of defenses against envy and greed. Self psychologically oriented therapists try to remain *inside* the patient's subjective

*Kernberg (1989): "Pathologic narcissism reflects libidinal investment not in a normal integrated self-structure but in a pathologic self-structure" (p. 723).

experience, while analysts influenced by ego psychology and object relations theory oscillate between internal and external positions (see Gardner, 1991).

I will not attempt a critical evaluation of Kohut's and Kernberg's contrasting theories, or those of other writers on this topic. Most therapists I know find they have patients for whom Kohut's formulations, both etiological and therapeutic, seem to fit and others for whom Kernberg's seem apt. Kernberg (1982) has suggested that Kohut's approach might be considered a subtype of supportive therapy, and therefore appropriate for narcissistic patients who are in the borderline-to-psychotic range. This idea is implicitly endorsed by many of my colleagues, who say they find Kohut's recommendations applicable to their more disturbed and depressed–depleted narcissistic clients. A complication of this view is that the narcissistically vulnerable people about whom Kohut originally wrote were in traditional analysis with him (several sessions a week using the couch) and so can be assumed to have been regarded by him as in the higher ranges of functioning. Because the jury is still out on the Kohut–Kernberg dispute, and because the interested reader can consult the original sources for the technical recommendations deriving from each conceptualization, I will mention only some general suggestions on the treatment of narcissism that exist outside this controversy.

I have already mentioned patience. Implicit in that attitude is an *acceptance of human imperfections* that make therapeutic progress a tedious and taxing business. The matter-of-fact assumption that we are all imperfect and resistant to change is very different from what the narcissistic person has internalized. Such a thesis is humane and realistic rather than critical and omnipotent. Some therapeutic mileage is already inherent in such a position. In particular, the therapist should embody a nonjudgmental, realistic attitude toward his or her own frailty.

One of Kohut's greatest technical contributions has been his attention to the consequences of the therapist's acknowledgment of errors, especially of lapses in empathy. From the standpoint of drive theory and ego psychology, a therapeutic mistake need not impel any activity in the analyst other than private reflection; as always, the patient is simply encouraged to associate to what happened and to report any reactions (see Greenson, 1967). Self psychologists have called our attention to how devastated a narcissistic person can be by a professional's failure of empathy, and how the only way to repair such an injury is by expressing regret. An apology both confirms the patient's perception of mistreatment (thereby validating his or her real feelings rather than furthering the insincere compliance with which narcissistic people are used to operating) and sets an example of maintaining self-esteem while admitting to shortcomings.*

It is critical that when one acknowledges one's inevitable errors, one does not become excessively self-critical. If the patient perceives that the therapist is in an agony of remorse, the message received is that mistakes should be rare and require stern self-censure—a delusion from which the narcissistic person is already suffering. It is better to take one's cue from Winnicott, who is reputed to have fielded a query about his rules for interpretation with the comment: "I make interpretations for two purposes. One, to show the patient that I am awake. Two, to show the patient that I can be wrong." Similarly, Arthur Robbins (1991), a psychoanalyst with expertise in art therapy and other expressive modes of treatment, describes his theory of technique as "Fuck-up therapy: I fuck up, and the patient corrects me."

Attempts to help a narcissistic patient also require a constant *mindfulness of the person's latent self-state*, however overwhelming the manifest one is. Because even the most arrogant, entitled narcissist is subject to excruciating shame in the face of what feels like criticism, therapists must take pains to frame sensitive interventions. Relatedness with narcissistic patients is always tenuous since they cannot tolerate being in circumstances where their fragile self-esteem is diminished. Their early reputation for being impossible to treat derived partly from analysts' experience with their abruptly terminating therapies of even several years' duration when their feelings were hurt.

I have mentioned the power of shame in the experience of the narcissistic person, and the importance of the therapist's discriminating between this affect and the sense of guilt. People with fragile self-esteem will go to great lengths to avoid acknowledging their role in anything negative that happens in their lives. Unlike people who easily feel guilty and handle their transgressions with efforts at reparation, narcissistically motivated people run from their mistakes and hide from those who would find them out. They induce in therapists either a disposition to confront them unempathically about their own contributions to their difficulties or a tendency to join them in bemoaning the bad deal they have gotten from others. Neither position is therapeutic, although the second is temporarily palliative to a person who otherwise may suffer chagrin bordering on mortification.

*Many of Kohut's recommendations about technique were foreshadowed by the counseling theories of Carl Rogers (see Stolorow, 1976). The one area in which Kohut went far beyond Rogers concerns the handling of errors by the therapist. Rogers's writings seemed to most readers to imply that perfect empathy, congruence, and authenticity are possible. Kohut had no such illusions.

The therapist faces the daunting task of expanding the narcissistic patient's awareness of and honesty about the nature of his or her behavior without stimulating so much shame that the person either leaves treatment or keeps secrets. One way to do this in the context of a person's complaints and criticisms about others is to ask, "Did you make your needs explicit?" The rationale for this query is that narcissistic people have deep shame about asking for anything; they believe that to admit a need exposes a deficiency in the self. They consequently get into interpersonal situations where they are miserable because another person does not effortlessly divine their needs and offer what they want without their undergoing what they see as the humiliation of asking. They then try to persuade the analyst that their problem is that the people they live with are insensitive. The question about articulating needs leads directly to the patient's belief that it is shameful to need someone and to an opportunity for the therapist to reeducate the person about human interdependency.

I commented earlier on the difference between selfobject and object transferences (in the older literature, these were referred to, respectively, as narcissistic and neurotic transferences). An implication of this difference is that the therapist cannot fruitfully investigate the transference reactions of narcissistic patients as one would those of other people. Whether one takes a more Kohutian or a more Kernbergian approach, the therapist should realize that despite the countertransference feeling that one means nothing to the patient, a narcissistic person actually needs the therapist *more* than do people without significant self-esteem deficits. It is a frequent surprise to therapists inexperienced with narcissistic patients to learn that the same person who renders them insignificant and impotent during therapy sessions is quoting them admiringly outside the consulting room. Even the arrogant, boastful, seemingly impervious patient betrays a deep dependency on the therapist by his or her vulnerability to feeling crushed when the therapist is insensitive. In working with narcissistic people, practitioners have to become accustomed to absorbing a great deal that they would address with other types of patients.

DIFFERENTIAL DIAGNOSIS

Injuries to self-esteem may lead anyone to behave temporarily like a narcissistic character. Moreover, all types of personality structure have a narcissistic function: They preserve self-esteem via certain defenses. But to qualify as characterologically narcissistic, one must have longstanding, automatic, and situation-independent patterns of subjectivity and behavior. Narcissistic personality organization seems currently overdiagnosed, perhaps especially by psychodynamic clinicians. The concept is often misapplied to people having situation-specific reactions and to psychopathic, depressive, obsessive compulsive, and hysterical personalities.

Narcissistic Personality versus Narcissistic Reactions

A primary caveat in diagnosing characterological narcissism has been suggested in the preceding material: Even more than with other psychological conditions to which all human beings are vulnerable, narcissistic concerns are ubiquitous and can easily be situationally incited. Kohut and Wolf (1978) referred to individuals who (like the Chinese graduate student mentioned in the Introduction to this part) confront circumstances that challenge their prior sense of identity and undermine their self-esteem as suffering from a "secondary narcissistic disturbance," not a narcissistic character disorder. It is an important distinction.

Any nonnarcissistic person can sound arrogant or devaluing, or empty and idealizing, under conditions that strain his or her identity and confidence. Medical school and psychotherapy training programs are famous for taking successful, autonomous adults and making them feel like incompetent children. Compensatory behaviors like bragging, opinionated proclamations, hypercritical commentary, or idealization of a mentor are to be expected under such circumstances. Phenomena like these are sometimes referred to in the psychoanalytic literature as comprising a "narcissistic defense" (e.g., Kernberg, 1984). That one is suffering with narcissistic issues does not make one a narcissistic personality. Where situational factors seem determinative of a narcissistic presentation, the interviewer should rely on historical and transferential data to infer the personality structure underneath the narcissistic injury.

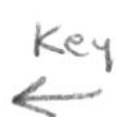

Narcissistic versus Psychopathic Personality

In the last section of the previous chapter, I mentioned the importance of discriminating between a predominantly sociopathic personality structure and one that is essentially narcissistic. Kohutian efforts at empathic relatedness, at least as they are conventionally put into practice, would be ineffective with psychopathic people because they do not emotionally understand compassionate attitudes; they scorn a sympathetic demeanor as the mark of weakness. The approach advocated by Kernberg, centering on the confrontation of the grandiose self, would be more respectfully assimilated by a psychopathically organized person, but as delineated in his articles on the topic (e.g., 1989), it lacks the necessary focus on the psychopath's battles for control and efforts to destroy. Kernberg regards antisocial trends as indicators of probable untreatability; he has consequently not developed recommendations about technique for this clinical population, as have therapists like Greenwald, Bursten, Groth (e.g., 1979), and Meloy, who have specialized in working with psychopathic clients.

Narcissistic versus Depressive Personality

The more depressed kind of narcissistic person can easily be misunderstood as having a depressive personality. The essential difference between the two groups is, to condense a great deal of clinical theory and observation into a simple image, that narcissistically depressed people are subjectively *empty*, whereas characterologically depressive people (those who used to be described as suffering depression of the more "melancholic" or guilty type) are subjectively *full*—of critical and angry internalizations. The narcissistic depressive feels devoid of a substantial self; the melancholic depressive feels the self is real but irreducibly bad. I will comment on these differences and their divergent therapeutic implications more in Chapter 11.

Narcissistic versus Obsessive Compulsive Personality

It is easy to misconstrue a narcissistic person as obsessive and/or compulsive on the basis of the attention to detail that may be part of the narcissistic quest for perfection. In the early days of psychoanalytic practice, fundamentally narcissistic people were often considered obsessive or compulsive because their presenting symptoms fell into one or both of those categories. They were then treated according to assumptions about the etiology of obsessive compulsive character that emphasized struggles for control and guilt over anger and fantasied aggression.

Narcissistic patients, who were empty more than angry, did not make much progress in that kind of therapy; they would feel misunderstood and criticized when the therapist seemed to harp on issues that were not central to their subjectivity. Although many people have both narcissistic and more classically obsessive concerns, those whose personalities were predominantly narcissistic tended to get little help from analytic therapy before the 1970s, when theories of the etiology and treatment of pathological narcissism radically extended our capacity to help people with disorders of the self. I know of a number of people treated analytically before that time who still bear grudges against their therapist and against psychoanalysis in general. In popular accounts of psychotherapy experiences one can find what seem to be examples of the effects of this misdiagnosis; David Viscott's (1972) depiction of his failed therapy with a "Dr. Frost," for instance, suggests that his analyst applied a style that may have been suitable for an obsessive person but was markedly unattuned to Viscott's hunger for empathic mirroring and affirmation of self. More details on this distinction and the implications of this diagnostic mistake will be found in Chapter 13.

Narcissistic versus Hysterical Personality

While the narcissistic versus obsessive compulsive personality differential is called for somewhat more frequently with men than with women, the need to distinguish between narcissism and hysteria comes up much more commonly with female patients. Because hysterically organized people use narcissistic defenses, they are readily misinterpreted as narcissistic characters. Women whose hysterical presentation includes considerable exhibitionistic behavior and a pattern of relating to men in which idealization is quickly followed by devaluation may appear to be basically narcissistic, but their concerns about self are gender specific and fueled by anxiety more than shame. Outside certain highly conflicted areas, they are warm, loving, and far from empty (see Kernberg, 1984).

The import of this differential lies in the contrasting therapeutic requirements for the two groups: Hysterical patients thrive with an attention to object transferences, whereas narcissistic ones require an appreciation of selfobject phenomena. In Chapter 14 I will go into more detail on this topic.

SUMMARY

This chapter has described the depleted subjective world of the person with a narcissistically organized character and the compensatory behaviors with which such a person tries to maintain a reliable and valued sense of self. I have emphasized the affects of shame and envy, the defenses of idealization and devaluation, and relational patterns of using and being used to equilibrate one's self-esteem and to repair damage to it. The narcissistic person's propensity for selfobject transferences was discussed, along with countertransference reactions in which a sense of unrelatedness prevails. Some implications for technique were derived from an appreciation of these special aspects of the narcissistic condition, although acknowledgment was made of current controversies in the psychoanalytic understanding of narcissism that make appropriate technique with this population a matter of some dispute. Finally, narcissistic character organization was distinguished from narcissistic reactions, from psychopathy, from depressive (melancholic) personality, from obsessive and compulsive character structure, and from hysteria.

SUGGESTIONS FOR FURTHER READING

There has been a voluminous psychoanalytic literature on narcissism since the 1970s, when Kohut (1971) published *The Analysis of the Self* and Kernberg (1975) offered an alternative conception in *Borderline Conditions and Pathological Narcissism*. Both these books contain so much jargon that they are almost impossible for someone new to psychoanalysis to read. More manageable alternatives include Alice Miller's (1975) *Prisoners of Childhood* (known in another edition as *The Drama of the Gifted Child*), Bach's (1985) *Narcissistic States and the Therapeutic Process*, and Morrison's (1989) *Shame: The Underside of Narcissism*. Morrison (1986) also edited a collection, available in paperback, titled *Essential Papers on Narcissism* that contains major psychoanalytic essays on the topic, most of which are excellent.

❖ 9 ❖
Schizoid Personalities

The person whose character is essentially schizoid is subject to widespread misunderstanding, based on the common misconception that schizoid dynamics are always suggestive of grave primitivity. Because the incontrovertibly psychotic diagnosis of schizophrenia fits people at the disturbed end of the schizoid continuum, and because the behavior of schizoid people is apt to be unconventional, eccentric, or even bizarre, nonschizoid others tend to pathologize those with schizoid dynamics—whether or not they are competent and autonomous, with significant areas of ego strength. In fact, schizoid people run the gamut from the hospitalized catatonic patient to the creative genius.

As with the other typological categories, a person may be schizoid at any level, from psychologically incapacitated to saner than average. Because the defense that defines the schizoid character is a primitive one (withdrawal into fantasy), it may be that healthy schizoid people are rarer than sicker ones, but I do not know of any research findings or disciplined clinical observations that support this assumption empirically.* Vocations like philosophical inquiry, spiritual discipline, theoretical science, and the creative arts attract people with this kind of character. At the high functioning end of the schizoid spectrum we might find people like Ludwig Wittgenstein, Martha Graham, and other admirably original and somewhat eccentric individuals.

*There is longstanding evidence that the most frequent premorbid personality type in those who become schizophrenic is schizoid (E. Bleuler, 1911; Nannarello, 1953; M. Bleuler, 1977; Peralta, Cuesta, & de Leon, 1991), but the converse idea, that all schizoid people are at risk of a psychotic break, has no empirical basis.

In 1980, with the publication of the DSM-III, conditions that most analysts would regard as different possibilities on the schizoid spectrum, or as minor variants on a general schizoid theme, appeared as discrete categories in the DSM. Complicated theoretical issues influenced this decision (see Lion, 1986), one reflecting differences of current opinion that echo old controversies about the nature of certain schizoid states (E. Bleuler, 1911; Kraepelin, 1919; Kretschmer, 1925; Schneider, 1959; Jaspers, 1963; Gottesman, 1991; Akhtar, 1992). Most analytic practitioners continue to regard the diagnoses of schizoid, schizotypal, and avoidant personality disorders as nonpsychotic versions of schizoid character, and the diagnoses of schizophrenia, schizophreniform disorder, and schizoaffective disorder as psychotic levels of schizoid functioning.

DRIVE, AFFECT, AND TEMPERAMENT IN SCHIZOID PERSONALITIES

Clinical experience suggests that temperamentally, the person who becomes schizoid is hyperreactive and easily overstimulated. Schizoid people often describe themselves as innately sensitive, and their relatives frequently mention their having been the kind of baby who shrinks from too much light or noise or motion. It is as if the nerve endings of schizoid individuals are closer to the surface than those of the rest of us. Controlled observation and research on temperament in children (Thomas, Chess, & Birch, 1970; Brazelton, 1982) have confirmed the reports of generations of parents that while most infants cuddle, cling, and mold themselves to the body of a warm caregiver, some newborns stiffen or pull back as if the adult has intruded on their comfort and safety. One suspects that such babies are constitutionally prone to schizoid personality structure, especially if there is a "poor fit" (Escalona, 1968) between themselves and their main caregivers.

In the area of drive as classically understood, the schizoid person seems to struggle with oral-level issues. Specifically, he or she is preoccupied with avoiding the dangers of being engulfed, absorbed, distorted, taken over, eaten up. A talented schizoid therapist in a supervision group I belonged to once described to the group members his vivid fantasy that the physical circle of participants constituted a huge mouth or a giant letter "C." He imagined that if he exposed his vulnerability by talking candidly about his feelings toward one of his patients, the group would close around him, making the "C" into an "O," and that he would suffocate and expire inside it.

While fantasies like those of my colleague invite the interpretation that they constitute projections and transformations of the fantasizer's own hunger (Fairbairn, 1941; Guntrip, 1961), the schizoid person does not experience appetitive drives as coming from within the self. Rather, the outer world feels full of consuming, distorting threats against security and individuality. Fairbairn's understanding of schizoid states as "love made hungry" addresses not the day-to-day subjective experience of the schizoid person but the dynamics underlying the opposite and manifest tendencies: to withdraw, to seek satisfactions in fantasy, to reject the corporeal world. Schizoid people are even apt to be physically thin, so removed are they from emotional contact with their own greed (cf. Kretschmer, 1925).

Similarly, schizoid people do not impress one as being highly aggressive, despite the violent content of some of their fantasies. Their families and friends often regard them as unusually gentle, placid people. A friend of mine, whose general brilliance and schizoid indifference to convention I have long admired, was described lovingly at his wedding by an older sister as having always been a "soft person." This softness exists in fascinating contradiction to his affinity for horror movies, true-crime books, and visions of apocalyptic world destruction. The projection of drive can be easily assumed, but this man's conscious experience—and the impression he makes on others—is of a sweet, low-keyed, lovable eccentric. Most analytic thinkers who have worked with people like my friend have inferred that schizoid clients bury both their hunger and their aggression under a heavy blanket of defense.

Affectively, one of the most striking aspects of many high-functioning individuals with schizoid dynamics is their *lack* of common defenses. They tend to be in touch with many emotional reactions at a level of genuineness that awes and even intimidates their acquaintances. It is common for the schizoid person to wonder how everybody else can be lying to themselves so effortlessly when the harsh facts of life are so patent. Part of the alienation from which schizoid people suffer derives from their experiences of not having their own emotional, intuitive, and sensory capacities validated—because others simply do not see what they do.The ability of a schizoid person to perceive what others disown or ignore is so natural and effortless that he or she may lack empathy for the less lucid, less ambivalent, less emotionally harrowing world of nonschizoid peers.

Schizoid people do not seem to struggle unduly with issues of shame or guilt. They tend to take themselves and the world pretty much as is without the internal impetus to make things different or to shrink from judgment. Yet they may suffer considerable anxiety about basic safety. When they feel overwhelmed, they hide—either literally with a hermit's reclusiveness or by retreat into their imagination (Kasanin & Rosen, 1933; Nannarello, 1953). The schizoid person is above all else an outsider, an onlooker, an observer of the human condition. The "split" that is implied in the etymology of the word schizoid exists in two areas: between the self and the outside world, and between the experienced self and desire (see Laing, 1965). When analytic commentators refer to split experience in schizoid people, they refer to a sense of estrangement from part of the self or from life; the defense mechanism of splitting, in which a person alternately expresses one ego state and then another opposite one, or divides the world defensively into all-good and all-bad aspects, is a different use of the word.

DEFENSIVE AND ADAPTIVE PROCESSES IN SCHIZOID PERSONALITIES

As noted previously, the pathognomonic defense in schizoid personality organization is withdrawal into an internal world of imagination. In addition, schizoid people may use projection and introjection, idealization, devaluation, and to a lesser extent, the other defenses that have their origins in a time before self and other were fully differentiated psychologically. Among the more "mature" defenses, intellectualization is the clear preference of most schizoid people. They rarely rely on mechanisms that blot out affective and sensory information, such as denial and repression; similarly, the defensive operations that organize experience along good-and-bad lines, such as compartmentalization, moralization, undoing, reaction formation, and turning against the self are not prominent in their repertoires. Under stress, schizoid individuals may withdraw from their own affect as well as from external stimulation, appearing blunted, flat, or inappropriate, often despite showing evidence of heightened attunement to affective messages coming from others.

The most adaptive and exciting capacity of the schizoid person is creativity. Most truly original artists have a strong schizoid streak—almost by definition, since one has to stand apart from convention to influence it in a new way. Healthier schizoid people turn their assets into works of art, scientific discoveries, theoretical innovations, or spiritual pathfinding, while more disturbed individuals in this category live in a private hell where their potential contributions are preempted by their terror and estrangement. The sublimation of autistic withdrawal into creative activity is a primary goal of therapy with schizoid patients.

OBJECT RELATIONS IN SCHIZOID CONDITIONS

The primary relational conflict of schizoid people concerns closeness and distance, love and fear. A deep ambivalence about attachment pervades their subjective life. They crave closeness yet feel the constant threat of engulfment by others; they seek distance to reassure themselves of their safety and separateness yet may complain of alienation and loneliness (Karon & VandenBos, 1981). Guntrip (1952), who depicted the "classic dilemma" of the schizoid individual as "that he can neither be in a relationship with another person nor out of it, without in various ways risking the loss of both his object and himself," refers to this dilemma as the "in and out programme" (p. 36). Robbins (1988) summarizes the dynamic as the message, "Come close for I am alone, but stay away for I fear intrusion" (p. 398).

Sexually, some schizoid people are remarkably apathetic, often despite being functional and orgasmic. The closer the other, the greater the worry that sex means enmeshment. Many a heterosexual women has fallen in love with a passionate musician, only to learn that her lover reserves his sensual intensity for his instrument. Similarly, some schizoid people crave unattainable sexual objects, while feeling vague indifference toward available ones. The partners of schizoid people sometimes complain of a mechanical or detached quality in their lovemaking.

Object relations theories of the genesis of schizoid dynamics have been, in my own view, burdened by efforts to locate the origins of schizoid states in a particular phase of development. The adequacy of the fixation–regression hypothesis in accounting for *type* of character structure is, as I have suggested previously, problematic, yet its appeal is understandable: It normalizes puzzling phenomena by considering them simple residues of ordinary infantile life. Klein (1946) thus traced schizoid mechanisms to a universal paranoid–schizoid position of early infancy. Other early object relations analysts followed suit in developing explanatory paradigms in which schizoid dynamics were equated with regression to neonatal experience (Fairbairn, 1941; Guntrip, 1971). Current theorists have tended to continue the developmental bias of the fixation–regression model, yet they differ about which early phase is the fixation point. For example, in the Kleinian tradition, Giovacchini (1979) regards schizoid disorders as essentially "prementational," while Horner (1979) assigns their origins to a later age when the child emerges from symbiosis.

Perhaps more productive speculations about the sources of schizoid personality lie in analytic observations about the kinds of rearing that influence youngsters in a schizoid direction. One type of relatedness that may encourage a child's withdrawal is an impinging, overinvested, overinvolved kind of parenting (Winnicott, 1965). The schizoid man with the smothering mother is a staple of recent popular literature and can also be found in scholarly work. A type of family background commonly observed by clinicians who have treated male patients with schizoid features is a seductive or boundary-transgressing mother and an impatient, critical father.*

The *content*, not just the degree, of parental involvement may also be relevant to the development of a pattern of schizoid aloofness and withdrawal. Numerous observers of the families of people who developed a schizophrenic psychosis have stressed the role of contradictory and confusing communications (Searles, 1959; Laing, 1965; Lidz & Fleck, 1965; Singer & Wynne, 1965a, 1965b; Bateson et al., 1969). It is possible that such patterns foster schizoid dynamics in general. A child raised with double-binding, emotionally dishonest messages could easily come to depend on withdrawal to protect the self from intolerable levels of confusion and anger. He or she would also feel deeply hopeless, an attitude often noted in schizoid patients (e.g., Giovacchini, 1979).

In apparent contrast to the parental-impingement theory of the development of schizoid features, there are also some reports of people for whom loneliness and relative neglect characterized their childhoods to such a degree that their preference for withdrawal, no matter how profoundly isolating, can be understood as their having made a virtue out of necessity.† It is typical of the literature on schizoid phenomena—an extensive literature because of the huge social cost of schizophrenia—that contrasting and mutually exclusive formulations can be found everywhere one looks (Sass, 1992). It is not impossible that both impingement and deprivation codetermine the schizoid problem: If one is lonely and deprived, yet the only kind of parenting available is unempathic and intrusive, a yearning–avoidant, closeness–

*Although recent editions of the DSM give no information on sex ratio for schizoid, schizotypal, and avoidant diagnoses, most therapists see more males than females with schizoid personalities. This accords with the psychoanalytic observation that because in most families the primary caregiver is female, with whom girls must identify and from whom boys must separate psychologically, women are more prone to disorders characterized by too much attachment (e.g., depression, masochism) and men to those expressing excessive isolation from others (e.g., psychopathy, schizoid conditions). See Dinnerstein (1976) and Chodorow (1978, 1989).

†Harry Stack Sullivan and Arthur Robbins, two analysts whose own schizoid trends prompted their efforts to interpret the schizoid experience to the larger mental health community, both report considerable early deprivation of companionship, and a consequent sense of loneliness and isolation (Mullahy, 1970; Robbins, 1988).

distance conflict would be inevitable. Masud Khan's (1963, 1974) studies of schizoid conditions emphasize the combination of "cumulative trauma" from failures of realistic maternal protection and "symbiotic omnipotence" inherent in the mother's intense overidentification.

THE SCHIZOID SELF

One of the most striking aspects of people with schizoid personalities is their disregard for conventional social expectations. In dramatic contrast to the narcissistic personality style covered in the previous chapter, the schizoid person may be markedly indifferent to the effect he or she has on others and to evaluative responses coming from those in the outside world. Compliance and conformity go against the grain for schizoid people, whether or not they are in touch with a painful subjective loneliness. Even when they see some expediency in fitting in, they tend to feel awkward and even fraudulent making social chitchat or participating in communal forms, regarding them as essentially contrived and artificial. The schizoid self always stands at a safe distance from the rest of humanity.

Many observers have commented on the detached, ironic, and faintly contemptuous attitude of many schizoid people (E. Bleuler, 1911; Sullivan, 1973; M. Bleuler, 1977). This tendency toward an isolated superiority may have its origins in fending off the incursions of an overcontrolling or overintrusive Other noted in the preceding etiological hypotheses. Even in the most seemingly disorganized schizophrenic patients, a kind of deliberate oppositionality has long been noted, as if the patient's only way of preserving a sense of self-integrity is in making a farce of every conventional expectation. Under the topic of "counter-etiquette," Sass (1992) comments on this phenomenon as follows:

> Cross-cultural research has shown . . . that schizophrenics generally seem to gravitate toward "the path of most resistance," tending to transgress whatever customs and rules happen to be held most sacred in a given society. Thus, in deeply religious Nigeria, they are especially likely to violate religious sanctions; in Japan, to assault family members. (p. 110)

One way of understanding these apparently deliberate preferences for eccentricity and defiance of custom is to assume that the schizoid person is assiduously warding off the condition of being defined—psychologically taken over and obliterated—by others.

Abandonment is thus a lesser evil than engulfment to people with schizoid character structure. Michael Balint (1945), in a famous essay with the evocative title "Friendly Expanses—Horrid Empty Spaces," contrasted two antithetical characterological orientations: The philobat (lover of distance), who seeks the comforts of solitude, and the "ocnophil" (lover of closeness), who when under stress gravitates *toward* others, seeking a shoulder to cry on.* Schizoid people are the ultimate philobats. Perhaps predictably, since human beings are often drawn to those with opposite and envied strengths, schizoid people tend to attract (and to be attracted to) warm, expressive, sociable people such as those with hysterical personalities. These proclivities set the stage for certain familiar and even comic problems in which the nonschizoid partner tries to resolve interpersonal tension by continually moving closer, while the schizoid person, fearing engulfment, keeps moving farther away (cf. Wheelis [1966] on the "illusionless" man and the visionary woman).

I do not wish to give the reader the impression that schizoid individuals are cold or uncaring. They may care very much about other people, yet still need to maintain a protective personal space. Some, in fact, gravitate to careers in psychotherapy, where they put their exquisite sensitivity to use safely in the service of others. Allen Wheelis (1956), who may be assumed to be in close touch with his own schizoid characteristics, wrote an eloquent essay on the attractions and hazards of a psychoanalytic career, stressing how people with a core conflict over closeness and distance may be drawn to the profession of analysis, a vocation that offers the opportunity to know others more intimately than anyone else ever will, while concealing the self behind the couch and the neutrality of one's interpretations.

For someone with schizoid dynamics, self-esteem is often maintained by individual creative activity. Issues of personal integrity and self-expression tend to dominate their self-evaluative concerns. Where the psychopath pursues evidence of personal power, or the narcissist seeks admiring feedback to nourish self-regard, the schizoid person wants confirmation of his or her genuine originality, sensitivity, and uniqueness. This confirmation must be internally rather than externally bestowed, and because of their high standards for creative endeavors, schizoid people are often rigorously self-critical. They may

*Scholars outside the psychoanalytic tradition have made comparable observations of differential preference for closeness or distance, as in the pursuer–distancer paradigm or the concept of approach–avoidance conflicts. It seems to be a universal tension and a central dimension of personality from almost anyone's perspective. See also Lachmann and Beebe (1989) and Livingston (1991).

take the pursuit of authenticity to such extreme lengths that their isolation and demoralization are virtually guaranteed.

Sass (1992) has compellingly described how schizoid conditions are emblematic of modernity. The alienation of contemporary people from a communal sensibility, reflected in the deconstructive perspectives of 20th-century art, literature, anthropology, philosophy, and criticism, has eerie similarities to schizoid and schizophrenic experience. Sass notes in particular the attitudes of alienation, hyperreflexivity (elaborate self-consciousness), detachment, and rationality gone virtually mad that characterize modern and postmodern modes of thought and art, contrasting them with "the world of the natural attitude, the world of practical activity, shared communal meanings, and real physical presences" (p. 354). His exposition also calls effectively into question numerous facile and oversimplified accounts of schizophrenia and the schizoid experience.

TRANSFERENCE AND COUNTERTRANSFERENCE WITH SCHIZOID PATIENTS

Although one would assume intuitively from their predilection for withdrawal that schizoid people would shun encounters as intimate as psychotherapy and psychoanalysis, they are in fact typically appreciative of and cooperative in the therapy process when treated with consideration and respect. The clinician's discipline in addressing the client's own agenda, and the safe distance created by the customary boundaries of treatment (time limitations, fee arrangements, ethical prohibitions against social or sexual relationships with clients, etc.), seem to decrease the schizoid person's fears about enmeshing involvements.

Schizoid clients approach therapy with the same combination of sensitivity, honesty, and fear of engulfment that typifies their other relationships. They may be seeking help because their isolation from the rest of the human community has become too painful, or because they have circumscribed goals related to that isolation, such as a wish to get over an inhibition against dating or pursuing other specific social behaviors. Sometimes the psychological disadvantages of their personality type are not evident to them; they may want relief from a depression or an anxiety state or another kind of symptom neurosis. At other times, they may arrive for treatment afraid—often rightly—that they are on the brink of going crazy.

It is not uncommon for a schizoid person to be tongue-tied and to feel empty and lost in the early phases of therapy. Long silences may have to be endured while the patient internalizes the safety of the setting. Eventually, however, unless a client is excruciatingly nonverbal or confusingly psychotic, most analytically oriented therapists enjoy treating people with schizoid character structures. As one would expect, they are often highly perceptive of their internal reactions, and they are grateful to have a place where the expression of them will not arouse alarm, disdain, or derision.

The initial transference–countertransference challenge for the therapist working with a schizoid patient is to find a way into the patient's subjective world without arousing too much anxiety about intrusion. Because schizoid people withdraw into detached and obscure styles of communication, it is easy to fall into a counterdetachment, in which one regards them as interesting specimens rather than as fellow creatures. Their original transference "tests," in the terms of control–mastery theory, involve efforts to see whether the therapist is concerned enough for them to tolerate their confusing, off-putting messages while maintaining the determination to understand and help. Naturally, they fear that the therapist will, like other people in their lives, withdraw from them emotionally and consign them to the category of hopeless recluse or amusing crackpot.

The history of efforts to understand schizoid conditions is replete with examples of "experts" objectifying the lonely patient, being fascinated at schizoid phenomena but keeping a safe distance from the emotional pain they represent and regarding the schizoid person's verbalizations as meaningless, trivial, or too enigmatic to bother to decode. The current psychiatric enthusiasm for physiological explanations of schizoid states is a familiar version of this disposition not to take the schizoid person's subjectivity seriously. As Sass (1992) has argued, efforts to understand biochemical and neurological contributions to schizoid and schizophrenic states do not obviate the continuing need to address the *meaning* of the schizoid experience to the patient. In *The Divided Self*, R. D. Laing (1965) reassesses a schizophrenic woman interviewed by Emil Kraepelin. The patient's words, which had been incomprehensible to Kraepelin, gain meaning when regarded from Laing's empathic perspective. Karon and VandenBos (1981) present case after case of helpable patients who might easily be dismissed as "management" projects by clinicians who are untrained or unwilling to understand them.

People who are characterologically schizoid and in no danger of a psychotic break—the majority of schizoid people—obviously provoke much less incomprehension and defensive detachment in their therapists than do hospitalized schizophrenics, the subject of most of the serious psychoanalytic writing on pathological withdrawal. But the same therapeutic requirements apply, in less extreme degree. The patient needs to be treated as if his or her internal experience, even if outlandish to others, has potentially discernable meaning and can constitute the basis for a nonthreatening intimacy with another person. The therapist must keep in mind that the aloofness of the schizoid client is an addressable defense, not an insurmountable barrier to connection. If the clinician can avoid acting on countertransference temptations either to prod the patient into premature disclosure, or to objectify and distance him or her, a solid working alliance should evolve.

Once a therapeutic relationship is in place, certain other emotional complexities may ensue. In my experience, the subjective fragility of the schizoid person is mirrored in the therapist's frequent sense of weakness or helplessness. Images and fantasies of a destructive, devouring external world may absorb both parties to the therapy process. Counterimages of omnipotence and shared superiority may also be present ("We two form a universe"). Fond perceptions of the patient as a unique, exquisite, misunderstood genius or underappreciated sage may dominate the therapist's inner responses, perhaps in parallel to the attitude of an overinvolved parent who imagined greatness for this special child.

THERAPEUTIC IMPLICATIONS OF THE DIAGNOSIS OF SCHIZOID PERSONALITY

The therapist who works with a schizoid patient must be open to a degree of authenticity and a level of awareness of emotion and imagery that would be possible only after years of work with patients of other character types. While I have known many practitioners who do well with most kinds of clients without having undergone a thoroughgoing personal analysis, I doubt that unless they are schizoid themselves, they can respond effectively to schizoid patients without having had extensive therapeutic exposure to their own inner depths.

Since most therapists have somewhat depressive psychologies, such that their fears of abandonment are stronger than fears of engulfment, they naturally try to move close to people they wish to help. Empathy with the schizoid patient's need for emotional space may consequently be hard to come by. A supervisor of mine once commented about my earnest and overly impinging efforts to reach a schizoid patient, "This man needs bicarbonate of soda, and you keep trying to feed him pumpkin pie." Emmanuel Hammer (1968) has commented on the effectiveness of simply moving one's chair further from the patient, thus giving nonverbal reassurance that the therapist will not intrude, hurry, take over, or smother.

In the early phases of therapy, interpretation should be avoided on the basis of the patient's fears of being treated intrusively. Comments and casual reactions may be gratefully accepted, but efforts to push the client beyond what he or she is expressing will disconcert or antagonize the schizoid person, increasing tendencies toward withdrawal. Susan Deri (1968) has emphasized the importance of phrasing one's remarks in the words or images just used by the patient in order to reinforce the person's sense of reality and internal solidity. Hammer (1990) further cautions against probing, quizzing, or treating the patient in a way that makes him or her feel like a "case."

Normalizing is an important part of effective therapy with schizoid people. The general technique of "interpreting up" was discussed in Chapter 4 with reference to people at the psychotic end of the psychotic–borderline–neurotic axis; it is also useful for schizoid patients at any level of psychological health because of their difficulty believing that their hyperacute reactions will be understood and appreciated. Even if they are demonstrably high functioning, most schizoid people worry that they are fundamentally aberrant, incomprehensible to others. They want to be fully known by the people they care about, but they fear that if they are completely open about their inner life, they will be exposed as freaks.

Even those schizoid people who are confident of the superiority of their perceptions are not indifferent to the effect they may have in alienating others. By behaving in a way that communicates that the schizoid person's inner world is comprehensible, the therapist helps him or her to internalize the experience of being accepted without being asked to submit to the agenda of another person. Eventually, enough self-esteem accrues so that even when other people fail to understand, the patient can appreciate that the difficulty may not lie in the grotesqueness of the client's sensibilities; it may instead reflect the limitations of others. The therapist's reframing of imaginal richness as talent rather than pathology is deeply relieving to schizoid people, who may have had their emotional reactions disconfirmed or minimized all their lives by less sensitive commentators.

One way to give a schizoid patient confirmation without being experienced as either engulfing or minimizing is to use artistic and literary sources of imagery to communicate understanding of the patient's issues. Robbins (1988), in the honorable and now mostly ignored Freudian tradition of talking about oneself in the context of discussing some psychological dynamism, describes the early part of his own psychoanalysis as follows:

> When there were many lengthy silences in which I had little sense of what to say or how to communicate my feelings regarding my life history, fortunately my analyst did not desert me. Sometimes he would offer me "bedtime stories" [Robbins had never been read to as a child] in the form of citing plays, literature, and movies that had some relevance to the diffuse threads and images I presented to him in treatment. My curiosity was aroused by the references, and I made a point of reading the material. The likes of Ibsen, Dostoyevsky, and Kafka became important sources of rich symbolic material that seemed to mirror and clarify my inner experiences. Literature, and later art, seemed to give symbolic form to what I was trying to express. Most importantly, this material provided a significant means of sharing emotionally with my analyst. (p. 394)

Robbins and his colleagues (Robbins et al., 1980; Robbins, 1989) have made extensive contributions to the creative arts therapies and have elaborated on the aesthetic dimension of psychoanalytic work with clients, aspects of therapy that hold particular promise for those who are schizoid.

Perhaps the most common obstacle to therapeutic progress with schizoid patients—once the therapy relationship is soundly in place and the work of understanding is proceeding—is the tendency for both therapist and patient to form a kind of emotional cocoon, where they understand each other perfectly and look forward to therapy sessions as a respite from a demanding world. Schizoid people have a tendency, with which an empathic therapist may unwittingly collude, to try to make the therapy relationship a substitute for, rather than an enhancer of, their lives outside the treatment room. A considerable length of time may go by before the therapist notices that although the patient develops rich insights in nearly every session, he or she has not gone to a social function, asked anybody out, improved a sexual relationship, or embarked on a creative project.

The generalization to the outside world of the schizoid client's attainment of a safe intimacy with the therapist can be a considerable challenge. The therapist confronts the dilemma of having been hired to foster better social and intimate functioning yet realizing that any reminders to the patient that he or she is not pursuing that goal may be received as intrusive, controlling, and unempathic with the need for space. This tension is analyzable eventually, and it may deepen the schizoid person's appreciation of how powerful is the conflict between desire for closeness and fear of it. As with most aspects of therapy, timing is everything.

Robbins (1988) has emphasized the importance to the schizoid patient of the therapist's willingness to act like, and to be seen as, a "real person," not just a transference object. In recent years, the "real" relationship that coexists with transference reactions has been rediscovered and stressed by many dynamically oriented practitioners (e.g., Paolino, 1981). This has particular relevance for the schizoid person, who has an abundance of "as if" relationships and needs the sense of the therapist's active participation as a human being: supporting risks in the direction of relationships, being playful or humorous in ways that were absent in the client's history, and responding to the patient with attitudes that counteract his or her tendencies to hide or to go through the motions of connecting emotionally with others. With schizoid people, one finds that the client's transference reactions are not only not obscured by a more responsive therapeutic style, they may even be more accessible to interpretation.

DIFFERENTIAL DIAGNOSIS

Schizoid psychology is easy to recognize, given the relative indifference of schizoid people to making a conventional impression on the interviewer. The central diagnostic challenge is assessing the strength of the client's ego. Less portentously, some obsessive and compulsive people, especially in the borderline-to-psychotic range, are easily misconstrued as more schizoid than they are.

Degree of Pathology

It is critical, first of all, to evaluate how disturbed a person in the schizoid range is. It is probably experience with the importance of this dimension that led the contributors to the recent editions of the DSM to give several alternative schizoid diagnoses, something they did not do for several other characterological conditions that also exist with a wide range of severity. Obviously, it is critical to consider possible psychotic processes in an intake interview; questions about hallucinations and delusions, attention to the presence or absence of disordered thinking, evaluation of the patient's capacity to distinguish ideas from actions, and, in puzzling instances, psychological testing are warranted with people who present with a schizoid style. Medication and/or hospitalization may be indicated when the results of such inquiries suggest psychosis.

Misunderstanding a schizophrenic person as a nonpsychotic schizoid personality can be a costly blunder. It is an equally unfortunate mistake, however, to assume that a patient is at risk of decompensation simply because he or she has a schizoid character. Schizoid people are often seen as sicker than they are, and for a therapist to make this error compounds the insults these clients have absorbed throughout a life in which their individuality may have always been equated with lunacy. (Actually, even with a psychotic patient, the therapist's stance that the client is not "just" a schizophrenic but a person with significant strengths, who can reasonably expect to be helped, is the most effective reducer of psychotic-level anxiety.)

Admiration for the high-functioning schizoid person's originality and integrity is a therapeutic attitude that is easy to adopt once one has accepted the fact that schizoid processes are not necessarily ominous. Some healthy schizoid individuals who have come about a problem not inextricably tied up with their personality will not want their eccentricities to be addressed. This is their right. Therapeutic knowledge of how to make a schizoid person comfortable and disclosive can still facilitate work on the issues that the patient does wish to confront.

Schizoid versus Obsessive and Compulsive Personalities

Schizoid people often isolate themselves and spend a great deal of time thinking, even ruminating, about the major issues in their fantasy life. They can also, because of their conflict about closeness, appear wooden and affectless, and respond to questions with intellectualization. Some have quirks of behavior that are or appear to be compulsive, or they have arranged their lives according to an idiosyncratic set of rituals. Consequently, they can be readily misunderstood as having an obsessive or obsessive compulsive personality structure. Many people combine schizoid and obsessive or compulsive qualities, but insofar as the two kinds of personality organization can be discussed as "pure" types, there are some important differences.

Obsessive individuals, in marked contrast to schizoid people, are usually quite social and, in similar contrast to the schizoid person's march to a unique drummer, may be highly concerned with respectability, appropriateness, the approval of their peers, and their reputation in the community. Obsessive people are also apt to be moralistic, observing carefully the mores of their reference group, whereas schizoid people are not particularly invested in conventional questions of right and wrong. People with obsessive compulsive personalities deny or isolate feelings unlike schizoid individuals, who identify them internally and pull back from relationships that invite their expression.

SUMMARY

I have emphasized how people with schizoid personalities preserve a sense of safety by avoiding intimacy with others from whom they fear engulfment and by escaping to internal fantasy preoccupations. When conflicted about closeness versus distance, schizoid people will opt for the latter, despite its loneliness, because closeness is associated with having the self taken over in noxious ways. Possible constitutional components include hypersensitivity and a consequent avoidance of stimulation. In addition to the use of autistic-like withdrawal into fantasy, the schizoid person employs other "primitive" defenses but also shows enviable capacities for authenticity and creativity. The impact of these tendencies on relations with other people was discussed, with attention to the patterns of family interaction that may have fostered the schizoid person's approach–avoidance conflict, namely the coexistence of deprivation and intrusion.

Relevant transference and countertransference issues include difficulties in the therapist's initial admission into the client's world, a tendency for the therapist to share the client's feelings of either helpless vulnerability or grandiose superiority, and temptations to be complicit with the patient's reluctance to move toward others. Treatment recommendations include maximal self-awareness in the therapist, as well as patience, authenticity, normalization, and a willingness to use one's "real" personality. Finally, the importance of assessing accurately a person's location on the schizoid continuum was stressed, and the schizoid character was differentiated from obsessive and compulsive personalities.

SUGGESTION FOR FURTHER READING

Most commentary on the schizoid condition is buried in writing on schizophrenia. An eloquent and absorbing exception is Guntrip's (1969) *Schizoid Phenomena, Object-Relations and the Self.*

❖ 10 ❖
Paranoid Personalities

Most of us have a clear mental image of a paranoid person and recognize the type when it is portrayed fictionally. Peter Sellers's brilliant performance in *Doctor Strangelove*, for example, captures the suspiciousness, humorlessness, and grandiosity that strike familiar chords in any of us who have paranoid acquaintances, or who recognize the comic elaboration of the paranoid streak we can all find in ourselves. Identifying less flagrant paranoid presentations requires a more disciplined sensibility. The essence of paranoid personality organization is the habit of dealing with one's felt negative qualities by projecting them; the disowned attributes then feel like external threats. The projective process may or may not be accompanied by a consciously megalomanic sense of self.

The diagnosis of paranoid personality structure implies to many people a serious disturbance in mental health, yet as I argued in Chapter 4 with special reference to paranoia, this type of organization exists on a continuum of severity from psychotic to normal (Freud, 1911; Shapiro, 1965; Meissner, 1978).* It may be that "healthier" paranoid people are rarer than "sicker" ones, but as was true for the subjects of the preceding three chapters, someone can have a paranoid character at any level of ego strength, identity integration, reality testing, and object relations. Recent DSM accounts of Paranoid

*As with the personality types discussed in Chapters 7 through 9, the defense that defines paranoia derives from a time before the child had clarity about internal versus external events, where self and object were thus confused. Paranoia by definition involves experiencing what is inside as if it were outside the self.

Personality Disorder give an excellent (though unempathic) description of nonpsychotic paranoia, rightly noting that our knowledge of it may be limited. A paranoid person has to be in fairly deep trouble before he or she seeks (or is brought for) psychological help; paranoid people are not disposed to trust strangers. In contrast to depressive, hysterical or masochistic people, for example, higher-functioning paranoid individuals tend to avoid psychotherapy unless they are in severe emotional pain or are causing significant upset to others.

People with normal-level paranoid characters often seek out political roles, where their disposition to oppose themselves to forces they see as evil or threatening can find ready expression. Many reporters covering the 1992 American presidential elections ascribed paranoid characteristics to Ross Perot, but even some of these amateur diagnosticians probably voted for him on the basis of his realistic competence. J. Edgar Hoover was another high-functioning public figure who appears to have had a strong paranoid element in his personality. At the other end of the developmental continuum, some serial murderers who killed their victims out of the conviction that the victims were trying to murder them, and Charles Manson of the California "hippie" cult, exemplify the destructiveness of projection gone mad; that is, paranoia operating without the moderating effects of more mature ego processes and without a solid grounding in reality.

I want to emphasize again what I mentioned in Chapter 5: Attributions of paranoia should not be made on the basis of an interviewer's belief that a person seeking help is wrong about the danger he or she is in. Some people who look paranoid are actually being stalked or persecuted—by Satanic or other marginal cults, for example, or by a rejected lover or a disaffected relative. (Some people who are diagnosably paranoid are *also* realistically imperiled; in fact, the off-putting qualities of many paranoid people make them natural magnets for mistreatment.) When interviewing for diagnostic purposes, one should never reject out of hand the possibility that the interviewee is legitimately frightened, or that those who are urging him or her to seek therapy have a personal stake in making the client look crazy.

Contrastingly, some individuals who are in fact paranoid do not appear to be. Nonparanoid associates in their social group—and the interviewer for that matter—may share their beliefs about the dangers of certain people, forces, or institutions (communism, capitalism, religious authorities, pornographers, the media, the federal government, patriarchy, racists, people of color—whatever is perceived as the obstacle to the triumph of good) and may therefore fail to discern that there is something internally generated and driven about their preoccupations (see Cameron, 1959). If Congressman Allard Lowenstein had fathomed the paranoid character of Dennis Sweeney, one of his protégés in the student movements of the 1960s and the man who later assassinated him in the grip of a delusion, he would have known better than to behave in a way that was interpretable as sexually seductive, and he would probably be alive today (see Harris, 1982). But Lowenstein and Sweeney had similar beliefs about what social evils required confrontation, and where Lowenstein's were not primarily projections, Sweeney's were.*

There are also people whose perceptions turn out to be very prescient, who are nevertheless paranoid. Howard Hughes had a consuming terror of the consequences of atomic testing in Nevada at a time when no one else was particularly concerned with nuclear contamination of the environment. Years later, as the toll exacted by radiation became clearer, he looked a lot less crazy to many. But the eventual vindications of his point of view do not make him less a paranoid; the events of his later life speak for the extent to which his own projections were the source of his suffering (Maheu & Hack, 1992). My aim in bringing up all these possibilities is to stress the importance of making informed, reflective diagnostic judgments instead of automatic, a priori assumptions—especially with clients whose grim, suspicious qualities make them hard to warm up to.

DRIVE, AFFECT, AND TEMPERAMENT IN PARANOID PERSONALITIES

Because they see the sources of their suffering as outside themselves, paranoid people in the more disturbed range are likely to be more dangerous to others than to themselves. They are much less suicidal than equally disturbed depressives, although they have been known to kill themselves to preempt someone else's (imagined) imminent destruction of them. The angry, threatening qualities of many paranoid people have prompted speculations that one contributant to a paranoid orientation is a high degree of innate aggression or irritability. It stands to reason that high levels of aggressive energy would be hard for a

*Social and political movements inevitably contain subgroups of paranoid participants whose fanaticism inspires disdain in those outside the movement and distress in those within it. If these elements are publicized as representative of the cause, other paranoid people become attracted to it—a phenomenon that has plagued grass-roots political organization in the media age.

young child to manage and integrate into a positively valued sense of self, and that the negative responses of caregivers to an obstreperous, demanding infant or toddler would reinforce his or her sense that outsiders are persecutory. Meissner (1978) has marshalled some empirical evidence (Chess, Rutter, Thomas, & Birch, 1963; Chess, Thomas, & Birch, 1967) connecting paranoia with an "active" symptomatic style in infancy (irregularity, nonadaptability, intensity of reaction, and negative mood) and with a thin stimulus barrier and consequent hyperexcitability (Bergman & Escalona, 1949; Brazelton, 1962).

Affectively, paranoid people struggle not only with anger, resentment, vindictiveness and the other more hostile feelings, they also suffer overwhelmingly from fear. Silvan Tomkins (e.g., 1963), whose theoretical work integrated empirical research to an extent unusual in psychodynamically sensitive writing, regarded the paranoid stance as a combination of fear and shame. The downward-left eye movements common in paranoid people (the "shifty" quality that even nonprofessionals notice) are physically a compromise between the horizontal-left direction specific to the affect of pure fear and the straight-down direction of uncontaminated shame (S. Tomkins, personal communication, 1972). Even the most grandiose paranoid person lives with the terror of harm from others and monitors each human interaction with extreme vigilance.

As for shame, that affect is as great a menace to paranoid people as to narcissistic ones, but the danger is experienced quite differently by each type of person. Narcissistic people, even of the most arrogant variety, are subject to conscious feelings of shame if they are unmasked in certain ways. Their energies go into efforts to impress others so that the devalued self will not be exposed to them. Paranoid people, contrastingly, use denial and projection so powerfully that no sense of shame remains accessible within the self. The energies of the paranoid person are therefore spent on foiling the efforts of those who are seen as bent on shaming and humiliating them. People with narcissistic character structures are afraid of revealing their inadequacies; those with paranoid personalities are afraid of other people's malevolence. This focus on the motives of others rather than on the nature of the self is, as anyone experienced with paranoid patients can testify, a formidable obstacle to therapy.

Also like narcissistic people, paranoid individuals are very vulnerable to envy. Unlike them, they handle it projectively. The degree of anger and intensity that they have to manage may account for some of the difference. Resentment and jealousy, occasionally of delusional proportions, darken their lives. Sometimes those attitudes are directly projected, taking the form of the conviction that "others are out to get me because of the things about me that they envy"; more often they are ancillary to the denial and projection of other affects and impulses, as when a paranoid man, oblivious to his own normal fantasies of infidelity, becomes convinced his wife is dangerously attracted to others. Frequently involved in this kind of jealousy is an unconscious yearning for closeness with a person of the same sex. Because paranoid people confuse such longings with erotic homosexuality (Ovesey, 1955; Karon, 1989), an orientation that frightens them, the wishes are abhorred and denied. These desires for care from a person of the same gender then resurface as the conviction that it is, for example, one's girlfriend rather than oneself who wants to be more intimate with a mutual male friend.

Finally, paranoid people are profoundly burdened with guilt, a feeling that is unacknowledged and projected in the same way that shame is. Some reasons for their deep sense of badness will be suggested below, along with ways of trying to relieve it therapeutically. Their unbearable burden of unconscious guilt is another feature of their psychology that makes paranoid clients so hard to help: They live in terror that when the therapist really gets to know them, he or she will be shocked by all their sins and depravities, and will reject them or punish them for their crimes. They are chronically warding off this humiliation, transforming any sense of culpability in the self into dangers that threaten from outside. They unconsciously expect to be found out, and they transform this fear into constant, exhausting efforts to discern the "real" evil intent behind anyone else's behavior toward them.

DEFENSIVE AND ADAPTIVE PROCESSES IN PARANOIA

By definition, projection dominates the psychology of the paranoid person. Depending on the patient's ego strength and degree of stress, it may be a psychotic, borderline, or neurotic level of projection. To review, the differences are as follows. In a frankly psychotic person, upsetting parts of the self are projected and fully believed to be "out there," no matter how crazy the projections may seem to others. The paranoid schizophrenic who believes that homosexual Bulgarian agents have poisoned his water is projecting his aggression, his wish for same-sex closeness, his ethnocentrism, and his fantasies of power. He does not find ways of making his beliefs fit with conventional notions of reality; he may be quite convinced that he is the only one in the world who sees the threat.

Because reality testing is (by definition) not lost in people at a borderline level of personality organization, paranoid patients in the borderline range project in such a way that those on whom disowned attitudes are projected are subtly provoked to feel those attitudes. This is projective identification: The person tries to get rid of certain feelings, yet retains empathy with them and needs to reassure the self that they are realistic. The borderline paranoid person works to make his or her projections "fit" the projective target. Thus the woman who disowns her hatred and envy announces to her therapist in an antagonistic manner that she can tell that the therapist is jealous of her accomplishments; interpretations given in a sympathetic spirit are reinterpreted by the client as evidence of envy-driven wishes to undermine and control, and soon the therapist, worn down by being steadily misunderstood, is hating the patient and envying her freedom to vent her spleen (Searles, 1959). This remarkable process torments therapists, who do not choose their profession expecting to have to endure such powerful negative feelings toward those they want to heal; it accounts for the general intolerance among many mental health professionals toward both borderline and paranoid patients.

In paranoid people at the neurotic level, internal issues are projected in a potentially ego-alien way. That is, the patient projects yet has some observing part of the self that eventually will be capable, in the context of a reliable relationship, of acknowledging the externalized contents of the mind as projection. People who, in an intake interview, describe themselves as paranoid are often in this category (though borderline and psychotic paranoid clients may sometimes talk this way also, in an effort to show that they know the jargon but without any real internal appreciation that their fears constitute projections).

A talented and healthy but characterologically paranoid patient of mine was subject to profound fears that I would sell him out in the service of my need to look good to others. For example, if a professional in the community who knew both of us were to criticize him to me, he was sure that I would somehow convey agreement. (Meanwhile, when he felt hurt in the transference, he had no reluctance to complain about me in ways that made some of my colleagues quite critical of my treatment of him.) Even before he was able to understand this fear as the projection of his own—unnecessarily hated—needs for acceptance and admiration, plus the projection and acting out of his defensive criticism, he was willing to consider that he might be putting something on me that I did not deserve.

The need of the paranoid person to handle upsetting feelings projectively entails the use of an unusual degree of denial and its close relative, reaction formation. All human beings project; indeed, the universal disposition toward projection is the basis for transference, the process that makes analytic therapy possible. But paranoid people do it in the context of such a great need to disavow upsetting attitudes that it feels like a whole different process from projective operations in which denial is not so integral. Freud (1911) accounted for paranoia, at least of the psychotic variety, by the successive unconscious operations of reaction formation ("I don't love you; I hate you") and projection ("I don't hate you; you hate me").

This is only one of several possible routes according to which the paranoid person emerges at a psychological place that may seem very far from the original, more humanly comprehensible attitudes that initiated the paranoid process (Salzman, 1960b). On this topic, Karon (1989) summarizes the ways in which a delusional paranoid person can handle wishes for same-sex closeness:

> If one considers the different ways in which one could contradict the feeling "I love him," one derives many typical delusions. "I do not love him, I love me (megalomania)." "I do not love him, I love her (erotomania)." "I do not love him, she loves him (delusional jealousy)." "I do not love him, he loves me (projecting the homosexuality, producing a delusional homosexual threat)." "I do not love him, I hate him (reaction formation)." And, finally, most common, projecting the delusional hatred as "He hates me, hence, it is alright for me to hate him (and if I hate him, I do not love him)." (p. 176)

Again, a significant difficulty in working with paranoid people concerns how long and convoluted is the distance between their basic affects and their defensive handling of them.

OBJECT RELATIONS IN PARANOIA

Clinical experience suggests that children who grow up paranoid have suffered severe insults to their sense of efficacy; more specifically, they have repeatedly felt overpowered and humiliated (Will, 1961; Tomkins, 1963; MacKinnon & Michels, 1971). In the family of Daniel Paul Schreber, from whose report of a paranoid psychosis Freud (1911) extracted a theory of paranoia, the father was a domineering patriarch who advocated, and insisted on his son's adopting, arduous physical regimes intended to toughen children up (Niederland, 1959).* Criti-

*See, however, Lothane's (1992) recent contrary evidence for the "soul murder" of Schreber not by his father, but by authorities he trusted and by the legal system of his era.

cism, capricious punishment, adults who cannot be pleased, and utter mortification are common in the backgrounds of paranoid people.

Those who rear children that become paranoid also frequently teach by example. A child may observe suspicious, condemnatory attitudes in parents, who emphasize—paradoxically, in view of their abusive qualities and the objectively kinder worlds of school and community—that family members are the only people one can trust. Paranoid people in the borderline and psychotic ranges tend to come from harsh homes where criticism and ridicule dominated familial relationships, or where one child, the future sufferer of paranoia, was the scapegoat—the target of the family members' hated and projected attributes, especially those in the general category of "weakness." Those in the neurotic-to-healthy range tend to come from families in which warmth and stability were combined with teasing and sarcasm.

Another contributant to paranoid personality organization is unmanageable anxiety—not necessarily of a paranoid variety—in a primary caregiver. A paranoid patient of mine came from a family in which the mother was so chronically nervous that she took a thermos of water with her everywhere she went (for her dry mouth) and described her body as having "turned into a cement block" from accumulated tension. Whenever her daughter would come to her with a problem, the mother would either deny it, because she could not bear any additional worries, or catastrophize about it, because she could not contain her anxiety. The mother was also confused about the line between fantasy and behavior and hence conveyed to her child that thoughts equalled deeds. The daughter got the message that her private feelings, whether loving or hateful, had a dangerous power.

For example, when once as an adult my patient told her mother that in reaction to her husband's arbitrariness she had challenged him, her mother first contended she was misreading him: He was a devoted husband, and she must be imagining anything objectionable coming from him. When my patient persisted with an account of the argument, her mother urged her to be careful, as he might beat her up or abandon her if provoked (she herself had been battered and then divorced by her husband). And when my patient went on to vent anger at how he had acted, she was begged to think about something else so that her negative thoughts would not make things worse. This well-meaning but very disturbed mother, who had had no comfort as a youngster, was incapable of comforting. In her daughter's formative years, her anxiety-soaked advice and dire predictions compounded the girl's fears. My client thus grew up being able to console herself only by drastic transformations of her feelings. When I began working with her, she had already seen several therapists who had been defeated by her bottomless need and relentless hostility. All of them had, appropriately, seen her as paranoid in either the psychotic or low-level borderline range. Her capacity to report transactions like the preceding to me, and to comprehend how destructive similar ones had been all her life, came only after many years of therapy.*

One can detect in the preceding example of distorted maternal responsiveness several different seeds of paranoia. First, both reality and the patient's normal emotional reactions to it were disconfirmed, instilling fear and shame rather than a sense of being understood. Second, denial and projection were modeled. Third, primitive omnipotent fantasies were reinforced, laying the foundation for a diffuse and overwhelming guilt. Finally, the interaction created additional anger while resolving none of the original distress, thus magnifying the patient's confusion about basic feelings and perceptions. In situations like this, where a person has been implicitly insulted (in this case, seen as unappreciative, incapable of managing feelings, dangerous), he or she must at some level feel even more aggravated than originally. But such a reaction may be judged as either incomprehensible or evil because the insulting party was only trying to help.

These kinds of mind-muddling transactions get replicated repeatedly in the adult relationships of paranoid people. Their internalized objects keep undermining both the paranoid person and those to whom he or she relates. If a child's primary source of knowledge is a caregiver who is deeply confused and primitively defended, who—in desperate attempts to feel safe or important—uses words not to express honest feeling but to manipulate, the child's subsequent human relations cannot be unaffected. The struggle of the paranoid person to understand what is "really" going on (Shapiro, 1965) is comprehensible in this light, as is the bewilderment, helplessness, and estrangement that occur in people dealing with paranoid friends, acquaintances, and relatives.

The mother's anxiety was not the only influence on this woman's psychology, of course. If she had had any significant caregiver capable of relating in a confirmatory way, her personality would probably not have developed in a paranoid direction. But her father, prior to abandoning his family when she was an older teenager, was frighteningly critical, explosive, and disrespectful of boundaries. The

*An adolescent prototype for this interaction was her telling her mother of her father's effort to molest her. Her mother managed both to insist that it had not happened and to blame it on her daughter's sexuality. For a detailed case history of this tormented yet persevering and ultimately recovering woman, see McWilliams (1986).

tendency of paranoid people to lash out rather than endure the anxiety of passively awaiting inevitable mistreatment ("I'll hit you before you hit me") is another well-known and unfortunate cost of this kind of parenting (Nydes, 1963). The presence of a frightening parent and the absence of people who can help the child process the resulting feelings (except by making them worse) is, according to many therapists who have successfully mitigated the condition, a common breeding ground for paranoia (MacKinnon & Michels, 1971).

Because of their orientation toward issues of power and their tendency to act out, paranoid people have some qualities in common with psychopathic ones. But a critical difference lies in their capacity to love. Even though they may be racked with suspicion about the motives and intentions of those they care about, paranoid individuals are capable of deep attachment and protracted loyalty. However persecutory or inappropriate they experienced their childhood caregivers, there was apparently enough availability and consistency in their early lives to preserve a sense of caring. The survival of this attitude is what makes empathically attuned therapy possible in spite of all their distortions, antagonisms, and terrors.

THE PARANOID SELF

The main polarity in the self-representations of paranoid people is an impotent, humiliated, and despised image of the self versus an omnipotent, vindicated, triumphant one. A tension between these two images suffuses their subjective world. Cruelly, neither position affords any solace: A terror of abuse and contempt goes with the weak side of the polarity, while the strong side brings with it the inevitable side effect of psychological power, a crushing guilt.

The weak side of this polarity is evident in the degree of fear with which paranoid people chronically live. They never feel fully safe and spend an inordinate amount of their emotional energy scanning the environment for dangers. The grandiose side is evident in their self-referential stance: Everything that happens has something to do with them personally. This is most obvious in psychotic levels of paranoia, instances in which a patient believes, say, that he or she is the personal target of an international spy ring or is receiving covert messages during television commercials about the incipient end of the world. But I have also heard high-achieving, reality-oriented clients ruminate about whether the fact that someone sat in their usual chair revealed a plot to harass and humiliate them. Incidentally, such clients often do not come across as paranoid in the intake interview, and it can be startling to the therapist to hear, after several sessions, the emergence of the organizing conviction that everything that happens to them reflects the significance to other people of their individual existence.

The megalomania of paranoid people, whether unconscious or overt, burdens them with unbearable guilt. If I am omnipotent, then all kinds of terrible things are my fault. The intimate connection between guilt and paranoia can be intuitively comprehended by any of us who have felt culpable and then worried about being exposed and punished. I notice that when one of my students is late turning in a paper, he or she avoids me whenever possible, as if the only thing on my mind is that transgression and my planned retribution. A women I was treating who was having an extramarital affair reported with amusement that while she was on a drive with her lover, holding hands in the car, she noticed a police vehicle ahead and pulled her hand away.

A complex and pervasive issue for many paranoid people is the combination of sexual identity confusion, longings for same-sex closeness, and associated preoccupations with homosexuality. A connection between paranoia and homosexual preoccupations has been frequently noted by clinicians (e.g., Searles, 1961) and has been confirmed by some empirical studies (e.g., Aronson, 1964). Paranoid people, even the minority of them who have acted on homoerotic feelings, may regard the idea of same-sex attraction as upsetting to a degree that is scarcely imaginable to the nonparanoid. To gay and lesbian people, who find it hard to see why their sexual orientation is perceived as so threatening, the homophobia of the paranoid is truly menacing. As the brief triumph of Nazism demonstrates, when paranoid trends are shared by a whole culture or subculture, the most horrific possibilities arise.*

The paranoid preoccupation with homosexuality has sometimes been explained as reflecting "unconscious homosexual impulses." This locution is misleading, in that it is not usually genital urges that stimulate homophobia; it is loneliness and the wish for a soulmate. As Karon (1989) has commonsensically explained:

*Students of the rise of Nazism (e.g., F. Stern, 1961; Gay, 1968; Rhodes, 1980) locate its psychological origins in the same kinds of events that clinicians have found in the childhoods of individual paranoid people. The crushing humiliation of Germany in World War I, and the subsequent punitive measures that created runaway inflation, starvation, and panic, with little responsiveness from the international community, laid the groundwork for the appeal of a paranoid leader and the organized paranoia that is Nazism. The homophobia of the Nazis is legendary, of course.

> Because as children we were comfortable with peers of the same sex before we became comfortable with opposite-sex peers, and because people of the same sex are more like us than people of the opposite sex, when we are withdrawn from everyone, we are attracted to someone of the same sex. Unfortunately, the patient becomes aware of this attraction, misinterprets it as homosexuality, and this sets off the defenses (p. 176)

In other words, at the core of the self-experience of paranoid people is a profound emotional isolation and need for what Sullivan (1953) called "consensual validation" from a "chum."

The main way in which paranoid people try to enhance their self-esteem is through exerting effective power against authorities and other people of importance. Experiences of vindication and triumph give them a relieving (although fleeting) sense of both safety and moral rectitude. The dreaded litigiousness of paranoid individuals derives from this need to challenge and defeat the persecutory parent. Some people with paranoid personalities provide devoted service to victims of oppression and mistreatment, because their disposition to battle unjust authorities and vindicate underdogs keeps them on the barricades far longer than other well-meaning social activists whose psychodynamics do not similarly protect them against burnout.

TRANSFERENCE AND COUNTERTRANSFERENCE WITH PARANOID PATIENTS

Transference in most paranoid patients is swift, intense, and negative. Occasionally, the therapist is the recipient of projected savior images, but more commonly he or she is seen as potentially disconfirming and humiliating. Paranoid clients approach a psychological evaluation with the expectation that the interviewer is out to feel superior by exposing their badness, or is pursuing some similar agenda that has nothing to do with their well-being. They tend to strike clinicians as grim, humorless, and poised to criticize. They may fix their eyes relentlessly on the therapist in what has been called the "paranoid stare."

Not surprisingly, interviewers respond with a sense of vulnerability and general defensiveness. Countertransference is usually either anxious or hostile; in the less common instance of being regarded as a savior, it may be benevolently grandiose. In any case, the therapist is usually aware of strong reactions, in contrast to the often subtler countertransferences that arise with narcissistic and schizoid patients.

Because of the combination of denial and projection that constitute paranoia, causing the repudiated parts of the self to be extruded, therapists of paranoid patients often find themselves consciously feeling the aspect of an emotional reaction that the client has exiled from consciousness. For example, the patient may be full of hostility, while the therapist feels the fear against which the hostility is a defense. Or the patient may feel vulnerable and helpless, while the therapist feels sadistic and powerful.

Because of the weight of these internal reactions in the therapist, and the extent to which they betray to a sensitive person the degree of suffering that a paranoid client is trying to manage, there is a countertransference tendency in most therapists to try to "set the patient straight" about the unrealistic nature of whatever danger the patient believes he or she is in. Most of us who have practiced for any length of time have had at least one client who seemed to be crying out for reassurance and yet, upon receiving it, became convinced that we were part of the conspiracy to divert him or her from a terrible threat. The therapist's powerlessness to give much immediate help to a person who is so unhappy and suspicious is probably the earliest and most intimidating barrier to establishing the kind of relationship that can eventually offer relief.

THERAPEUTIC IMPLICATIONS OF THE DIAGNOSIS OF PARANOIA

The first challenge a therapist faces with a paranoid patient is creating a solid working alliance. Although establishing such a relationship is necessary (and sometimes challenging) for the successful treatment of any client, it is particularly important in work with paranoid people because of their difficulty trusting. A beginning student of mine, asked about his plan for working with a very paranoid woman, commented, "First I'll get her to trust me. Then I'll work on assertiveness skills." Wrong. When a paranoid person truly trusts the therapist, the treatment is over, and it has been a huge success. But the student was right in one sense: There has to be some initial embracing by the client of the *possibility* that the therapist is well-intentioned and competent. And this takes not only considerable forbearance from the therapist, it takes some capacity for comfort talking about the negative transference and conveying that the degree of hatred and suspicion aimed at the clinician is to be expected. The therapist's unflustered acceptance of powerful degrees of hostility contributes to the patient's sense of safety from retribution, mitigates fear that hatred destroys, and exemplifies how aspects of the self that the patient has regarded as evil are simply ordinary human qualities.

The technique part of this chapter will be longer than most comparable sections because effective therapeutic procedure with paranoid clients differs substantially from what most of us regard as "standard" psychoanalytic practice. Although it has in common the goals of understanding at the deepest level, bringing into consciousness the unknown aspects of the self, and promoting the most thoroughgoing possible acceptance of one's full humanity, it accomplishes these ends differently. For example, interpretation "from surface to depth" is usually impossible with paranoid clients because so many radical transformations of their original feelings have preceded their manifest preoccupations. A man who longs for support from someone of his gender, who has unconsciously misread that yearning as sexual desire, denied that, projected it on to someone else, displaced it, and become overwhelmed with fears that his wife is having an affair with his friend will not have his real concerns addressed if the therapist encourages him to associate to the idea of his wife's infidelity.

"Analyzing resistance before content" can be similarly ill-fated. Commenting on actions or statements made by a paranoid client only makes him or her feel judged or scrutinized like a laboratory guinea pig (Hammer, 1990). Analysis of the defenses of denial and projection elicits only more Byzantine uses of the same defenses. The conventional aspects of psychoanalytic technique, such as exploring rather than answering questions, bringing up aspects of a patient's behavior that may be expressing an unconscious or withheld feeling, calling attention to slips, and so forth, were designed to increase patients' access to internal material and to support their courage to talk more openly about it (Greenson, 1967). With paranoid people, such practices boomerang. If the standard ways of helping clients to open up elicit only further elaborations of a paranoid sensibility, how can one help?

First, one can call on a sense of humor. Most experts (e.g., MacKinnon & Michels, 1971) have advised against joking in the treatment of paranoia lest the patient feel teased and ridiculed. This caution is warranted, but it does not rule out the therapist's modeling an attitude of self-mockery, amusement at the world's irrationalities, and other nonbelittling forms of wit. Humor is indispensable in therapy—perhaps especially with paranoid clients—since jokes are a time-honored way to discharge aggression safely. Nothing relieves both patient and therapist more than glimpses of light behind the gloomy stormcloud that envelopes a paranoid person. The best way to set the stage for mutual enjoyment of humor is to laugh at one's own foibles, pretensions, and mistakes. Paranoid people miss nothing; no defect in the therapist is safe from their scrutiny. A friend of mine claims to have perfected the "nose yawn," a priceless asset to the conduct of psychotherapy, but I would bet my couch that even he could not fool a good paranoid. The woman whose history I described earlier in this chapter has *never* failed to notice my yawning, no matter how immobile my face. I reacted to her initial confrontations about this with apologetic admissions that she had found me out again, and with whining self-pity about not being able to get away with anything in her presence. This kind of reaction, rather than the heavy, humorless exploration of what her fantasy was when she thought I was yawning, has expedited our work together.

Naturally, one stands ready to apologize if one's wit is mistaken for ridicule, but the idea that work with hypersensitive patients must be conducted in an atmosphere of oppressive seriousness is unnecessarily fussy. Especially after a reliable working alliance has been established, something that may take months or years, a modicum of judicious teasing, in an effort to make omnipotent fantasies ego alien, can be very helpful to a paranoid person. Jule Nydes (1963), who had an enviable gift for working with difficult clients, cites the following interventions:

> One patient . . . was convinced that his plane would crash while en route to a well earned vacation in Europe. He was startled and relieved when I remarked, "Do you think God is so merciless that He would sacrifice the lives of a hundred other people simply to get at you?"
>
> Another such example is that of a young woman . . . who developed strong paranoid fears shortly before her forthcoming marriage which she unconsciously experienced as an outstanding triumph. This was at the time the "mad bomber" was planting his lethal weapons in subway cars. She was certain that she would be destroyed by a bomb, and so she avoided the subway. "Aren't you afraid of the 'mad bomber'?" she asked me. And then before I could reply she sneered, "Of course not. You ride only in taxicabs." I assured her that I rode the subways and that I was unafraid for the very good reason that I knew the "mad bomber" was out to get her, not me. (p. 71)

Hammer (1990), who stresses the importance of indirect, face-saving ways of sharing insights with paranoid patients, recommends the following joke as a way to interpret the drawbacks of projection:

> A man goes toward his neighbor's house to borrow a lawnmower, thinking how nice his friend is to extend him such favors. As he

> walks along, however, doubts concerning the loan begin to gnaw at him. Maybe the neighbor would rather not lend it. By the time he arrives, the doubts have given way to rage, and as the friend appears at the door the man shouts, "You know what you can do with your damn lawnmower; shove it!" (p. 142)

Humor, especially willingness to laugh at oneself, is probably therapeutic in that to the patient it represents being "real," rather than playing a role and pursuing a secret game plan. The histories of paranoid people may be so bereft of basic authenticity that the therapist's direct emotional honesty comes as a revelation about how people can relate to each other. With some reservations cited below, having to do with maintaining clear boundaries, I recommend being very forthcoming with paranoid clients. This means responding to their questions honestly rather than withholding answers and investigating the thoughts behind the inquiry; it is my experience that when the manifest content of a paranoid person's concern is respectfully addressed, he or she becomes more rather than less willing to look at the latent concerns represented in it.

Second, one can "go under" or "sidestep" or "do an end run around" (depending on one's favorite metaphor) the complex paranoid defense to the affects against which it has been erected. In the preceding hypothetical case of the man consumed with ruminations about his wife's possible infidelity, one could be helpful by commenting on how lonely and unsupported he seems to feel. It is startling to see how fast a paranoid harangue can disappear if the therapist simply lets it run its course, avoiding all temptations to address the content of a convoluted defensive process, and then engages empathically with the disowned, projected feelings from which the angry preoccupation originally sprang.

Often the best clue to the original feeling being defended against is one's countertransference; paranoid people are usefully imagined as actually projecting their unacknowledged attitudes *physically* into the therapist. Thus, when the patient is in an unrelenting, righteous, powerful rage, and the therapist feels resultingly threatened and helpless, it may be deeply affirming for the client to be told, "I know that what you're in touch with is how angry you are, but I sense that in addition to that anger, you're coping with profound feelings of fear and helplessness." Even if one is wrong, the client hears that the therapist wants to understand what is creating such severe degrees of upset.

Third, one can frequently help patients suffering from an increase in paranoid reactions by identifying what has happened in their recent experience to upset them. Such precipitants usually involve separation (a child has started school, a friend has moved away, a parent has not answered a letter), failure, or—paradoxically—success (failures are humiliating; successes involve omnipotent guilt and fears of punishment). One of my patients tends to go on long paranoid tirades, during which I can usually figure out what he is reacting to only after 20 or 30 minutes. If I assiduously avoid confronting his paranoid operations and instead comment on how he may be underestimating how bothered he is by something that he mentioned in passing, his paranoia tends to lift without any analysis of that process at all. Educating people to notice their states of arousal and look for precipitants often preempts the paranoid process altogether.

One should usually avoid direct confrontation of the content of a paranoid idea. Paranoid people are acutely perceptive about emotion and attitude; where they get mixed up is on the level of interpretation of the *meaning* of these manifestations (Sullivan, 1953; Shapiro, 1965; Meissner, 1978). When one challenges their interpretations, they tend to believe that one is telling them they are crazy for having seen what they saw, rather than that they have misconstrued its implications. Hence, although it is tempting to offer alternative interpretations, if one does this too readily, the patient feels dismissed, disparaged, and robbed of the astute perceptions that stimulated the paranoid interpretation.

When a paranoid client is brave enough to ask outright whether the clinician agrees with his or her understanding of something, the therapist can offer other interpretive possibilities with suitable tentativeness ("I can see why you thought the man intended to cut you off, but another possibility is that he'd had a fight with his boss and would have been driving like a maniac no matter who was on the road"). Notice that the therapist in this example has not substituted a more benevolent motive for the paranoid person's self-referential one ("perhaps he was swerving to avoid hitting an animal") because if paranoid people think one is trying to pretty up intentions that they *know* are debased, they will get more anxious rather than less. Note also that the comment is made in the tone of a throw-away line, so that the patient can either take it or leave it. With paranoid patients one should avoid any interventions that invite them to explicitly accept or reject the therapist's ideas. From their perspective, acceptance equals a humiliating submission and rejection invites retribution.

Fourth, one can make repeated distinctions between thoughts and actions, holding up the most heinous fantasies as examples of the remarkable, admirable, creative perversity of human nature. The therapist's capacity to feel pleasure in hostility, greed, lust, and similar less-than-stellar tendencies without acting them out helps the patient to reduce fears of an out-of-control, evil core. Lloyd Silverman (1984) has stressed the general value of going beyond interpretation of feelings and fantasies to the recommendation that one enjoy them, a particularly important dimension of work with paranoid people. Sometimes without this aspect of treatment, patients get the idea that the purpose of therapy is to help them purge themselves of such feelings rather than to help them embrace them as part of the human condition.

When one of my daughters was a preschooler, a nursery-school teacher promulgated the idea that virtue involved "thinking good thoughts and doing good deeds." This troubled her. She was much relieved when I commented that I disagreed with her teacher and felt that thinking bad thoughts was a lot of fun, especially when one could do good deeds in spite of those thoughts. For months afterward, especially when she was trying not to abuse her infant sister, she would get a mischievous expression on her face and announce, "I'm doing good deeds and thinking very bad thoughts!" Although she was a much quicker study than a person with a lifetime of confusion about fantasy and reality, what I was trying to teach her is the same message that is healing to paranoid clients.

Fifth, one must be hyperattentive to boundaries. Whereas one might sometimes lend a book out or spontaneously admire a new hairstyle with another kind of patient, such behaviors are rife with complication when enacted with a paranoid person. Paranoid clients are perpetually worried that the therapist will step out of role and use them for some end unrelated to their psychological needs. Even those who develop intensely idealizing transferences and insist that they want a "real" friendship with the therapist—perhaps especially these clients—react with terror if one acts in a way that seems uncharacteristically self-extending.

Consistency is critical to a paranoid person's sense of security; inconsistency stimulates fantasies that wishes have too much power. Exactly what the individual therapist's boundaries are (e.g., how missed sessions or phone calls to the therapist's home are handled) matters less than how reliably they are observed. It is much more therapeutic for a paranoid person to rage and grieve about the limits of the relationship than to worry that the therapist can actually be seduced or frightened out of his or her customary stance. While a surprising deviation that speaks for the therapist's caring can light a spark of hope for a depressive person, it will ignite a blaze of anxiety in a paranoid patient.

On this topic, I should mention the risk of pseudoerotic transference storms in paranoid clients. Same-sex therapists have to be even more carefully professional that opposite-sex ones, on account of the vulnerability of many paranoid people to homosexual panic, but both may find themselves suddenly the target of an intense sexualized hunger or rage. The combination of extreme psychological deprivation and cognitive confusion (affection with sex, thoughts with action, inside with outside) often produces eroticized misunderstandings and fears. The best the therapist can do is to restore the therapeutic frame, tolerate the outburst, normalize the feelings behind the eruption, and differentiate between those feelings and the behavioral limits that make psychotherapy possible.

Finally, it is critical that one convey both personal strength and unequivocal frankness to paranoid clients. Because they are so full of hostile and aggressive strivings, so confused about where thoughts leave off and actions begin, and so plagued with feelings of destructive omnipotence, their greatest worry in a therapy relationship is that their evil inner processes will injure or destroy the therapist. They need to know that the person treating them is stronger than their fantasies. Sometimes what matters more than what is said to a paranoid person is how confidently, forthrightly, and fearlessly the therapist delivers the message.

Most people who have written about the actual experience of treating paranoid people (as opposed to the much larger literature on theories about the origins of paranoid processes) have stressed respect, integrity, tact, and patience (Fromm-Reichmann, 1950; Arieti, 1961; Searles, 1965; MacKinnon & Michels, 1971; Karon, 1989; Hammer, 1990). Some, especially those who have worked with psychotic clients, have recommended endorsing the patient's view of reality, in order to create enough affirmation for him or her to start shedding the paranoid constructions that therapist and client now seem to share (Lindner, 1955; Spotnitz, 1969). Most writers, however, feel one can convey respect for the client's distortions, and avoid injurious critiques of them, without going that far.

Because of their excruciating sensitivity to insult and threat, it is not possible to treat paranoid patients without some debacles. Sometimes the therapy work seems like an endless exercise in damage control. Moreover, in the short run, one has to tolerate a protracted feeling of standing alone, since people with paranoid psychologies are not inclined to confirm, by verbal acknowledgment or visible appreciation, one's exertions in the service of understanding. But a devoted, reasonably humble, honest practitioner can make a radical difference over the years with a paranoid person, and will find beneath all the client's rage and indignation a deep well of warmth and gratitude.

DIFFERENTIAL DIAGNOSIS

The diagnosis of paranoid personality structure is usually easy to make, except, as noted previously, in instances in which a person is high functioning and trying to keep the extent of his or her paranoia hidden from the interviewer. As with schizoid clients, attention to the possibility of psychotic processes in a manifestly paranoid patient is warranted.

Paranoid versus Psychopathic Personality

In Chapter 7 I commented on the differential importance of guilt as a central dynamic in the respective psychologies of paranoid and antisocial people. I should also mention love. If a paranoid person feels that you and he or she share basic values, and that you can be counted upon in adversity, there is virtually no limit to the loyalty and generosity of which he or she is capable. Projective processes are common in antisocial people, but where psychopaths are fundamentally unempathic, paranoid people are deeply object related. The main threat to long-term attachment in paranoid people is not lack of feeling for others but rather experiences of betrayal; in fact, they are capable of cutting off a relationship of 30-years' duration when they feel wronged. Because they connect with others on the basis of similar moral sensibilities and hence feel that they and their love objects are united in an appreciation of what is good and right, any perceived moral failing by the person with whom they are identified feels like a flaw in the self that must be eradicated by banishing the offending object. But a history of aborted relationships is not the same thing as an inability to love.

Paranoid versus Obsessive Personality

Obsessive people share with paranoid individuals a sensitivity to issues of justice and rules, a rigidity and denial around the "softer" emotions, a preoccupation with issues of control, a vulnerability to shame, and a penchant for righteous indignation. They also scrutinize details and may misunderstand the big picture because of their fixation on minutia. Further, obsessional people in the process of decompensating into psychosis may slide gradually from irrational obsessions into paranoid delusions. Many people have both paranoid and obsessional features.

People in these respective diagnostic categories differ, however, in the role of humiliation in their histories and sensitivities; the obsessive person is afraid of being controlled but lacks the paranoid person's fear of physical harm and emotional mortification. Obsessive patients are much more likely to try to cooperate with the interviewer despite their oppositional qualities, and therapists working with them do not suffer the degree of anxiety that paranoid patients induce. Standard psychoanalytic technique is usually helpful to obsessive clients; rage reactions to conventional clarifications and interpretations in a patient one has believed to be obsessional may be the first sign that his or her paranoid qualities predominate.

Paranoid versus Dissociative Personality

Most people with multiple personality disorder have an alter personality that carries the paranoia for the personality system and may impress an interviewer as representative of the whole person. Because emotional mistreatment is implicated in the etiologies of both paranoia and dissociation, the coexistence in individual people of these processes is common. In Chapter 15 I will discuss the diagnosis of dissociative disorders thoroughly enough that it will be clear how to discriminate an individual with a paranoid personality from a dissociative person with a paranoid alter personality or paranoid tendencies.

SUMMARY

I have described the manifest and latent qualities of people whose personalities are predominantly paranoid, stressing their reliance on projection. Possible etiological variables include innate aggressiveness or irritability, and consequent susceptibilities to fear, shame, envy, and guilt. I considered the role of formative experiences of threat, humiliation, and projective processes in the family system, and anxiety-ridden, contradictory messages in the development of this type of personality organization, and I described the paranoid person's sense of self as alternately helplessly vulnerable and omnipotently destructive, with ancillary preoccupations resulting from a core fragility in identity and self-esteem. The intensity of transference and countertransference processes, especially those involving rage, was discussed.

Technical extrapolations include recommendations that therapists of paranoid patients should demonstrate a good-humored acceptance of self and an amused appreciation of human foibles; work with affect and process rather than defense and content; identify specific precipitants of symptomatic upset, avoiding frontal assaults on paranoid interpretations of experience; distinguish between ideas and actions; preserve boundaries; and convey attitudes of personal power, authenticity, and respect. Finally, people with predominantly paranoid psychologies were differentiated from those with psychopathic, obsessive, and dissociative types of personality organization.

SUGGESTIONS FOR FURTHER READING

The most comprehensive book on paranoia may be Meissner's (1978) *The Paranoid Process*. But Shapiro's (1965) chapter on the paranoid style is better written, shorter, and livelier.

❖11❖

Depressive and Manic Personalities

In this chapter I will discuss people with character patterns shaped by depressive dynamics. I will also address briefly the psychologies of those whose personalities are characterized by the denial of depression; that is, those who have been called manic, hypomanic, and cyclothymic. While people in the latter diagnostic groups approach life with strategies antithetical to those used unconsciously by depressive people, the basic organizing themes, expectations, wishes, fears, conflicts, and unconscious explanatory constructs of depressive and manic people are similar.

As is well known, many people experience alternating manic and depressive states of mind; those with psychotic-level conditions used to be described as having a "manic–depressive" illness. The current preference is to call them "bipolar." The former term carried implications of delusion and suicidality, yet many people who never become psychotic experience marked cycles of mania and dysthymia. People who are predominantly depressive, those who are predominantly manic, and those who swing from one pole to the other all exist at every point on the developmental continuum.*

*It may be that "almost all" hypomanic characters are borderline (Kernberg et al., 1989), yet I have known several hypomanic people, and have treated a few, who depended heavily on denial and other archaic operations but who also had too integrated an identity and too keen a self-observing capacity to be considered borderline.

DEPRESSIVE PERSONALITIES

An unnecessary impediment to our collective professional understanding of depressive psychology, in the view of many analytic commentators (e.g., Frances & Cooper, 1981; Kernberg, 1984), was created when the formulators of the DSM-III elected to put all depressive and manic conditions under the heading of "Mood Disorders." By doing so, and in the process dispensing with the category of depressive personality, they emphasized the affective aspects of dysthymic conditions at the expense of imaginal, cognitive, behavioral, and sensory components that are equally important in the phenomenology of depression. Their decision also had the effect of diverting our attention from an understanding of the defensive processes that characterize depressive people even when they are not in a clinically depressed state.*

There is no doubt about what a clinical depression looks like, and many of us have had the bad luck to have suffered one. The unremitting sadness, lack of energy, anhedonia (inability to enjoy ordinary pleasures), and vegetative disturbances (problems in eating, sleeping, and self-regulating) are unmistakable. Freud (1917a) was the first writer to compare and contrast depressive ("melancholic") conditions with normal mourning; he observed that the significant difference between the two states is that in ordinary grief reactions the *external world* is experienced as diminished in some important way (e.g., it has lost a valuable person), whereas in depressive conditions, what feels lost or damaged is a part of the *self*. In some ways, then, depression is the opposite of mourning; people who grieve normally do not get depressed, even though they are pervasively sad during the period that follows bereavement or loss.

The cognitive, affective, imaginal, and sensate processes that are so striking in a sudden clinical depression (especially in one suffered by a person without strong dysthymic inclinations) operate in a chronic, organizing, self-perpetuating way in the psyches of those of us with depressive personalities (Laughlin, 1956, 1967). Given the intended audience of this book, the phrase "those of us" may be particularly apposite, since, if professional impressions may be trusted, a substantial proportion of psychotherapists are characterologically depressive. We

*I have been told by colleagues privy to the discussions from which the newer nosology emerged that some committee members expected analytic practitioners to diagnose their characterologically depressive patients as "300.4" (Dysthymic Disorder) on *Axis II*, the characterological axis of a full diagnostic work-up, but when I have done this for insurance or peer-review purposes, the diagnosis has been rejected. Such is the power of our formal categories to shape our attitudes toward psychopathology and our capacities to imagine different ways to understand people.

naturally empathize with sadness, we understand wounds to self-esteem, we seek closeness and resist loss, and we ascribe our therapeutic successes to our patients' efforts and our failures to our personal limitations.

Greenson (1967), in commenting on the connection between a depressive sensibility and the requisite qualities of successful therapists, went so far as to argue that analysts who have not suffered a serious depression may be handicapped in their work as healers. Greenson might reasonably have considered himself an exemplar of someone at the healthy end of the depressive continuum, along with more visibly anguished historical figures like Abraham Lincoln. At the highly disturbed end of the spectrum one finds the delusional and ruthlessly self-hating mental patients who, until the discovery of antidepressive medicines, could absorb years of a devoted therapist's efforts and still believe uncritically that the best way to save the world was to destroy the self.*

DRIVE, AFFECT, AND TEMPERAMENT IN DEPRESSION

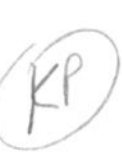

That one can inherit a vulnerability to depression has been suggested by studies of family histories, twins, and adoptees (Wender et al., 1986; Rice et al., 1987). Depression clearly runs in families, although no one can yet confidently evaluate the extent to which the transmission of depressive tendencies is genetically determined versus the extent to which depressed parents behave in ways that set up their children for dysthymic reactions.

Freud (1917a) speculated, and Abraham (1924) subsequently elaborated, that an important precursor to depressive inclinations is the experience of premature loss. In line with the classical theory that people who are either overindulged or deprived become fixated at the infantile stage during which this happened, depressive individuals were understood as having been weaned too soon or too abruptly, or as having suffered some other early frustration that overwhelmed their capacities to adapt (see Fenichel, 1945). The "oral" qualities of people with depressive characters influenced this construction; it was noted that depressive people were often overweight, that they usually liked

*For a poignant glimpse of such a person, and of the pain both suffered and inflicted by her, see the depiction of Frances Fonda (Henry's first wife and Jane and Peter's mother) in Henry Fonda's (1981) autobiography. Note especially Robert Knight's anguished letter of condolence to Mr. Fonda after his wife's success in killing herself (pp. 208–209). William Styron's (1990) *Darkness Visible* should also be required reading for those seeking a deep appreciation of the experience of extreme depression.

eating, smoking, drinking, talking, kissing, and other oral gratifications, and that they tended to describe their emotional experience in analogies about food and hunger. The idea that depressive people are orally fixated remains popular among psychoanalysts, probably as much because of the intuitive appeal of such a formulation as because of its theoretical status. When one of my supervisors commented that I see everybody as hungry, thus confronting my tendency to project my depressive issues on all my clients, I was able to start discriminating between those who needed to be emotionally fed and those who needed to be asked why they had not learned to cook.

An early psychodynamic way of describing a depressive process, and one that has been thoroughly popularized, illustrates the application of drive theory to specific clinical problems. It was noted (Freud, 1917a) that people in depressed states aim most of their negative affect away from others and toward the self, hating themselves out of all proportion to their actual shortcomings. At a time when psychological motivation was translated into libido and aggression, this phenomenon was described as "sadism (aggression) against the self" or as "anger turned inward." Because of its clinical promise, this formulation was embraced eagerly by Freud's colleagues, who began trying to help their patients to identify things that had angered them so that the pathological process could be reversed. It fell to later theorists to explain *why* a person would have learned to turn angry reactions against the self and what functions would be served by maintaining such a pattern.

The aggression-inward model is consistent with observations that depressive people seldom feel spontaneous or unconflicted anger on their own behalf. Instead, they feel guilt. Not the denied and defensively reinterpreted guilt of the paranoid person, but a conscious, ego-syntonic, pervasive sense of culpability. The author William Goldman once quipped to an interviewer, "When I'm accused of a crime I didn't commit, I wonder why I have forgotten it." Depressive people are agonizingly aware of every sin they have committed, every kindness they have neglected to extend, every selfish inclination that has crossed their minds.

Sadness is the other major affect of people with a depressive psychology. Evil and injustice distress them but rarely produce in them the indignant anger of the paranoid, the moralization of the obsessive, the undoing of the compulsive, or the anxiety of the hysterical person. The sorrow of someone who is clinically depressed is so palpable and arresting that in the public mind—and evidently now in the professional one as well—the terms sadness and depression have become virtually synonymous. As previously mentioned, since many people who are free of dysthymic symptoms have depressive personalities, and since grief and depression are in at least one respect mutually exclusive conditions, this equation is misleading; yet even a psychologically robust, high-spirited person with a depressive character will convey to a perceptive listener the hint of an inner melancholy. Monica McGoldrick's (1982) brilliant depiction of the Irish, a group famous for having a song in the heart and a tear in the eye, captures the ambience of a whole ethnic subculture with a depressive soul.

Unless they are so disturbed that they cannot function normally, most depressive people are easy to like and admire. Because they aim hatred and criticism inward rather than outward, they are usually generous, sensitive, and compassionate to a fault. Because they give others the benefit of any doubt, and strive to preserve relationships at any cost, they are natural appreciators of therapy. In the section on technique I shall discuss how to prevent these appealing qualities from working to their detriment.

DEFENSIVE AND ADAPTIVE PROCESSES IN DEPRESSION

The most powerful and organizing defense used by depressive people is introjection.* Clinically, it is the most important operation to understand in order to modify a person's depressive psychology. As psychoanalytic clinical theory developed, simpler energic concepts (aggression-in versus aggression-out) yielded to reflections on the internalization processes that Freud had begun to describe in "Mourning and Melancholia" (1917a) and that Abraham had noted as the depressive person's "identification with the lost love-object." As analysts began emphasizing the importance of incorporative processes in depression (Rado, 1928; Klein, 1940; Bibring, 1953; Jacobson, 1971; Blatt, 1974), they added immeasurably to our therapeutic power in the face of dysthymic misery.

In working with depressive patients, one can practically hear the internalized object speaking. When a client says something like, "It must be because I'm selfish," a therapist can ask, "Who's saying that?"

*Two kinds of depression, often labeled "introjective" (guilty) and "anaclitic" (dependent) (Blatt, 1974), keep emerging as conceptually separable in research done by both analytic and cognitive investigators (Blatt & Bers, 1993). When introjective dynamics solidify into personality, the result is the psychology described here; when anaclitic patterns permeate character, they define the depressive type of narcissistic person discussed in Chapter 8.

and be told, "My mother" (or father, or grandparent, or older sibling, or whoever is the introjected critic). Often the therapist feels as if he or she is talking to a ghost, and as if therapy, to be effective, will have to include an exorcism. As this example shows, the kind of introjection that characterizes depressive people is the unconscious internalization of the more hateful qualities of an old love object. His or her positive attributes are generally remembered fondly, while negative ones are felt as part of the self (Klein, 1940).

As I noted in Chapter 2, the internalized object does not have to be a person who in reality was hostile, critical, or negligent (though this is often the case, and it encumbers therapy with extra challenges) in order for the patient to have experienced the object that way and internalized such images. A young boy who feels deserted by a father who loves him very much—perhaps he suddenly had to work two jobs to make ends meet or was hospitalized for a serious illness—will feel hostility over his abandonment but will also yearn for him and feel self-rebuke for not having appreciated him sufficiently when he was around. Children project their reactions on to love objects that desert them, imagining that they left feeling angry or hurt. Then such images of a malevolent or injured abandoner, because they are too painful to bear and because they interfere with hopes for a loving reunion, are driven out of awareness and experienced as a bad part of the self.

A child thus emerges from experiences of traumatic or premature loss with an idealization of the lost object and a relegation of all negative affect into his or her sense of self. These well-known depressive dynamics create a pervasive feeling that one is bad, has driven away a needed and benevolent person, and must work very hard to prevent one's badness from provoking future desertions. The reader can see that this formulation is not inconsistent with the older anger-inward model; in fact, it accounts for why someone could get into the habit of handling hostile feelings in precisely this way. If one emerges from painful separations believing that it is one's badness that drove the beloved objects away, one may try very hard to feel nothing but positive affects toward those who are loved. The resistance of depressive people toward acknowledging ordinary and natural hostilities is comprehensible in this context, as is the upsetting and much-remarked phenomenon of the person who stays with an inconsiderate or abusive partner, believing that if only he or she were somehow good enough, the partner's mistreatment would stop.

Turning against the self (A. Freud, 1936; Laughlin, 1967), another commonly observed defense mechanism in depressive people, is a less archaic outcome of the introjective dynamics described above. Introjection as a concept covers the more total experience of feeling incomplete without the object and taking him or her into one's sense of self in order to feel whole, even if that means taking into one's self-representation the sense of badness that comes from painful experiences with the object. Turning against the self gains a reduction in anxiety, especially separation anxiety (if one believes it is one's anger and criticism that ensure abandonment, one feels safer directing it against the self), and also maintains a sense of power (if the badness inheres in me, I can change this disturbing situation).

Children are existentially dependent. If those on whom they must depend are unreliable or badly intentioned, they have a choice between facing that reality and living in chronic fear or denying it, believing that the source of their unhappiness lies within themselves, and thereby preserving a sense that self-improvement can alter their circumstances. People will usually favor any kind of suffering over helplessness. Clinical experience attests resoundingly to the human propensity to prefer the most irrational guilt to an acknowledgment of impotence. Turning against the self is a predictable outcome of an emotionally insecure history.

Idealization is the other defense important to note in depressive patients. Because their self-esteem has been reduced in response to their experiences, the admiration with which they view others is correspondingly increased. Self-perpetuating cycles of holding others in excessively high regard, then feeling diminished in comparison, then seeking idealized objects to compensate for the diminution, feeling inferior to those objects, and so on, are typical for depressive people. This idealization differs from that of narcissistic people in that it organizes around moral concerns rather than status and power.

OBJECT RELATIONS IN DEPRESSION

The above section on ego processes in depressive patients suggests some important themes in their object relations. First, there is the role of early and/or repeated loss. The striking affective correspondences between depression and mourning have prompted theorists at least as far back as Freud to look for the origins of dysthymic dynamics in painful, premature experiences of separation from a love object. And such experiences have been easy to find in the histories of depressive clients. Despite the failure of empirical studies to illuminate such a relationship, analysts continue to connect depressive psychology to early loss (Jacobson, 1971; Altschul, 1988). Early loss is not always concrete, observable, and empirically verifiable (e.g., death of a parent); it may be more internal and psychological, as in the case of a child who yields to a caregiver's pressure to renounce dependent behaviors before he or she is emotionally ready to do so.

Erna Furman's (1982) deceptively modest essay "Mothers Have to Be There to Be Left" explores this second kind of loss. In a respectful but trenchant critique of classical ideas about the mother's responsibility to wean infants when they are ready to accept the loss of a need-gratifying object, Furman stresses that unless they are hurried, children wean themselves. The striving for independence is as primary and powerful as the wish to depend; separation is naturally sought by youngsters who are confident of the availability of the parent if they need to regress and "refuel" (Mahler, 1972a, 1972b). Furman's recasting of the separation process in terms of the child's natural movement forward challenges a persistent Western notion (reflected in older psychoanalytic thinking and in many popular books on child rearing) that parents must titrate frustrations because left to themselves, youngsters will prefer regressive satisfactions.

According to Furman, who has devoted a distinguished career to understanding children, it is ordinarily the mother, not the baby, who feels keenly the loss of a gratifying instinctual satisfaction at weaning—and by analogy at other times of separation. Along with her pleasure and pride in her child's growing autonomy, she suffers some pangs of grief. Normal children appreciate these pangs; they expect their parents to shed a tear on the first day of school, at the first prom, at graduation. The separation–individuation process eventuates in depressive dynamics, Furman believes, only when the mother's pain about her child's growth is so great that she either clings and induces guilt ("I'll be so lonely without you") or pushes the child away counterphobically ("Why can't you play by yourself?!"). Children in the former situation are left feeling that normal wishes to be aggressive and independent are hurtful; in the latter case, they learn to hate their natural dependent strivings. Either way, an important part of the self is experienced as bad.

Not just the experience of early loss but circumstances that conspire to make it difficult for the child to understand realistically what happened, and to grieve normally, will engender depressive tendencies. One such circumstance is developmental. Two-year-olds are simply too young to fathom *that* people die and *why* they die, and they are incapable of appreciating complex interpersonal motives such as "Daddy loves you, but he is moving out because he and Mommy don't get along." The world of the 2-year-old is still magical and categorical. At the height of conceiving things in gross categories of good and bad, the toddler whose parent disappears will generate assumptions about badness that are impossible to counteract with reasonable educative comments. A major loss in the separation–individuation phase virtually guarantees some depressive dynamics.

Other circumstances include family members' neglect of their children's needs when they are beset by difficulties and their ignorance of the degree to which children require explanations that counteract their self-referential and moralistic interpretations. Judith Wallerstein's long-term research on the outcome of divorce (Wallerstein & Blakeslee, 1989) has demonstrated that along with lack of abandonment by the noncustodial parent, the best predictor of a nondepressive adaptation to parental divorce is the child's having been given an age-appropriate, accurate explanation of what went wrong in the marriage.

Another circumstance that encourages depressive tendencies is a family atmosphere in which mourning is discouraged. When parents and other caregivers model the denial of grief, or insist (e.g., after an acrimonious divorce) that the child join in a family myth that everyone is better off without the lost object, or need the child to reassure them that he or she is not in pain, mourning goes underground and eventually takes the form of the belief that there is something wrong in the self. Sometimes children feel intense, unspoken pressures from an emotionally overburdened parent to protect the adult from further grief, as if acknowledging sorrow were equivalent to falling apart. The child cannot fail to conclude that grief is dangerous and that needs for comfort are destructive.

Sometimes in a family system the prevailing morality is that mourning and other forms of self-care and self-comfort are "selfish" or "self-indulgent," or "just feeling sorry for yourself," as if such activities were prima facie contemptible. Guilt-induction of this sort, and associated admonishments to a stricken child to stop whining and get over it, instill both a need to hide any vulnerable aspects of the self and, out of identification with the critical parent, an eventual hatred of those aspects of oneself. Many of my depressive patients were called names whenever they could not control their natural regressive reactions to family difficulties; as adults, they abused themselves psychologically in parallel ways whenever they were upset.

The combination of emotional or actual abandonment with parental criticism is particularly likely to create depressive dynamics. A patient of mine lost her mother to cancer when she was 11 and was left with a father who repeatedly complained that her unhappiness was aggravating his ulcer and hastening his death. Another client was called a sniveling baby by her mother when she cried because, at age 4, she was being shipped away to overnight camp for several weeks. A depressed man I worked with whose mother was severely depressed and unavailable emotionally during his early years was told he was selfish and insensitive for wanting her time, and that he should be grateful she was not sending him to an orphanage. In such instances it is easy to see that angry reactions to emotional abuse by the parent would have felt too dangerous to the child, who already feared rejection.

Some of the depressive patients I have worked with appear to have been the most emotionally astute person in their family of origin. Their reactivity to situations whose emotional implications the other family members were better at denying got them branded "hypersensitive" or "overreactive," labels they continued to carry internally and to connect with their general sense of inferiority. Alice Miller (1975) described how families can unwittingly exploit the emotional talent of a particular child, with the result that the child eventually feels valued only for serving a particular family function. If the child is also scorned and pathologized for the possession of emotional gifts, depressive dynamics will be even stronger than if he or she is simply used as a kind of family therapist.

Finally, a powerful causative factor in depressive dynamics is significant depression in a parent, especially in a child's earliest years. Biologically inclined theorists have tended to attribute to genetic processes the fact that dysthymic illnesses run in families, but analytically oriented writers have been more cautious. A seriously depressed mother with no one to help out will give a baby only the most custodial kind of care, no matter how sincerely she wishes to help it start life on the best possible footing. The more we learn about infants, the more we know about how critical their earliest experience is in establishing their basic attitudes and expectations (Spitz, 1965; Brazelton, 1980; Greenspan, 1981; Stern, 1985). Children are deeply bothered by a parent's depression; they feel guilty for making normal demands, and they come to believe that their needs drain and exhaust others. The earlier their dependence on someone who is deeply depressed, the greater is their emotional privation.

Numerous different pathways can thus lead to a depressive accommodation. Both loving and hateful families can breed depressive dynamics out of infinitely varied combinations of loss and insufficient psychological processing of that loss. In a society where adults fail to make enough time to listen sensitively to the concerns of children, where people move their residence routinely, where divorce is common, and where painful emotions can be ignored because drugs will artificially counteract them, it is not surprising that our rates of youthful depression and suicide have skyrocketed, that counterdepressive compulsions like substance abuse and gambling are on the rise, that we are seeing an explosion of popular movements in which the "lost child" or the "child within" is rediscovered, and that self-help groups that reduce feelings of isolation and fault are widely sought. Human beings seem not to have been designed to handle as much instability in their relationships as contemporary life provides.

THE DEPRESSIVE SELF

People with depressive psychologies believe that at bottom they are bad. They lament their greed, their selfishness, their competition, their vanity, their pride, their anger, their envy, their lust. They consider all these normal aspects of experience to be perverse and dangerous. They worry that they are inherently destructive. These anxieties can take a more or less oral tone ("I'm afraid my hunger will destroy others"), or an anal-level one ("My defiance and sadism are dangerous"), or a more oedipal dimension ("My wishes to compete for and win love are evil").

Depressive people have made sense out of their experiences of unmourned losses by the belief that it was something in them that drove the object away. The fact that they *felt* rejected has been converted into the unconscious conviction that they *deserved* rejection, that their faults provoked it, and that future rejection is inevitable if anyone comes to know them intimately. They try very hard to be "good," but they fear being exposed as sinful and discarded as unworthy. One of my patients became convinced at one point that I would refuse to see her again after hearing about her childhood death wishes toward a younger sibling. She, like many sophisticated psychotherapy clients today, knew at the conscious level that such wishes are an expectable part of the psychology of the displaced child, yet in her deeper experience she was still awaiting condemnation.

The guilt of the depressive person is at times unfathomable. Some guilt is simply part of the human condition, and is appropriate to our complex and not entirely benign natures, but depressive guilt has a certain magnificent conceit. In someone with a psychotic depression it can emerge as the blatant conviction that some disaster was caused by one's personal sinfulness—police departments are accustomed to delusional depressives calling up to claim responsibility for highly publicized crimes that they could not possibly have committed—but even in expansive, high-functioning, nonclinically depressed adults with a depressive character structure similar ideas will emerge in psychotherapy. "Bad things happen to me because I deserve them" is a consistent undercurrent theme of depressive clients. They may even have a paradoxical kind of self-esteem based on the grandiose idea that "No one is as bad as I am."

Because they are in a state of constant readiness to believe the worst about themselves, depressives can be very thin-skinned. Criticism may devastate them; in any message that includes mention of their shortcomings they will tend to hear only that part of the communication. When criticism is intended constructively, as in an evaluation at work, they tend to feel so exposed and wounded that they miss or minimize any complimentary facets of their informant's report. When they are subject to genuinely mean-spirited attacks, they are incapable of seeing beyond any grains of truth in the content to the fact that no one deserves to be treated abusively, no matter how legitimate are their persecutor's complaints.

Depressive people often handle their unconscious dynamics by helping others, by philanthropic activity, or by contributions to social progress that have the effect of counteracting their guilt. It is one of the great ironies of life that it is the most realistically benevolent people who seem most vulnerable to feelings of moral inferiority. Many individuals with depressive personalities are able to maintain a stable sense of self-esteem and avoid depressive episodes by doing good. In researching characterological altruism (McWilliams, 1984), I found that the only times my charitable subjects had experienced depression were when circumstances had made it temporarily impossible for them to carry on their humanitarian activities.

Psychotherapists, as previously noted, often have significant depressive dynamics. They seek opportunities to help others so that their anxieties about their destructiveness will be kept at bay. Since it is hard to help people psychologically, at least as fast as we would all wish, and since we cannot avoid inflicting temporary pain on patients in the service of their growth, feelings of exaggerated responsibility and disproportionate self-criticism are common in beginning therapists. Supervisors can confirm, in fact, how often such dynamics get in the way of their trainees' expeditious learning of their craft.* One of my depressive patients, a therapist, responded to any setback with a client,

*Not only do depressively organized people get attracted to careers in psychotherapy but, in addition, most training introduces a period of "normal" depression. In the program where I teach, for example, I have noticed that whatever their individual personalities, students tend to go through a depressive period some time around their second year. Graduate training in general is a breeding ground for dysthymic reactions, since one has the worst of both parent and child roles (one is expected to be adult, responsible, autonomous, and original, yet one gets no power; one is dependent on one's "elders" in the field, yet one has no accompanying promise of protection and comfort). Training in therapy additionally confronts people with the fact that learning an art is very different from mastering a content area. Students who come to our program as stars of their undergraduate departments find the transition to self-exposure and critical feedback on their work to be emotionally jarring.

especially if it provoked negative feelings in her, with a search for her own role in the problem—to such a degree that she ignored opportunities to learn about the ordinary vicissitudes of working with that particular kind of patient. The fact that therapy is a two-person process, where intersubjectivity is a given, was converted by her into a quest for self-purification and a terror that she was somehow basically unsuited to helping people.

Women seem to be more at risk of depressive solutions to emotional problems than men. In the last two decades feminist theorists (e.g., Chodorow, 1978, 1989; Gilligan, 1982; J. B. Miller, 1984; Surrey, 1985) have accounted for this phenomenon by reference to the fact that the primary caregiver in most families is female. Male children consequently attain a sense of gender identity from being different from the mother, and females derive it from identification with her. An outcome of this imbalance in early parenting is that men use introjection less, as their masculinity is confirmed by separation rather than by fusion, and women use it more, because their sense of femaleness comes from connection.

TRANSFERENCE AND COUNTERTRANSFERENCE WITH DEPRESSIVE PATIENTS

Depressive clients are ordinarily easy to love. They attach quickly to the therapist, ascribe benevolence to his or her aims even when fearing criticism, are moved by empathic responsiveness, work hard to be "good" in the patient role, and appreciate bits of insight as if they were morsels of life-sustaining food. They tend to idealize the clinician (as morally good, in contrast to their subjective badness), but not in the empty and emotionally unconnected way typical of more narcissistically structured patients. Healthier depressive people are highly respectful of the therapist's status as a separate, real, and caring human being, and they try hard not to be burdensome. Even borderline and psychotic depressives are palpably seeking love and connection, and they ordinarily induce a natural caring response.

At the same time, depressive people project on to the therapist their internal critics, the introjects that have variously been referred to in the psychoanalytic literature as constituting a "sadistic" or "harsh" or "primitive" superego (Freud, 1917a; Abraham, 1924; Rado, 1928; Klein, 1940; Schneider, 1950). It can be a startling experience to see a patient writhe in miserable anticipation of disapproval when confessing some minor crime of thought. Depressive clients are subject to the chronic belief that the therapist's concern and respect would vanish if he or she *really* knew them. This belief can persist over months and years, even in the face of their having volunteered every negative thing they can think of about themselves, and having consequently encountered only steadfast acceptance from the therapist.

As depressive patients progress in therapy, they project their hostile attitudes less and experience them more directly in the form of anger and criticism toward the therapist. At this point in treatment, their negativity often takes the form of communications that they do not really expect to be helped and that nothing the therapist is doing is making a difference. It is important to tolerate this phase of treatment without taking their criticisms too personally and to console oneself that in the process, they are getting out from under all the self-directed complaining that was previously keeping them unhappy.

State-of-the-art psychopharmacology now enables us to work with depressive people at all levels of disturbance (see Karasu's [1990] synopsis of indications for pharmacotherapy) and to analyze the above dynamics even in psychotic clients. Before the discovery of the antidepressive properties of lithium and other chemicals, many patients with borderline and psychotic structure were so firmly convinced of their badness, and so sure of the therapist's inevitable hatred of them, that they could not tolerate the pain of attachment. Sometimes they would commit suicide after years of treatment because they could not bear to start feeling hope and thereby risk another devastating disappointment.

Healthier depressive clients have always been easy to work with because their convictions about their basic flaws are mostly unconscious and are ego alien when brought into awareness. People who are more troubled usually need medication to reduce the intensity of their depressive feelings. The ruthless, implacable states of self-loathing by which borderline and psychotic depressives can be possessed are infrequent in medicated patients. It is as if their depressive dynamics have been made chemically ego dystonic. The shadows of self-hatred that remain after they are established on an appropriate medication can be addressed as one would analyze pathological introjects with neurotic-level depressive people.

Countertransference with depressive individuals runs the gamut from benign affection to omnipotent rescue fantasies, depending upon the severity of the patient's depressive issues. Such reactions constitute a complementary countertransference (Racker, 1968); the therapeutic fantasy is that one can be God, or the Good Mother, or the sensitive, accepting parent that the client never had. These longings can be understood as a response to the patient's unconscious belief that the cure for depressive dynamics is unconditional love and total understanding. (There is a lot of truth in this idea, but as I will spell out shortly, it is also dangerously incomplete as a therapeutic approach.)

There is also a concordant countertransference familiar to therapists of depressive patients: One feels demoralized, incompetent, blundering, hopeless, and in general "not good enough" to help the client. Depressive attitudes are contagious. I first became aware of this when I was working in a mental health center and (naively) scheduled four severely depressed people in a row. By the time I came shambling to the office coffee pot after the fourth session, the clinic secretaries were offering me chicken soup and a shoulder to cry on. It is thus easy for therapists, especially depressive ones, to respond internally to introjective misery as Lou Grant used to on "The Mary Tyler Moore Show": "Yeah, life's a bitch, and then you die." Or with the inference that one is just an inadequate therapist. These feelings can be mitigated if one is fortunate enough to have plentiful sources of emotional gratification in one's personal life (see Fromm-Reichmann, 1950). They also tend to diminish over one's professional lifetime as it becomes incontrovertible that one has succeeded in helping even relentlessly dysthymic patients.

THERAPEUTIC IMPLICATIONS OF THE DIAGNOSIS OF DEPRESSION

The most important condition of therapy with a depressed or depressively organized person is an atmosphere of acceptance, respect, and compassionate efforts to understand. Most writings about psychotherapy—whether they express a general humanistic stance, a psychodynamic orientation, or a cognitive-behavioral preference—emphasize a style of relatedness that is particularly adapted to the treatment of depressive clients. Although a basic tenet of this book is that this generic therapeutic attitude is insufficient to the task of therapy for some diagnostic groups (e.g., psychopathic and paranoid), I want to stress how critical it is to helping depressive people. Because they have radar for the slightest verification of their fears of criticism and rejection, a therapist working with depressive patients must take special pains to be nonjudgmental and emotionally constant.

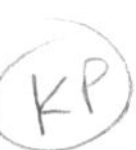

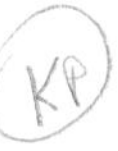

Analyzing the client's undercurrent presumptions about inevitable rejection, and understanding his or her counteractive efforts to be "good" in order to forestall it, constitute much of the work with depressive people. For higher-functioning patients, the famous analytic couch is particularly useful because it brings such themes quickly into focus.* A young woman I once treated (who had no manifest depressive symptoms but whose character was depressively organized) was an expert at reading my expressions. When we worked face to face, she so rapidly disconfirmed expectations that I was critical and rejecting that she was not even aware she had had any such apprehensions. Neither was I; she was so skilled at this monitoring that my usual mindfulness of someone's searching gaze was not aroused. When her decision to use the couch deprived her of eye contact, she was amazed to find herself suddenly hesitant to talk about certain topics because of the conviction that I would not approve of her.

Even in situations or with clients where use of the couch is not an option, there are ways of sitting and talking that minimize patients' opportunities for visual search so that they can get in touch with how chronic and automatic is their vigilance. One of my colleagues had long resisted my encouragement to ask a particularly discerning depressive client of hers to use the couch. She was finally persuaded when nature intervened on my side of the argument. One evening when she was working with this man, an electrical storm knocked out the power in her office, and they decided to continue the session in the dark. Without opportunities for visual checking, this client and his therapist made the same discovery that my depressive patient did.

For obvious reasons, effective therapy requires opposite conditions with more disturbed depressive patients. Their presumptions of their unlovability and terrors of rejection are so profound and ego syntonic that without the freedom to scrutinize the therapist's face and invalidate their worst fears, they will be too anxious to talk freely. The therapist may have to log a great deal of time demonstrating acceptance before even the *conscious* expectations of rejection in a depressive client can become open to scrutiny and eventual invalidation.

It is imperative with depressive patients to explore and interpret their reactions to separation, even to the separation of brief silence from the therapist. (Long silences are to be avoided; they arouse the patient's

*Freud began asking patients to lie on the couch for a most prosaic reason: He got tired of being stared at. He quickly learned, however, that there were serendipitous benefits to this innovation. The supine posture relaxes people, inducing a more flowing kind of consciousness (now understood as a mild trance state, comparable to that evoked in light hypnosis and transcendental meditation [Edelstein, 1981]); it also highlights transference reactions. The illumination of the transference is the main reason that analysts continue to use the couch, but it is also still true that when one is treating an accomplished "scanner," it is a relief to be out of visual contact. It allows the therapist the freedom to respond internally to the patient's material without self-consciousness: to fantasize, to respond affectively, even to weep without worrying that the patient will be distracted from internal processes by the therapist's emotional reactivity.

feelings of being uninteresting, valueless, adrift, hopeless.) Depressive people are deeply sensitive to abandonment and are unhappy being alone. More important, they experience loss—usually unconsciously, but especially those in the psychotic range, sometimes consciously—as evidence of their badness. "You must be going away because you're disgusted with me," or "You're leaving to escape my insatiable hunger," or "You're taking off to punish me for my sinfulness" are all variants on the depressive theme of basic iniquity and unlovability. Hence it is critical not only to be attuned to how bothersome ordinary losses are to a depressive patient—this will come up naturally in anticipation of the therapist's vacations or when the therapist cancels a session—but also to how he or she interprets them.

Harold Sampson (1983) cites research in which two matched depressed women were treated analytically over a similar period, the first by a model stressing empathy, acceptance, and the grieving of unmourned losses; the second according to control–mastery notions that unconscious guilt and pathogenic beliefs about the self must also be addressed. In interviews held a year after termination, each woman was asked to assess her treatment. The first was full of gratitude toward her therapist, whose devoted care she depicted in warm and idealizing ways. But she was also still depressed. The second patient said she lacked vivid memories of her analysis, although she thought it had been helpful, and seemed considerably less invested in singing her analyst's praises. She also impressed the interviewers as self-confident and serene, and she was now living a highly satisfying life.

This finding underscores the importance of unearthing self-referential fantasies, not just facilitating mourning over present and past separations. It shows that while basic nonjudgmental acceptance may be a necessary condition of therapy with a depressive person, it is not a sufficient one. This discovery also raises important issues about short-term individual therapy with depressive clients. Treatments that are arbitrarily limited to a certain number of sessions may provide welcome comfort during a painful episode of clinical depression, but the time-limited experience may be ultimately assimilated by the depressive person as another relationship that was traumatically cut short—further evidence that the patient is not good enough to inspire attachment.

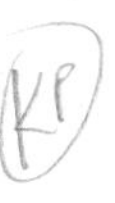

Alternatively or additionally, a compulsorily brief treatment may be taken in as substantiating the patient's assumption that he or she is pathologically dependent, since shortened therapies are often presented by clinic personnel as the treatment of choice. The depressive conclusion that "this obviously works for other patients but not for a bottomless pit like me" will undermine self-esteem even if in the short term the treatment improves the person's mood. In working with depressive clients under conditions that require a forced termination, it is thus especially important to predict preemptively the patient's expectable interpretation of the meaning of the loss.

One tendency I have noted in beginning therapists treating depressive clients is a disposition to avoid taking vacations or imposing cancellations that are not rescheduled out of a wish to spare the patient unnecessary pain. In fact, most of us in the field probably started out being neurotically flexible and generous in an effort to protect our depressive patients from suffering. But what depressive people really need is not uninterrupted care. What they need is the experience that the therapist *returns* after a separation. Specifically, they need to know that their hunger did not permanently alienate the therapist and that their anger at being abandoned did not destroy the relationship. One cannot learn these lessons without enduring a loss in the first place.

On being encouraged to get in touch with anger and other negative feelings, depressive patients will frequently explain that they cannot take the risk of noticing hostility toward the therapist because "How can I get angry at someone I need so much?" It is important that the therapist not join in this elliptical thinking. (Unfortunately, because their underlying beliefs are similar to those of the patient, therapists with depressive sensibilities may regard such remarks as making perfect sense.) One should point out instead that the question contains the unexamined assumption that anger drives people apart. It often comes as a revelation to depressive individuals that the freedom to admit negative feelings increases intimacy, whereas being false or out of touch produces isolation. Anger interferes with normal dependency only if the person one is depending upon has pathological reactions to it—a circumstance that defines the childhood experience of many depressive clients but not the possibilities for adult relationships with more resilient people.

Therapists often find that their efforts to mitigate their depressive patients' sense of badness are either ignored or received paradoxically. Supportive comments to a person immersed in self-loathing may provoke increased depression. The mechanism by which the patient converts positive feedback into self-attack goes something like this: "Anyone who *really* knew me could not possibly say such positive things. I must have duped this therapist into thinking I am okay. I'm bad for misleading such a nice person. Furthermore, any support from this direction cannot be trusted because this therapist can be easily fooled." Hammer (1990) is fond of quoting Groucho Marx here, who used to insist that he would not be interested in joining any country club that would have him for a member.

If praise backfires, what can one do to improve the self-esteem of a depressive person? The ego psychologists had a very useful prescription: Don't support the ego; attack the superego. For example, if a man is berating himself for the crime of envying a friend's success, and the therapist responds that envy is a normal emotion, and that especially since the patient did not act it out, he might congratulate himself rather than running himself down, the patient may respond with silent skepticism. But if the therapist says, "So what's so terrible about that?" or teases him for trying to be purer than God, or tells him good-naturedly to "Join the human race!" the patient may be able to take the message in. When interpretations are put in a critical tone, they are more easily tolerated by depressive people ("If she's criticizing me, there must be some truth in what she says, since I know I'm bad in *some* way"), even when what is being criticized is a critical introject.

Another aspect of sensitive treatment of depressive patients is the therapist's willingness to appreciate, as developmental achievements, behaviors that would signify resistance in other clients. For example, many therapy patients express their negative reactions to treatment by canceling sessions or failing to bring a check. Depressive people work so hard to be good that they are usually exemplary in the patient role—so much so that their compliant behavior may be legitimately considered part of their pathology. One can make small dents in a depressive mentality by interpreting a client's cancellation or temporary nonpayment as a triumph over the fear that the therapist will retaliate at the slightest sign of opposition. One is tempted with excessively cooperative patients just to relax and appreciate one's luck, but if a depressive person never behaves in adversarial or selfish ways in treatment, the therapist should bring that pattern up as worthy of investigation.

Overall, therapists of characterologically depressive patients must permit and even welcome the client's removing their halo. It is nice to be idealized, but it is not in the patient's best interest. Therapists in the earliest days of the psychoanalytic movement knew that it signified progress when a depressed patient became critical or angry with the clinician; while they understood this more or less hydraulically, contemporary analysts appreciate it from the standpoint of self-valuation. Depressive patients need eventually to leave the "one-down" position and to see the therapist as an ordinary, flawed human being. Retaining idealization inherently retains an inferior self-image.

Finally, where one's professional circumstances permit, it is more important with depressive patients than with others to leave decisions about termination up to them. It is also advisable to leave an open door for further treatment and to analyze ahead of time any inhibitions the client may have about asking for help in the future (one often hears that coming back for a psychological "tune-up" would be admitting defeat, or that the therapist might be disappointed with a less than complete "cure"). Since the causes of dysthymia so frequently include irreversible separations—which forced the growing child to cut all ties and suppress all regressive longings, instead of feeling secure in the availability of an understanding parent—the termination phase with depressive patients must be handled with special care and flexibility.

DIFFERENTIAL DIAGNOSIS

The two characterological dispositions most commonly confused with depressive psychology are narcissism (of the depleted rather than the grandiose variety) and masochism. Misdiagnoses are more often made in the direction of construing as depressive someone who is more basically either narcissistic or masochistic than in the direction of misunderstanding an essentially depressive person as either of the other types. The tendency of therapists to misread a patient as depressive when his or her personality is more appropriately conceptualized in one of these other ways seems to me attributable to two factors. First, depressively inclined therapists may project their own dynamics on to nondepressive patients. Second, people with either narcissistic or masochistic personality structure typically have some symptoms of clinical depression, especially dysthymic mood. Either diagnostic mistake can have unfortunate clinical consequences.

Depressive versus Narcissistic Personality

In Chapter 8 I described people with depressed–depleted forms of narcissistic personality. They differ from the depressively organized subjects of this chapter in that their inner experience is shame, emptiness, meaninglessness, boredom, and existential despair, whereas the more "melancholic" type of depressive picture that analysts denote by the term depressive personality includes feelings of guilt, sinfulness, destructiveness, hunger, and self-hatred. It is as if the narcissistically organized person lacks a sense of self, while the depressive one has a very clear sense of self—but a painfully negative one. Narcissistically depressed people tend to have selfobject transferences, while those with depressive personalities have object transferences. Countertransference with the former is vague, irritated, affectively shallow; with the latter it is much clearer and more powerful, usually involving rescue fantasies.

The technical implications of this differential are subtle but important. Explicitly sympathetic, encouraging reactions can be comforting to a narcissistically organized person, but they may further demoralize a depressively structured individual in the paradoxical manner described above. Attacking the presumed superego—even in gentle ways such as commenting on possible self-reproach—will not help a person whose basic structure is narcissistic because self-attack is not part of the narcissistic dynamism. Interpretations that redefine affective experience in the direction of anger rather than more passive emotional responses will similarly fizzle with narcissistic patients since their main state of feeling is shame, not self-directed hostility. Such interpretive efforts may, however, relieve and even energize melancholic clients, whose responsiveness can make the old anger-in-versus-anger-out formulations look uncannily apt.

Interpretive reconstructions that emphasize critical parents and injurious separations will generally fall on deaf ears with narcissistic clients, no matter how depressed they are, because rejection and trauma are rarely pathogenic of narcissistic dynamics. But they may be gratefully received by depressive patients as an alternative to their long-standing habit of attributing all their pain to their personal shortcomings. With a narcissistic person, attempts to work conventionally "in the transference" may be shrugged off, belittled, or absorbed into an overall idealization, but a depressive patient will appreciate this approach and make good use of it. Overall, this differential equates to the metaphorical understanding of narcissistic clients as pathologically empty and depressive ones as pathologically filled with hostile introjects. Therapy must be tailored to these contrasting subjective worlds.

Depressive versus Masochistic Personality

Depression and the self-defeating patterns that analytically oriented practitioners refer to as masochism are closely connected, since both orientations are adaptations to unconscious guilt. They coexist so frequently, in fact, that Kernberg (e.g., 1984), in acknowledgment of Laughlin's (1967) seminal observations, considers the "depressive–masochistic personality" one of three standard neurotic-level kinds of character organization. In spite of their frequent coexistence and synergism, I have preferred to differentiate carefully between depressive and masochistic psychologies. An organizing principle of this text has been to attend to those differences among people that have an established conceptual status in the psychoanalytic tradition and that have significant implications for psychotherapy technique. In Chapter 12 I will explore the differences between predominantly depressive and predominantly masochistic personalities and elaborate on the implications of those differences for treatment.

MANIC AND HYPOMANIC PERSONALITIES

Mania is the flip side of depression. People with hypomanic personalities have an essentially depressive organization, which is counteracted by the defense of denial. Because most people who maintain a degree of mania suffer from episodes in which their denial fails and their depression surfaces, the term "cyclothymic" has sometimes been used to describe their psychology. In the second edition of the DSM (DSM-II; American Psychiatric Association, 1968), both depressive and cyclothymic personality disorders were accepted diagnoses.

Hypomania is not a state that simply contrasts with depression; point for point, it is the polar opposite of it. The hypomanic individual is elated, energetic, self-promoting, witty, and grandiose. Akhtar (1992) summarizes:

> The individual with hypomanic personality is overtly cheerful, highly social, given to idealization of others, work-addicted, flirtatious, and articulate, while covertly he is guilty about his aggression toward others, incapable of being alone, defective in empathy, unable to love, corruptible, and lacking a systematic approach in his cognitive style. (p. 193)

People in a manic state or with a manic personality are famous for grand schemes, racing thoughts, and extended freedom from ordinary physical requirements, such as food and sleep. They seem constantly "up"—until exhaustion eventually sets in. Because the person experiencing mania literally cannot slow down, drugs like alcohol, barbiturates, and opiates that depress the central nervous system may be highly attractive. Many comics and humorists appear to have hypomanic personalities; their relentless wit can sometimes be quite wearing. Sometimes the dysthymic side of a very funny person is more visible, as with Mark Twain or Ambrose Bierce or Lenny Bruce, all of whom suffered serious depressive episodes.

DRIVE, AFFECT, AND TEMPERAMENT IN MANIA

Manic people are notable for high energy, excitement, mobility, distractibility, and sociability. They are often great entertainers, storytellers, punsters, mimics—treasures to their friends, who nevertheless sometimes complain that because they turn all serious remarks into occasions for humor, they are hard to get close to emotionally. When negative affect appears in people with manic and hypomanic psychologies, it manifests not as sorrow and disappointment, but as anger, sometimes in the form of episodes of sudden, uncontrolled rage.

Like their counterparts in the depressive realm, they strike psychoanalytically inclined observers as organized along oral lines (Fenichel, 1945): They may talk nonstop, drink recklessly, bite their nails, chew gum, smoke, gnaw on the insides of their mouth. Especially at the disturbed end of the manic continuum, many are overweight. Their perpetual motion suggests considerable anxiety, despite their often markedly elevated mood. The emotional pleasure they display and, by contagion, bestow, has a somewhat fragile, undependable quality; their acquaintances often harbor vague worries about their stability. While happiness is a familiar condition for the manic person, a calm serenity may be an emotional state completely outside his or her experience (Akiskal, 1984).

DEFENSIVE AND ADAPTIVE PROCESSES IN MANIA

The core defenses of manic and hypomanic people are denial and acting out. Denial is conspicuous in their tendency to ignore (or to transform into humor) events that would distress or alarm most other people. Acting out occurs mainly in the form of flight: They run from situations that might threaten them with loss. They may also escape painful affects by other kinds of acting out, including sexualization, intoxication, provocation, and even acts that appear psychopathic, such as theft (hence, some analysts have questioned the stability of the reality principle in manic clients [Katan, 1953]). Manic people also devalue, a process isomorphic with the depressive tendency to idealize, especially when they contemplate making loving attachments that they fear will disappoint.

For a manic person, anything that distracts is preferable to emotional suffering. People with manic propensities, especially those with more severe disturbance and those in a temporarily psychotic state, may also use the defense of omnipotent control; they may feel invulnerable, immortal, convinced of the assured success of some grandiose scheme. Acts of impulsive exhibitionism, rape (usually of a spouse or intimate), and authoritarian control are not unknown among manic people during a psychotic break.

OBJECT RELATIONS IN MANIA

In the histories of manic people, perhaps even more strikingly than in those of depressives, one finds a pattern of repeated traumatic separations with no opportunity for the child to process them emotionally. Deaths of important people who went unmourned, divorces and separations that no one addressed, and family relocations for which there was no preparation litter the childhoods of the manic. One hypomanic man I worked with had moved 26 times during his first 10 years; more than once he arrived home after school to find the moving van in the driveway.

Criticism and abuse, emotional and sometimes physical, are also common in the backgrounds of manic and hypomanic individuals. I have already discussed this combination of traumatic separation and emotional neglect and mistreatment as it applies to depressive outcomes; it may be that in the histories of manic people the losses were more extreme, or that attention to their emotional significance by the child's caregivers was even scarcer than it is in the backgrounds of depressive people. Otherwise it is hard to explain the need for a defense as extreme as denial.

THE MANIC SELF

One of my manic patients described herself as a spinning top. She was keenly aware of her need to keep moving lest she have to feel something painful. Manic people are frightened of attachment, because to care about someone means that losing him or her will be devastating. The manic continuum from psychotic to neurotic structure loads more heavily in the borderline and psychotic areas because of the primitivity of the processes involved; a consequence of this is that many manic, hypomanic, and cyclothymic people are at risk of the subjective experience of self-disintegration that self psychologists refer to as fragmentation. Manic individuals are afraid that if they do not keep moving, they will fall apart.

Self-esteem in people with manic structure may be maintained, somewhat tenuously, by a combination of success at avoiding pain and elation at captivating others. Some manic individuals are masterful at attaching other people to themselves emotionally without reciprocating an investment of comparable depth. Because they are often brilliant and witty, their friends and colleagues—especially those holding the common but fallacious belief that intelligence and severe psychopathology are mutually exclusive—can be nonplussed to learn of their psychological vulnerabilities. Suicide attempts and flagrantly psychotic behavior can suddenly invade a manic fortress if some loss becomes too painful to deny.

TRANSFERENCE AND COUNTERTRANSFERENCE WITH MANIC PATIENTS

Manic clients can be winsome, insightful, and fascinating. They also tend to be confusing and exhausting. Once while working with a hypomanic young woman, I became aware of the fantasy that my head was in a clothes dryer, the kind in the laundromat that whirl garments in full view but too fast to track. Sometimes in an initial interview one is aware of a nagging feeling that with such a turbulent history, the patient should be showing more emotionality in recounting it. At other times one is aware of somehow not being able to put all the pieces together.

The most dangerous countertransference tendency in therapists working with hypomanic people is underestimation of the degree of suffering and potential disorganization that lie beneath their engaging presentation. What may appear to be a congenial observing ego and a reliable working alliance may be the operation of manic denial and defensive charm. More than one therapist has been shocked by the results of projective testing with an appealing hypomanic patient; the Rorschach in particular often picks up a level of psychopathology that no one on the intake team suspected.

THERAPEUTIC IMPLICATIONS OF THE DIAGNOSIS OF MANIA OR HYPOMANIA

One's primary concern with a hypomanic patient must be the prevention of flight. Unless the therapist discusses this in the first session, interpreting the person's defensive need to escape from meaningful attachments (which will be evident from the history) and contracting with the client to remain for a certain period after feeling the impulse to bolt, there will be no therapy because there will be no patient. One does this as follows:

> "I notice that every important relationship in your life has been disrupted abruptly, usually at your initiative. There's no reason why that won't also happen in *this* relationship—especially because in therapy so many painful things get stirred up. When

life gets painful, your pattern is to flee. I want you to make a deal with me up front that no matter how reasonable it seems, if you suddenly decide to break off your therapy at any point, you'll come back for at least six more sessions,* so that we can understand in depth your decision to go and have a chance to process the ending in an emotionally appropriate way."

This may be the first time the patient has been confronted with the fact that there *is* an emotionally appropriate way to end relationships; that is, one has to deal with grief and other expectable feelings that surround endings. A constant focus on the denial of grief and negative emotions in general should inform the therapy work. Most analysts (e.g., Kernberg, 1975) have considered the prognosis for hypomanic patients to be guarded at best, even when the therapist takes every precaution to prevent flight, because of these clients' extreme difficulties tolerating grief. Sometimes more manifestly "sick" manic patients are easier to help, because the degree of their psychological discomfort supports their motivation to stay in treatment.

With more disturbed manic patients, as with more seriously ill depressive ones, psychotropic medicine has been a godsend. Current psychiatric sophistication makes it possible to adjust type and dosage of medication to the specific needs of the patient; the days when lithium was the only effective drug for mania are long gone. I have found it important, however, to be sure that the prescribing physician takes a careful, individualized approach to each patient; manic clients are as variable as anyone else and often have idiosyncratic physical sensitivities, addictions, and allergies. A dependable relationship with their physician as well as their psychotherapist, and a mutually supportive relationship between these practitioners, supports their recovery. Contrary to some conventional wisdom, psychotherapy is valuable and effective with manic patients; without it, they fail to work through their experiences of ungrieved loss and to learn how to love with less fear. They also stop taking their medicine.

Healthier hypomanic people tend to come to therapy later in life, when their energies and drives have lessened, and when they can see clearly in retrospect how fragmented and unsatisfying their histories are. They sometimes come for individual help after a long stint of work on an addiction in a 12-step program, when their self-destructiveness has lessened and they want to make sense of their life. Like narcissistic

*This quantity is arbitrary. The therapist can pick any number of sessions that seems reasonable and that the patient can imagine tolerating. It can certainly be mutually negotiated.

clients of the grandiose type, with whom they share some defensive patterns, older hypomanic people are sometimes easier to help than their younger counterparts (Kernberg, 1984). But they still need to contract against premature flight. The dearth of literature on the psychotherapeutic treatment of hypomanic personalities may reflect the fact that many therapists learn the hard way that they should have made such an agreement.

Some considerations applicable to the treatment of paranoid patients also apply to hypomanic ones. Frequently one must "go under" a defense; for example, aggressively confronting denial and naming what is denied rather than inviting the patient to explore this intrinsically rigid, inflexible defense. The therapist must appear strong and devoted. He or she should interpret upward, educating the hypomanic person about normal negative affect and its lack of catastrophic effects.

Because of manic terrors of grief and self-fragmentation, therapy should move slowly. The clinician who demonstrates deliberateness offers a spinning client a different model of how to live in the world of feelings. Treatment should also be conducted in an especially forthright tone. In their efforts to avoid psychic pain, most manic people have learned to say whatever works. Emotional authenticity is a struggle for them. The therapist must therefore inquire periodically whether they are telling the truth, as opposed to explaining away, entertaining, or temporizing. Like paranoid people, hypomanic clients need a therapist who is active and incisive, and who lacks cant, hypocrisy, and self-deception.

DIFFERENTIAL DIAGNOSIS

The main obstacle to accurate assessment of hypomanic clients was noted in the section on transference and countertransference: Therapists tend to misperceive these initially appealing people as having less primitive defenses, more ego strength, and better identity integration than they do, a mistake that may alienate a sensitive hypomanic person after only one interview. Manically organized clients outside the psychotic range are most commonly diagnosed as hysterical, narcissistic, or compulsive. Those with psychotic symptoms are most frequently misunderstood as schizophrenic.

Hypomanic versus Hysterical Personality

Because of their charm, their seeming capacity to engage warmly, and their apparent insightfulness, hypomanic clients, especially women, can be misunderstood as hysterical. This error risks losing the patient quickly, since the technical stance appropriate to people with hysterical organization makes the hypomanic person feel insufficiently "held" and only superficially understood. The unconscious conviction that anyone who seems to like them has been duped exists in manically structured people just as in depressive ones; it will issue in devaluation of and flight from the therapist unless addressed directly in ways that would be contraindicated with a hysterically structured patient. Evidence of abruptly ended relationships with people of both sexes, a history of traumatic and unmourned losses, and absence of the hysterical person's concern with gender and power are some of the areas that differentiate hypomanic from hysterical people.

Hypomanic versus Narcissistic Personality

Because grandiosity is a central feature of manic functioning, it is easy to misconstrue a hypomanic or cyclothymic person as the more grandiose kind of narcissistic patient—again, in remarkable parallel to confusions between genuinely depressive (melancholic) patients and the depressed–depleted type of narcissistic person. A good history should highlight the disparity; narcissistically structured people lack the turbulent, driven, catastrophically fragmented backgrounds of most hypomanic clients.

Again, the intrapsychic difference is between subjective emptiness in the narcissistic person and the presence of savagely negative introjects—managed by denial—in the hypomanic one. Although an arrogant narcissistic person can be difficult to treat, and resists attachment in many ways, the threat of immediate flight is minimal. Misconstruing a hypomanic individual as narcissistic can thus cost one a patient. The two groups have an affinity, however, in that both become more accessible therapeutically when older; moreover, analysts who understand grandiose narcissism in introjective terms (e.g., Kernberg, 1975) advocate a similar approach to each type of client.

Hypomanic versus Compulsive Personality

The driven qualities of the hypomanic person invite comparison with characterological compulsivity. Both compulsive and hypomanic people are ambitious and demanding, and on this basis, they have sometimes been compared (Cohen, Baker, Cohen, Fromm-Reichmann, & Weigart, 1954; Akiskal, 1984). Their similarities are mostly superficial, however. Akhtar (1992), contrasting the hypomanic person with the compulsive client (whom he construes, following Kernberg, as being by definition at the neurotic level of personality organization), summarizes:

> Unlike the hypomanic, the compulsive individual is capable of deep object relations, mature love, concern, genuine guilt, mourning, and sadness. . . . The compulsive is capable of lasting intimacy but is modest and socially hesitant. The hypomanic, on the contrary, is pompous, loves company, and rapidly develops rapport with others only to lose interest in them soon afterward. The compulsive loves details, which the hypomanic casually disregards. The compulsive is tied down by morality and follows all rules, while the hypomanic, like the "perverse character" (Chasseguet-Smirgel, 1985), cuts corners, defies prohibitions, and mocks conventional authority. (pp. 196–197)

Thus, as is the case with the distinction between hypomania and hysteria, it is critical to notice the difference between the internal meaning and the manifest content of behavior.

Mania versus Schizophrenia

A manic person in a psychotic condition can look very much like a schizophrenic in an acute hebephrenic episode. This differential is important for medication purposes. Popular impressions aside, the fact that someone is overtly psychotic does not equate to his or her being schizophrenic. To determine the nature of a person's disorganization, especially with younger patients having an initial psychotic break, it is important to take a good history (from the client's family if the client is too delusional to talk), to assess underlying flatness of affect and to evaluate the capacity to abstract. The conditions we sometimes call "schizoaffective" comprise psychotic-level reactions that have both manic–depressive and schizophrenic features and consequently require especially sensitive pharmacological treatment.

SUMMARY

In this chapter I have discussed patients who are organized characterologically along depressive lines, whatever their experience with the disorders of mood that we know as clinical depression. In terms of drive, emotion, and temperament, I emphasized orality, unconscious guilt, and exaggerated sorrow or joy, depending on whether the patient is depressively or manically inclined. The ego processes of introjection, turning against the self, and idealization in predominantly depressive structure, and the ego processes of denial, acting out, and devaluation in predominantly manic organization, were detailed. Object relations were understood in terms of traumatic loss, inadequate mourning, and parental depression, criticism, abuse, and misunderstanding. Images of the self as irredeemably bad were discussed. Emphasis was placed on the appealing qualities of depressive and manic people in the sections on transference and countertransference, with associated rescue wishes and potential demoralization of the therapist.

Technical suggestions included, in addition to a sustained empathic attitude, the vigorous interpretation of explanatory constructs, persistent exploration of reactions to separation, attacks on the superego, and in manic patients, flight-prevention contracts and a persistent demand for honest self-expression. Diagnostically, depressive clients were distinguished from narcissistically organized people with depressive overtones and from masochistically oriented patients; hypomanic and manic clients were differentiated from hysterical, narcissistic, compulsive, and schizophrenic people.

SUGGESTIONS FOR FURTHER READING

Laughlin's (1967) chapter on the depressive personality is excellent, though hard to find these days. Gaylin's (1983) anthology on depression contains a first-rate summary of psychoanalytic thinking on depression. The only recent essay I know of on the hypomanic personality is in Akhtar's (1992) *Broken Structures*. Again, Fenichel (1945) is worth reading on both depressive and manic conditions for those who are not put off by his somewhat arcane terminology.

❖12❖ Masochistic (Self-defeating) Personalities

People who seem to be their own worst enemies pose fascinating questions for students of human nature. When someone's history is filled with decisions and actions antithetical to that person's well-being, we find it hard to grasp. Freud saw self-defeating behavior as the most vexing problem addressed by his theory, since he had founded it (in conformance with the biological theory of his day [see Sulloway, 1979]) on the premise that organisms try to maximize pleasure and avoid pain. He emphasized how in normal development, infantile choices are determined by the pleasure principle, later modified by the reality principle (see Chapter 2). Because some choices seem at face value to observe neither the pleasure nor the reality principle, Freud did a lot of stretching and revising of his own metapsychology to account for self-defeating or "masochistic" behavior patterns (Freud, 1905, 1915a, 1916, 1919, 1920, 1923, 1924).*

*For one thing, he eventually postulated a "death instinct" of equal power with the life-promoting libidinal drive, a principle akin to Aristotle's notion of anabolism and catabolism as primary natural processes. This construct has been of interest to students of metapsychology, but most therapists regard it as too abstract to be clinically useful. Further, most contemporary analysts believe that masochistic behavior can be explained without recourse to such an experience-distant concept, whatever its epistemic status.

Early psychoanalytic theory needed to account for the erotic practices of those who, like the Austrian writer Leopold von Sacher-Masoch, sought orgasm via torment and humiliation. Sexual excitement in suffering pain had already been named after Sacher-Masoch, just as pleasure in inflicting it had been named after the Marquis de Sade (Krafft-Ebing, 1900). To Freud, who emphasized the ultimate sexual origins of most behavior, it followed naturally to apply the term masochism to ostensibly nonsexual patterns of self-created pain (see LaPlanche & Pontalis, 1973; Panken, 1973).

To distinguish a general pattern of suffering in the service of some ultimate goal from the narrow sexual meaning of masochism, Freud (1924) coined the phrase "moral masochism." By 1933 the concept was accepted widely enough that Wilhelm Reich included the "masochistic character" in his compilation of personality types, stressing patterns of suffering, complaining, self-damaging and self-depreciating attitudes, and an inferred unconscious wish to torture others with one's pain. Moral masochism and masochistic personality dynamics have intrigued analysts for a long time (Reik, 1941; Fenichel, 1945; Menaker, 1953; Berliner, 1958; Laughlin, 1967; Schafer, 1984; Asch, 1985; Grossman, 1986; Kernberg, 1988).

When contemporary writers refer to masochism without a specific sexual referent, they usually mean moral masochism. Like other phenomena covered in this book, morally masochistic behavior is not necessarily pathological, even though it is, in the narrowest sense, self-abnegating. Sometimes morality dictates that we suffer for the sake of something worthier than our short-term individual comfort (see de Monchy, 1950; Brenner, 1959; Kernberg, 1988). This is the spirit in which Helena Deutsch (1944) observed that motherhood is inherently masochistic. Most mammals, in fact, put the welfare of their young ahead of their personal survival. This may be "self-defeating" for an individual animal but not for the offspring and the species. Even more praiseworthy instances of masochism occur when people risk their lives, health, and safety in the service of a greater social good, like the survival of their culture or values. Some people—Mahatma Gandhi and Mother Teresa come to mind—for whom strong masochistic trends in their personalities can be assumed, have demonstrated heroic, even saintly devotion to causes greater than their individual selves.

Outside the range of moral masochism, the term "masochistic" is sometimes used to refer to nonmoralized patterns of self-destructiveness, as with people who are accident-prone, or with those who mutilate or otherwise harm themselves deliberately but without suicidal intent. Implied in this use of the word is that there is some method behind the self-destructive person's apparent madness, that some objective is being pursued that makes physical suffering pale, in the mind of the self-injurer, when evaluated next to the emotional relief being sought through these improbable means. Self-cutters, for example, will typically explain that the sight of their own blood makes them feel alive and real, and that the anguish of feeling nonexistent or alienated from sensation is profoundly worse than any temporary physical discomfort.

Masochism thus exists in varying degrees and tones. Self-destructiveness can characterize anyone from the psychotic self-mutilator to the Chevy Chase-like bumbler. Moral masochists range from the Christian martyrs of legend to the Jewish mothers of lore. Everyone behaves masochistically under certain circumstances (see Salzman, 1960a; Baumeister, 1989), often to good effect. Children learn on their own that one way to get attention from caregivers is to get themselves in trouble. A colleague of mine described his initiation into the dynamics of normal masochism when his 7-year-old daughter, angry at him for not having spent any time with her, announced her intention to go upstairs and break all her toys.

A modus operandi of moral triumph through self-imposed suffering may become so habitual in a person that he or she may be legitimately seen as having a masochistic character. Richard Nixon, for instance, has been regarded as a moral masochist by many observers (see Wills, 1970) on the basis of his aggrieved, self-righteous tone, his predilection to present himself as suffering nobly, and his questionable judgment in situations in which his welfare has been at stake (e.g., his failure to destroy the Watergate tapes that eventually destroyed his presidency).

I want to stress here that the term masochism as used by psychoanalysts does not connote a love of pain and suffering. The person who behaves masochistically endures pain and suffering in the hope, conscious or unconscious, of some greater good. When an analytic observer comments that a battered wife is behaving masochistically in staying with an abusive man, the commentator is not accusing her of liking to be beaten up. The implication is rather that her actions betray a belief that tolerating abuse either accomplishes some goal that justifies her suffering (such as keeping her family together), or averts some even more painful eventuality (such as complete abandonment), or both. The remark also suggests that her calculation is not working, that her staying with an abuser is objectively more destructive or dangerous than her leaving would be, yet she continues to behave as if her ultimate well-being were contingent on her enduring mistreatment.*

Masochistic and depressive character patterns overlap considerably, especially at the neurotic-to-healthy level; most people with either structure have aspects of the other. Kernberg (1984, 1988) regards the depressive–masochistic personality as one of the most common types of neurotic character. I am emphasizing the *differences* between the two psychologies because, especially at the borderline and psychotic levels, they require significantly contrasting therapeutic styles. Much damage can be done when, with the best intentions, a therapist misunderstands a predominantly masochistic person as basically depressive, and vice versa.

DRIVE, AFFECT, AND TEMPERAMENT IN MASOCHISM

In interesting contrast with depressive conditions, self-defeating patterns have not been subject to extensive empirical research, possibly because the concept of masochism has not been widely embraced beyond the psychoanalytic community. Consequently, little is known about constitutional contributions to masochistic personality organization. Except for Krafft-Ebing's conclusion that sexual masochism is genetic and some speculations about the role of oral aggression (e.g., L. Stone, 1979), few hypotheses have been made about innate temperament. Clinical experience suggests that the person who becomes characterologically masochistic may be (as may also be true of those who develop a depressive character) more constitutionally sociable or object-seeking than, say, the withdrawing infant who inclines toward a schizoid style.

The possibility of individual constitutional vulnerability to masochism is thus still an open question. A related biological topic that has claimed much more professional attention, and that seems much clearer at least at the phenomenological level, concerns gender. There is an impression among many practitioners and researchers (e.g., Galenson, 1988) that childhood trauma and maltreatment create contrasting

*I emphasize this because in the discussions about whether the DSM-III-R should include a masochistic diagnosis in the Personality Disorders section (tentatively labeled "Self-defeating Personality Disorder"), it became apparent that practitioners who are unfamiliar with or unfriendly to the psychodynamic tradition regard the attribution of masochism as equivalent to accusing people so diagnosed of enjoying pain—of "blaming the victim" as if he or she consciously provoked abuse for the sake of some perverted form of enjoyment.

dispositions in children of different sexes. Namely, abused girls tend to develop a masochistic pattern, while abused boys are more likely to identify with the aggressor and to develop in a more sadistic direction. Like all generalizations, this one admits of many exceptions—masochistic men and sadistic women are not rare. But perhaps the greater physical strength of adult men, and the anticipation of that advantage by little boys, disposes males to master trauma by proactive means and leaves their sisters with a disposition toward stoicism, self-sacrifice, and moral victory through physical defeat—time-honored weapons of the weak. If there are also biological and chemical processes that influence this intriguing divergence, we are still in the dark as to how they operate.

The affective world of the masochistically organized person is very similar to that of the depressive one, with a critical addendum. Conscious sadness and deep unconscious guilt feelings predominate, but in addition, most masochistic people can easily feel anger, resentment, and even indignation on their own behalf. In such states of feeling, self-defeating people have more in common with those disposed to paranoia than with their depressive counterparts. In other words, masochistic people see themselves as suffering, but unfairly; as victimized or just ill-starred, cursed through no fault of their own (as in "bad karma"). Unlike those with simply depressive themes, who are at some level resigned to their unhappy fate because it is all they think they deserve, masochistic people may rail against it like Shakespeare's lover who troubled deaf Heaven with his bootless cries.

DEFENSIVE AND ADAPTIVE PROCESSES IN MASOCHISM

Like depressive people, masochistic ones employ the defenses of introjection, turning against the self, and idealization. In addition, they rely heavily on acting out (by definition, since the essence of masochism lies in self-defeating actions). Moral masochists also use moralization (again, definitionally) to cope with their inner experiences. For reasons that I will cover shortly, people with self-defeating personalities are more active in general than depressive people, and their behavior reflects their need to *do* something with their depressive feelings that counteracts states of demoralization, passivity, and isolation.

The hallmark of masochistic personality is defensive acting out in ways that risk harm. Most unconsciously driven, self-defeating actions include the element of an effort to master an expected painful situation (R. M. Loewenstein, 1955). If one is convinced that, for example, all authority figures will sooner or later capriciously punish those who depend on them, and if one is in a chronic state of anxiety waiting for this to happen, then provoking the expected punishment will relieve the anxiety and provide reassurance about one's power: At least the time and place of one's suffering is self-chosen. Therapists with a control–mastery orientation (e.g., Suffridge, 1991) refer to this behavior as "passive-into-active transformation."

Freud (1920) was initially impressed with the power of what he called the *repetition compulsion* in instances of this type. Life is unfair: Those who suffer most in childhood usually suffer most as adults, and in scenarios that uncannily mirror their childhood circumstances. To add insult to injury, the adult situations seem to observers to be of the sufferer's own making, though that is hardly the conscious experience of that person. As Sampson, Weiss, and their colleagues have pointed out, repetitive patterns characterize everyone's behavior; if one is lucky enough to have had a safe and affirming childhood, one's personal schemata are hardly visible, since they fit comfortably with realistic opportunities in life and tend to reproduce emotionally positive situations. When one has had a frightening, negligent, or abusive background, the need to recreate those circumstances in order to try to master them psychologically can be not only visible but tragic.

A self-cutting patient I treated for many years eventually located the sources of her masochism in early abuse by her mother, including once when this deeply disturbed woman had, in a blind rage, cut my patient with a knife. As memories came back, and as she grieved over her prior helplessness and began discriminating between present and past realities, her self-mutilation gradually ceased. But not before she had scarred her skin irreversibly and had created traumatic scenes for other people. Because she was at the psychotic level of personality organization, the work was slow and precarious, though ultimately successful.

A much healthier woman I worked with used to announce her latest financial extravagances to her frugal, obsessive compulsive husband whenever their relationship began to feel warm and comfortable. This would reliably send him into a fury. We figured out together that this provocative habit revealed an unconscious conclusion she had drawn as a child that whenever things are calm, a storm is about to break. When her marriage was going well, she would begin unconsciously to worry that like her explosive father, her husband was about to destroy their happiness with an outburst. She was thus behaving in a way that she viscerally knew would bring it on, in order to get it over with and begin a pleasant interlude.

Unfortunately, from her husband's standpoint she was not reinstating pleasure, she was causing pain.

Reik (1941) explored several dimensions of masochistic acting out, including: (1) provocation (as in the preceding vignette); (2) appeasement ("I'm already suffering, so please withhold any further punishment"); (3) exhibitionism ("Pay attention: I'm in pain"); and (4) deflection of guilt ("See what you made me do!"). Most of us use minor masochistic defenses frequently for one or more of these reasons. Therapists in training who approach supervision in a flood of self-criticism are often using a masochistic strategy to hedge their bets: If my supervisor thinks I made a major error with my client, I've already shown that I'm aware of it and have been punished enough; if not, I get reassured and exonerated.

Self-defeating behavior is usually very object related: It has a way of engaging others and sometimes involving them in the masochistic process. Once in a therapy group I belonged to, a member kept bringing the group's criticism down upon himself in a relentlessly predictable way, of which he seemed naively unaware. When confronted with the evidence that his whining, self-abasing stance evoked exasperation and attack from others, he became uncharacteristically subdued and admitted, "I'd rather be hit than not touched at all." I will say more about this dynamic in the section on object relations.

Moralization can be an exasperating defense in masochistic clients. Often they are much more interested in winning a moral victory than in solving a practical problem. It took me weeks of work to get one self-defeating patient to consider writing a letter to the IRS that would get her the large refund to which she was legally entitled. She spent her therapy hours trying to convince me that the IRS had handled her tax return ineptly—which was emphatically true but completely beside the point if the point was to get her money back. She much preferred my sympathetic indignation to my attempts to help her get recompensed. Left to herself, she would have gone on collecting and bemoaning injustices rather than eliminating one.

Part of the dynamic here seems to be a special way of handling the depressive conviction that one is bad. The need to get listeners to validate that it is *others* who are guilty can be great enough to overwhelm the practical objectives to which most people give priority. One reason that children with a stepparent—even a kind and well-meaning one—tend to behave masochistically (acting resentful or defiant, and inciting punitive responses) may pertain to unconscious guilt. Youngsters who have lost a parent tend to worry that their badness drove him or her away. Preferring a sense of guilty power to helpless impotence, they try to convince themselves and others that it is the substitute parent who is bad, thus deflecting attention from their own felt wrongdoing. They provoke until the stepparent's behavior supports their conviction.

These dynamics may explain why it is often hard to influence a stepfamily system in a purely behavioral way. The agenda of an angry and guilt-driven party may have much more to do with continuing to suffer (so that someone else is seen as culpable) than with improving the family atmosphere. This phenomenon is of course not exclusive to children or to reconstituted families. Any elementary-school teacher has a reservoir of anecdotes about biological parents who presented themselves as long-suffering martyrs to their child's misbehavior yet could not implement any suggestions for improving it. One gets the feeling that their need to be confirmed in a perception of the child as bad, and in their own role as enduring stolidly, outranks other considerations.

Another defensive process that should be mentioned here is denial. Masochistically organized people frequently demonstrate by their words and behavior that they are suffering, or that someone is abusing them, yet they may deny that they are feeling any particular discomfort and protest the good intentions of the perpetrator. "I'm sure she means well and has my best interests at heart," one of my clients once remarked about an employer who obviously disliked him and had humiliated him in front of all his colleagues. "How did you feel about her treatment of you?" I asked. "Oh, I figured she was trying to teach me something important," he responded, "so I thanked her for her efforts."

OBJECT RELATIONS IN MASOCHISM

Emmanuel Hammer is fond of saying that a masochistic person is a depressive who still has hope. What he means is that in the etiology of masochistic as opposed to depressive conditions, the deprivation or traumatic loss that led to a depressive reaction was not so devastating that the child simply gave up on the idea of being loved (see Spitz, 1953; Berliner, 1958; Salzman, 1962; Lax, 1977; I. Bernstein, 1983). Many parents who are barely functional can nevertheless be jarred into action if their child is hurt or endangered. Their children learn that although in general they feel abandoned and therefore worthless, if they are suffering enough, they may get some care (Thompson, 1959). One young woman I saw for an intake procedure had an extraordinary history of injury, illness, and misfortune. She had also had a psychotically depressed mother. When I asked for her earliest memory, she cited an incident from age 3 when she had knocked over an iron, burned herself, and received a rare infusion of maternal solace.

Usually the history of a masochistic person sounds like the history of a depressive one, with major unmourned losses, critical or guilt-inducing caregivers, role reversals where the child feels responsible for the parents, instances of trauma and abuse, and depressive models (Dorpat, 1982). Yet if one listens carefully, one also hears a theme of people being there for the patient when he or she was in deep enough trouble. Where depressive people feel that there is no one there for them, masochistic ones feel that if only they can sufficiently demonstrate their need for sympathy or care, they may not have to endure complete emotional abandonment.

Esther Menaker (e.g., 1953) was one of the first analysts to describe how the origins of masochism lie in unresolved dependency issues and fears of being alone. "Please don't leave me; I'll hurt myself in your absence" is the essence of many masochistic communications, as it was in the example of my colleague's daughter who planned to destroy all her toys (see also Berliner, 1958). In a fascinating research project on the psychologies of severely and repeatedly battered women, the ones that women's shelter personnel tear their hair out over because they keep returning to partners who barely stop short of killing them, my former student Ann Rasmussen (1988) learned that these gravely endangered people fear abandonment much more than they fear pain or even death. She notes:

> When separated from their batterers, most of the subjects fell into an abyss of such acute despair that they succumbed to Major Depressions and could barely function. . . . Many described being incapable of feeding themselves, getting out of bed, and interacting with others. As one subject put it, "when we were apart I didn't know how to get up in the morning . . . my body forgot how to eat, each bite was like a rock in my stomach." The depths to which they sank when alone were unrivaled by any states of distress they experienced when with their abusive mates. (p. 220)

It is not uncommon to learn from masochistic patients that the only time a parent was emotionally invested in them was when they were being punished. An association of attachment and pain is inevitable under these circumstances. Teasing, that peculiar combination of affection and cruelty, can also breed masochism (Brenman, 1952). Especially when punishment has been excessive, abusive, or sadistic, the child learns that suffering is the price of relationship. And children crave relationship even more than physical safety. Victims of childhood abuse usually internalize their parents' rationalization for the mistreatment, because it feels better to be beaten than to be neglected. Another subject in Rasmussen's (1988) study confided:

> I have had the feeling I wished I was little again. I wish I was still up under my mother's care. I wish I could be whipped now, because whipping is a way of making people listen and to know in the future. If I had a mother to whip me more, I could keep myself in line. (p. 223)

One other aspect of the history of many people whose personalities become masochistically structured is that they have been powerfully rewarded for enduring tribulation gallantly. When she was 15, a woman I know lost her mother to cancer of the colon. The mother lived at home in the months she was dying, wasting away in an increasingly comatose and incontinent state. Her daughter took over the role of nurse, changing the dressings on her colostomy, washing the bloody sheets daily, and turning her mother's body to prevent bedsores. The mother's mother, deeply touched by such devotion, expounded fulsomely on how brave and unselfish her granddaughter was, how God must be smiling on her, how uncomplainingly she gave up normal adolescent pursuits to care for her dying mother. All this was true, but the long-term effect of her having received so much reinforcement for self-sacrifice, and so little encouragement to take some time off to meet her own needs, set her up for a lifetime of masochism: She handled every subsequent developmental challenge by trying to demonstrate her generosity and forbearance. Others reacted to her as tiresomely self-righteous, and they chafed at her repeated efforts to mother them.

In their everyday relationships, self-defeating people tend to attach to friends of the misery-loves-company variety, and if they are of the moral masochistic variety of sufferer, they gravitate toward those who will validate their sense of injustice. They also tend—battered spouses being only the most extreme example—to recreate relationships in which they are treated with insensitivity or even sadism. Some sadomasochistic attachments seem to be a result of the self-defeating person's having chosen a mate with a preexisting tendency to abuse; in other instances it appears that he or she has connected with an adequately kind partner and brought out the worst in him or her.

Nydes has pointed out (1963; cf. Bak, 1946) that people with masochistic personalities have certain commonalities with paranoid people, and that some individuals swing cyclically from masochistic to paranoid orientations. The source of this affinity is their common orientation to *threat*. Both paranoid and self-defeating people feel in constant danger of attacks on their self-esteem, security, and physical well-being. The paranoid solution in the face of this anxiety is something like "I'll attack you before you attack me," while the masochistic response is "I'll attack myself first so you don't have to do it." Both masochistic and paranoid people are unconsciously preoccupied with the relationship between power and love. The paranoid person sacrifices love for the sake of a sense of power; the masochistic one does the reverse. Especially at the borderline level of personality organization, these different solutions may present as alternating ego states, leaving a therapist confused as to whether to understand the patient as a frightened victim or a menacing antagonist.

Masochistic dynamics may permeate the sexual life of someone with a self-defeating personality (Kernberg, 1988), but many characterologically masochistic people are not sexual masochists (in fact, while their masturbation fantasies may contain masochistic elements in order to magnify excitement, they are often turned off sexually by any note of aggression in their partner). Conversely, many people whose particular sexual history gave them a masochistic erotic pattern are not self-defeating personalities. One unfortunate legacy of early drive theory, which connected sexuality so intimately with personality structure at the conceptual level, has been a glib assumption that sexual dynamics and personality dynamics are always isomorphic. Often, they are. But perhaps luckily, people are frequently more complex.

THE MASOCHISTIC SELF

The self-representation of the masochistic person is also comparable, up to a point, with that of the depressive: unworthy, guilty, rejectable, deserving of punishment. In addition, there may be a pervasive and sometimes conscious sense of being needy and incomplete rather than simply bereft, and a belief that one is doomed to be misunderstood, unappreciated, and mistreated. People with a moral-masochistic personality structure often impress others as grandiose and scornful, exalted in their suffering and scornful of those lesser mortals who could not endure equivalent tribulation with so much grace. Although this attitude makes moral masochists look as if they are enjoying their suffering, a better formulation would be that they have found a compensatory basis in it for supporting their self-esteem (Stolorow, 1975; Kohut, 1977; Schafer, 1984; Cooper, 1988).

Sometimes when masochistic clients are recounting instances of mistreatment by others, one sees traces of a sly smile on their otherwise aggrieved features. It is easy to infer that they are feeling some sadistic pleasure in defaming their tormenters so soundly. This may be another source of the common assumption that self-defeating people enjoy their misery. It is more accurate to say that they derive some secondary gain from their attachment-through-suffering solutions to their interpersonal dilemmas. They fight back by not fighting back, exposing their abusers as morally inferior for showing their aggression, and savoring the moral victory that this stratagem achieves. Most therapists are familiar with clients who complain piteously about mistreatment by a boss, relative, friend, or mate, yet when encouraged to do something to remedy their situation, look disappointed, change the subject, and switch their grievances to another arena. When self-esteem is enhanced by bearing misfortune courageously, and is diminished by acting on one's own behalf ("selfishly" or "self-indulgently" in the moral lexicon of masochistic people), it is difficult to reframe an unpleasant situation as requiring corrective measures.

Unlike most depressively organized people, who tend to retreat into loneliness, masochistic people handle their felt badness by projecting it onto others and then behaving in a way that elicits evidence that the badness is outside rather than inside. This is another way in which self-defeating patterns and paranoid defenses are similar. Masochistic people usually have less primitive terror than paranoid ones, however, and do not require as many defensive transformations of affect in order to eject their unwanted aspects. And unlike paranoids, who may be very reclusive, they need other people close at hand to be the repositories of their disowned sadistic inclinations. A paranoid person can resolve anxiety by attributing projected malevolence to vague forces or distant persecutors, but a masochistic one attaches it to someone right at hand, whose observable behavior demonstrates the rightness of the projector's belief in the moral turpitude of the object.

TRANSFERENCE AND COUNTERTRANSFERENCE WITH MASOCHISTIC PATIENTS

Masochistic clients tend to reenact with a therapist the drama of the child who needs care but can only get it if he or she is demonstrably suffering. The therapist may be seen as a parent who must be persuaded to save and comfort the patient, who is too weak, threatened, and unprotected to handle life's exigencies without help. If the client has gotten into some truly disturbing, dangerous situations, and seems clueless as to how to get extricated, it is not uncommon for a therapist to feel that before treatment can begin, the person's safety must be secured. In less extreme examples of masochistic presentations, there is still some communication of helplessness in the face of life's mistreatment, along with evidence that the only way the client knows how to cope with difficulty is by trying to be tolerant, stoic, or even cheerful in the face of misfortune.

The patient's subjective task is thus to persuade the therapist that he or she (1) *needs* to be rescued and (2) *deserves* to be rescued. Coexisting with these aims is the fear that the therapist is an uncaring, distracted, selfish, critical, or abusive authority who will expose the client's worthlessness, blame the victim for being victimized, and abandon the relationship. The rescue agendas and fears of maltreatment may be either conscious or unconscious, ego syntonic or ego alien, depending on the client's level of personality structure. In addition, self-defeating people live in a state of dread, almost always unconscious, that an observer will discern their shortcomings and reject them for their sins. To combat such fears, they try to make obvious both their helplessness and their efforts to be good.

There are two common countertransferences to masochistic dynamics: countermasochism and sadism. Usually both are present. The most frequent pattern of practitioner response, especially for newer therapists, is first to be excessively (and masochistically) generous, trying to persuade the patient that one appreciates his or her suffering and that one can be trusted not to attack. Then, when that approach only seems to make the patient more helpless and wretched, the therapist notices ego-alien feelings of irritation, followed by fantasies of sadistic retaliation toward the client for being so intractably resistant to help.

Because therapists often have depressive psychologies, and because it is easy—especially early in treatment—to misunderstand a predominantly masochistic person as a basically depressive one, clinicians often seek to do for the patient what would be helpful to *them* if they were in the patient role. They emphasize in their interpretations and their conduct that they are available, that they appreciate the extent of the person's unhappiness, and that they will take extra pains to be of help. Therapists have been known to reduce the fee, schedule extra sessions, take phone calls around the clock, and make other special accommodations in the hope of increasing a therapeutic alliance with a patient who is stuck in a dismal morass. Such actions, which might facilitate work with a depressive person, are counterproductive with a masochistic one in that they invite regression. The patient learns that self-defeating practices pay off: The more pronounced the suffering, the more giving the response. The therapist learns that the harder he or she tries, the worse things get—a perfect mirror of the masochistic person's experience of the world.

I have observed in myself and my students that we all learn the hard way how to work with masochistic clients, how to avoid acting out masochistically and suffering upsetting sadistic reactions to people for whom we would rather feel sympathy. Most therapists recall vividly the client with whom they learned to set limits on masochistic regression rather than to reinforce it. In my own case, I am embarrassed to report that in the flush of a rescue fantasy toward one of my first deeply disturbed patients, a paranoid–masochistic young man in the psychotic range, I was so eager to prove I was a good object that, on hearing his sad story about how there was no way for him to get to work anymore, I lent him my car. Not surprisingly, he drove it into a tree.

In addition to the common inclination to support rather than confront masochistic reactions, therapists usually find it hard to admit to sadistic urges. Because feelings that go unacknowledged are likely to be acted out, this inhibition can be dangerous. The sensitivity of contemporary consumers of mental health services to the possibility of therapists' blaming the victim is probably not accidental; it may well derive from the sense of many former patients that they were subjected to unconscious sadism from therapists when they were in a vulnerable role. If one has extended oneself to the point of resentment with a client who only becomes more dysphoric and whiny, it gets easy to rationalize either a punitive interpretation or a rejection ("Perhaps this person needs a different therapist").

Masochistic clients can be infuriating. There is nothing more toxic to a therapist's self-esteem than a patient who sends the message, "Just try to help me—I'll only get worse." This negative therapeutic reaction (Freud, 1937) has long been known to reflect unconscious masochistic dynamics, but understanding that intellectually and going through it emotionally are two different things. It is hard to maintain an attitude of benign support in the face of someone's stubbornly self-abasing behavior (see Frank et al. [1952] on the "help-rejecting complainer").

Even in writing this chapter I am aware of slipping into a mildly affronted tone as I try to describe the masochistic process; some analysts writing about self-defeating patients have sounded outright contemptuous (e.g., Bergler, 1949). The ubiquity of such feelings highlights the need for carefully formulated therapeutic strategies. Masochistic and sadistic countertransference reactions need not burden treatment unduly, though a therapist who denies feeling them will almost certainly run into trouble.

THERAPEUTIC IMPLICATIONS OF A DIAGNOSIS OF MASOCHISM

Beginning early in the 20th century, Freud and many of his followers wrote about masochistic dynamics, describing their origins and functions, their unconscious objectives, and their hidden meanings. The first person to write specifically about technique with characterologically masochistic people, however, was Esther Menaker. In "The Masochistic Factor in the Psychoanalytic Situation" (1942), she observed that many aspects of classical treatment, such as the patient's lying supine while the analyst looks on and the analyst's interpreting in an authoritative manner, could be experienced by masochistic clients as replicating humiliating interactions of a dominant–submissive nature. She recommended technical modifications such as face-to-face treatment, emphasis on the real relationship as well as on the transference, and avoidance of all traces of omnipotence in the analyst's tone. Without the excision of all such potentially sadomasochistic features of the therapy situation, Menaker felt that patients would be at risk of feeling only a repetition of subservience, compliance, and the sacrifice of autonomy for closeness.

This argument still holds, though perhaps more in the spirit than the letter of Menaker's recommendations. Her remarks about the couch, for example, have become somewhat moot, since in contemporary psychoanalytic practice, only high-functioning patients would be encouraged to lie down and free associate (and presumably the neurotic-level masochistic person would have a strong enough observing ego to appreciate that relaxing on a couch does not equate to accepting a humiliating defeat). But her stress on the centrality of the real relationship stands. Because the masochistic person urgently needs an exemplar of healthy self-assertion, the quality of the therapist as a human being, expressed in the way he or she structures the therapeutic collaboration, is critical to the prognosis of a self-defeating patient—more so than for people with most other kinds of personalities. The therapist's unwillingness to be exploited or to extend generosity to the point of inevitable resentment may open up whole new vistas to someone who was brought up to sacrifice all self-regarding concerns for the sake of others. Hence, the first "rule" for treating self-defeating clients is not to model masochism.

Years ago, one of my supervisors, knowing I had a commitment to serving people of limited means, told me that it was fine to let most kinds of patients run up a bill if they suffered financial reverses, but that I should never be lenient in this way with a masochistic client. As I am constitutionally incapable of taking good advice until I make the mistake that illuminates its wisdom, I disregarded his warning in the case of a diligent, earnest, and personally appealing man who convincingly described a money crisis that seemed outside his control. I offered to "carry" him until he got back on his feet financially. He proceeded to get more and more incompetent with money, I got more and more aggrieved, and eventually we had to rectify my mistake with a headache of a plan for repayment. I have not made this error since, but I notice that my students typically learn this piece of technique through bitter experience, just as I did. It would not be so upsetting if the therapist were the only one who paid the price of misguided generosity, but as the harm to the patient becomes obvious, one's confidence as a healer can suffer as much as one's pocketbook.

It is thus no service to self-defeating clients to demonstrate "therapeutic" self-sacrifice. It makes then feel guilty and undeserving of improvement. They can scarcely learn how to exert their prerogatives if the therapist models self-effacement. Rather than trying to give a masochistic person a break with the fee, one should charge an amount that is adequate recompense for the skill needed to work with a challenging dynamic, and then receive payment in the spirit of feeling entitled to it. Nydes would intentionally show masochistic patients his pleasure in being paid, fondling their bills happily or folding their checks with obvious relish.

The resistance of most therapists to showing appropriate amounts of self-concern and self-protectiveness, despite the clear need of masochistic patients to see and to stop hating those aspects of themselves, probably comes not only from possible internal inhibitions about self-interest—always a good bet with therapists—but also from accurate forebodings that self-defeating patients will react to the display of such qualities with anger and criticism. In other words, one will be punished for selfishness, in the same way most masochistic people were punished by their early objects. This is true. It is also to be hoped for. Self-destructive people do not need to learn that they are tolerated when they are smiling bravely; they need to find out that they are accepted even when they are losing their temper.

Moreover, they need to understand that anger is natural when one does not get what one wants and can be simply understood as such by others. It does not have to be fortified with self-righteous moralism and exhibitions of suffering. Masochistic people believe they are entitled to feel hostility only when they have been clearly wronged, a presumption that costs them countless hours of unnecessary psychological exertion. When they feel some normal level of disappointment, frustration, or anger, they must either deny or moralize in order not to feel shamefully selfish. When a therapist acts self-concerned, and treats his or her masochistic patients' reactive outrage as natural and interesting, some of these patients' most cherished and pathological internal categories get reshuffled.

For this reason, most experienced therapists advise "No *rachmones*" (no expressions of sympathy) with masochistic patients (Nydes, 1963; Hammer, 1990). This does not mean that one blames them for their difficulties, or returns sadism for their masochism, but it does mean that instead of communications that translate into "You poor thing!," one tactfully asks, "How did you get yourself into that situation?" The emphasis should always be on the client's capacity to improve things. These ego-building, noninfantilizing responses tend to irritate self-defeating people, who believe that the only effective way to elicit warmth is to demonstrate helplessness; thus such interventions provide opportunities for the therapist to welcome the expression of normal anger and to show understanding for the patient's negative feelings.

Similarly, one should not rescue. One of my most disturbed masochistic patients, whose symptoms ranged from bulimia to multiple addictions to anxieties of psychotic proportions, used to go into a paralysis of panic whenever she feared that an expression of her anger had alienated me. On one such occasion, she became so frantic that she persuaded the staff of the local mental health center to hospitalize her and signed herself in for 72 hours. Within half a day, having calmed down and now wanting no part of an inpatient experience, she got a psychiatrist to agree that if she obtained my permission, she could be discharged early. "You knew you were signing yourself in for 3 days when you did this," I responded, "so I would expect you to keep your commitment." She was livid. But years later, she confided that that had been the turning point in her therapy, because I had treated her like a grown-up, a person capable of living with the consequences of her actions.

In the same vein, one should not buy into guilt and self-doubt. One can feel powerful pressure from masochistic clients to embrace their self-indicting psychology. Guilt-provoking messages are often strongest around separations. A person whose self-destructiveness escalates just when the therapist is about to take a vacation (a common scenario) is unconsciously insisting that the therapist is not allowed to enjoy something without agonizing over how it is hurting the patient. Behaviors that translate into "Look what you made me suffer!" or "Look what you made me do!" are best handled by empathic reflection of the client's pain, combined with a cheerful unwillingness to let it rain on one's parade.

Setting an example that one takes care of oneself without feeling guilt about the neurotic reactions of others may elicit moralistic horror from masochistic people, but it simultaneously inspires them to experiment with being a bit more self-respectful. I originally learned this while working with a group of young mothers whose shared masochism was formidable (McWilliams & Stein, 1987). My co-leader was the target of oppressive nonverbal broadcasts that her upcoming vacation was wounding the group members. These messages were delivered with disingenuous maternal reassurances that she should not feel too bad about forsaking them. In response, she announced that she did not feel the slightest bit guilty, and that she was looking forward to having a good time and not having to think about the group at all. The women became incensed but were animated and honest again, as if pulled out of a quagmire of deadness, hypocrisy, and passive aggression.

Timing, of course, is critical. If one comes on too strong too fast, before a reliable working alliance is in place, the patient will feel criticized and blamed. The art of conveying a sympathetic appreciation that the suffering of masochistic people is truly beyond their conscious control (despite its appearing to be self-chosen) and at the same time adopting a confrontational stance, one that respects their ability to make their volition conscious and change their circumstances, cannot be taught in a textbook. But any reasonably caring practitioner develops an intuition about how and when to confront, and about how, when one's inevitable mistakes increase the patient's pain (Wolf, 1988), to apologize without excessive self-recrimination.

In addition to behaving in ways that counteract the pathological expectations of masochistic patients, the therapist should actively interpret evidence for irrational but prized unconscious beliefs such as "If I suffer enough, I'll get love," or "The best way to deal with my enemies is to demonstrate that they are abusers," or "The only reason something good happened to me was that I was sufficiently self-punitive." It is common for self-defeating people to have magical beliefs that connect assertiveness or confidence with punishment, and self-abasement with eventual triumph. One finds in most religious practices and folk traditions a connection between suffering and reward, and masochistic people often support their pathology uncritically with these ideas. Such beliefs may console us, softening our outrage about suffering that may be both capricious and unambiguously destructive. However, when these ideas get in the way of taking action when it might be effective, they do more harm than good.

Among the greatest contributions of control–mastery theory to psychoanalytic understanding is its emphasis on pathogenic beliefs (e.g., Weiss, 1992) and on the client's repeated efforts to test them. In addition to passing these tests by such means as the refusal to act masochistically in the role of therapist, the clinician must help the client become aware of what the tests are, and what they reveal about his or her underlying ideas about the nature of life, human beings, the pursuit of happiness, and so on. This part of treatment, though not as emotionally challenging as controlling one's countertransferences, is the hardest to effect. Omnipotent fantasies behind masochistic behaviors die hard. One can always find evidence in random events that one's successes have been punished and one's sufferings rewarded. The therapist's persistance in exposing irrational beliefs often makes the difference between a "transference cure"—the temporary reduction of masochistic behaviors based on idealization of and identification with the therapist's self-respecting attitude—and a deeper and lasting movement away from self-abnegation.

DIFFERENTIAL DIAGNOSIS

Masochistic patterns are common to all psychopathology. We would not ordinarily consider something pathological if it were not harmful to the self in some way. Thus, by definition, there is a masochistic component in all the personality configurations discussed in this book—at least when they approach a pathological level of defensive rigidity or developmental arrest sufficient to establish them as character "disorders" rather than simply "character." But the masochistic function of any type of pattern is not identical to masochism as an organizing personality theme. The types of individual psychology most easily confused with the kind of characterological masochism covered here are depressive and dissociative psychologies.

Masochistic versus Depressive Personality

Many people have a combination of depressive and masochistic dynamics, and are appropriately regarded as depressive–masochistic characters. Most, however, have the balance between these elements weighted in one direction or the other. It is important to discriminate between these two depressively toned psychologies because the optimal therapeutic style for each type of personality differs. The predominantly depressive person needs above all else to learn that the therapist will not judge, reject, or abandon, and will, unlike the internalized objects that maintain depression, be particularly available when he or she is suffering. The more masochistic person needs to find out that self-assertion, not helpless suffering, can elicit warmth and acceptance, and that the therapist, unlike the parent who could be brought to reluctant attention if a disaster was in progress, is not particularly interested in the details of the patient's current misery.

If one treats a depressive person as masochistic, one may provoke increased depression and even suicide, as the client will feel both blamed and abandoned. If one treats a masochistic person as depressive, one may reinforce self-destructiveness. At the most concrete level, most experienced practitioners have found that when antidepressant medication is given to someone with a masochistic personality, even if symptoms of clinical depression are present, the medicine does very little other than to feed the patient's pathogenic belief that he or she needs authorities and their magic in order to feel better.

When seeing a person with both depressive and masochistic tendencies, the therapist must keep assessing whether a more depressive or more masochistic dynamic is active in the work at hand, so that the tone of his or her interventions is appropriate to the primary defensive process in the patient.

Masochistic versus Dissociative Psychology

Over the past two decades there has been an explosion in our knowledge about dissociation. Acts that we used to understand exclusively according to general theories of masochism have been reinterpreted in more specific ways for patients with a history of traumatic and sadistic abuse. A surprisingly large group of people are subject to dissociated states in which they repeat prior harm to themselves. The most dramatic exemplar of a vulnerability to dissociated self-injury is the client with multiple personality disorder who switches ego states by self-hypnotic means and then engages in a reenactment of early tortures. Investigation usually reveals the existence of an alter personality, identified with the original tormentor, for whom the main personality is amnestic.

The general dynamic in such cases is indeed masochistic, but if the therapist misses the fact that the self-injury was carried out by an alter personality when the person the therapist knows as the patient was not in control of the body, interpretations will be futile. Chapter 15 covers treatment suggestions for dissociative people; for now the reader should note that especially in more bizarre cases of self-harm, the patient should be asked matter-of-factly if he or she remembers doing it.* If the client does recall inflicting the injuries, one should then inquire about the degree to which he or she felt depersonalized or disembodied. Until such a patient has access to the state of mind in which a self-destructive act was committed, interventions aimed at reducing dissociation take priority over interpretations of masochism.

SUMMARY

I have given a brief history of the concept of moral masochism and related self-defeating patterns, distinguishing them from lay conceptions of masochism as joy in pain. I mentioned gender predispositions (to masochism in women and sadism in men) while stressing that masochistic personality organization is common in people of both sexes. Emotional components of masochism include the main depressive affects plus anger and resentment, and relevant ego processes include the depressive defenses plus acting out, moralization, and denial. Masochistic relationships parallel early experiences with objects who attended to the growing child negligently or abusively, yet with occasional warmth when he or she was suffering. Masochistic self-representation is similar to that of the depressive person, with the addition of self-esteem regulation through enduring mistreatment bravely.

Transferences of self-defeating patients were understood as reflecting wishes to be valued and rescued; countertransferences of masochism and sadism were discussed. Treatment recommendations include attention to the real relationship (specifically the therapist's modeling of healthy self-regard), respect for the patient's capability and responsibility for problem solving, and persistence in exposing, challenging, and modifying pathogenic beliefs. Finally, masochism was distinguished from depressive and dissociative psychologies.

SUGGESTIONS FOR FURTHER READING

Reik's (1941) study of moral masochism, though dated in some aspects, is still worth reading and is not so mired in difficult metapsychology

*If abuse was inflicted by an alter personality, it will usually not be remembered. Dissociative clients are rattled by forgetting, however, and will not volunteer that they do not recall hurting themselves. They "cover" their amnesia by appearing to go along with the therapist's assumption that they recollect what they did.

that a beginner in this area would be put off. Stolorow's (1975) essay will bring the reader up to date on masochism from a more contemporary, self psychology perspective. Lax's (1977) study of masochistic women is a valuable contribution of recent years, as is Cooper's (1988) article on the narcissistic–masochistic character. An edited volume on masochism by Glick and Meyers (1988) includes several good essays, most of which concern characterological patterns.

> or extreme demands, these personality characteristics may congeal into symptomatic behavior that will then be ritualized. (p. 10)

He might have added that Wilhelm Reich (1933) depicted them as "living machines," on the basis of their rigid intellectuality (Shapiro, 1965). Woodrow Wilson or Hannah Arendt or Martin Buber could be considered representative of a high-functioning person in this diagnostic group, while Mark Chapman, whose obsession with John Lennon led to a compulsion to assassinate him, might be seen as at the psychotic end of the obsessive compulsive continuum.

DRIVE, AFFECT, AND TEMPERAMENT IN OBSESSIVE AND COMPULSIVE PERSONALITIES

Freud (1908) believed that obsessive and compulsive people had been rectally hypersensitive in infancy, physiologically and constitutionally. Contemporary analysts have not found such an assumption necessary to account for obsessional dynamics, but most would agree that "anal" issues color the unconscious worlds of obsessional people. Freud's (1909, 1913, 1917b, 1918) emphasis on fixation at the anal phase of development (roughly 18 months to 3 years), particularly on aggressive urges as they become organized during that period, was novel, seminal, and far less outlandish than debunkers of psychoanalysis would have it.

First, Freud noted that many of the features that typically hang together in people with obsessive compulsive personalities—cleanliness, stubbornness, concerns with punctuality, tendencies toward withholding—are the salient issues in a toilet-training scenario. Second, he found anal imagery in the language, dreams, memories, and fantasies of obsessive compulsive patients.* Third, he had clinical evidence that the people he treated for obsessions and compulsions had been pushed toward bowel control prematurely or harshly or in an atmosphere of parental overinvolvement (Fenichel, 1945).† Connec-

*The earliest memory of one obsessive man I treated was of sitting on the toilet refusing to "produce." The reader can probably infer his attitude in response to the invitation to free associate.

†The rectal sphincter does not mature until around 18 months. Hence, the authoritative advice to middle-class parents early in the 20th century to start toilet training in their child's first year was disastrous. It promoted coercion in the name of parental diligence and transformed a benign process of mastery into a dominance–submission contest. If one considers the popularity in that era of giving enemas to young children, an intrinsically traumatic procedure usually rationalized in the name of "hygiene," one cannot fail to be impressed with the sadistic implications of the culturally sanctioned rush toward premature anal control.

tions between anality and obsessionality have since been repeatedly supported by empirical research (e.g., Noblin, Timmons, & Kael, 1966; Fisher, 1970; Rosenwald, 1972; Tribich & Messer, 1974; Fisher & Greenberg, 1985) as well as by clinical reports attesting to obsessive compulsive preoccupations with the anal issues of dirt, time, and money (MacKinnon & Michels, 1971). Classical formulations about obsessive and compulsive dynamics that center on early body experience are very much alive and well (see Shengold's [1987] *Halo in the Sky* for a brilliant contemporary exploration of anality). Though for some reason, American theorists have been less interested recently in the anal phase than analysts in France (e.g., Grunberger, 1979; Chasseguet-Smirgel, 1984).

Freud reasoned that toilet training usually constitutes the first situation in which the child must renounce what is natural for what is socially acceptable. The responsible adult and the child who is being trained too early or too strictly or in an atmosphere of lurid parental overconcern enter a power struggle that the child is doomed to lose. The experience of being controlled, judged, and required to perform on schedule creates angry feelings and aggressive fantasies, often about defecation, that the child eventually feels as a bad, sadistic, dirty, and shameful part of the self. The need to feel in control, punctual, clean, and reasonable, rather than out of control, erratic, messy, and caught up in emotions like anger and shame, becomes important to the maintenance of identity and self-esteem. The kind of harsh, all-or-nothing superego created by these kinds of experiences manifests itself in a rigid ethical sensibility that Ferenczi (1925) wryly called "sphincter morality."

The basic affective conflict in obsessive and compulsive people is rage (at being controlled) versus fear (of being condemned or punished), but what strikes therapists working with them is that affect is muted, suppressed, unavailable, or rationalized (MacKinnon & Michels, 1971). Words are used to conceal feelings, not to express them. Any therapist can recall instances of asking an obsessional client how he or she *felt* about something and getting back what he or she *thought*. An important exception to the rule of concealed affect in this diagnostic group concerns rage: Anger is acceptable to the obsessional person if it is seen as reasonable and justified. Righteous indignation is thus tolerable, even admired; being annoyed because one did not get what one wanted is not. Therapists frequently feel the presence of normal irrational anger in an obsessive person, but the patient typically hides it—despite sometimes being able to acknowledge intellectually that some instance of behavior (forgetting the check for the third time, or interrupting the therapist in midsentence, or pouting) could denote a passive aggressive or hostile attitude.

Shame is the other exception to the general picture of affectlessness in obsessive compulsive people. They have high expectations for themselves, project them on to the therapist, and then feel embarrassed to be seen falling short of their own standards for proper thoughts and deeds. Shame is generally conscious, at least in the form of mild feelings of chagrin, and if gently treated, can usually be named and investigated by the therapist without the protest and denial that are usually evoked by questions about other feelings.

DEFENSIVE AND ADAPTIVE PROCESSES IN OBSESSIVE AND COMPULSIVE PERSONALITIES

As the preceding paragraphs imply, the organizing defense of predominantly obsessive people is *isolation* (Fenichel, 1928). In compulsive people, the main defensive process is *undoing*. Those who are obsessive and compulsive employ both isolation and undoing. Higher-functioning obsessional people do not usually use isolation in its most extreme forms; they instead prefer maturer versions of the separation of affect from cognition: rationalization, moralization, compartmentalization, and intellectualization. Finally, people in this clinical group rely heavily on *reaction formation*. Less definingly but as an adjunct to the preceding mechanisms, obsessional people at all developmental levels also use *displacement*, especially of anger, in circumstances in which by diverting it from its original source to a "legitimate" target, they can own such a feeling without shame.

Cognitive Defenses against Drives, Affects, and Wishes

Obsessional people overvalue cognition and mentation. They tend to consign feelings to a devalued realm associated with childishness, weakness, loss of control, disorganization, and dirt. They are consequently at a significant disadvantage in situations where emotions, physical sensations, and fantasy have a powerful and legitimate role. The widow who ruminates ceaselessly about the details of her husband's funeral, keeping a stiff upper lip and converting all mourning into frenetic busyness, not only fails to process her grief effectively but also deprives others of the consolations of offering comfort. Obsessional people in executive positions deny themselves adequate release and recreation, and hurt their employees by making drivenness the company rule.

People with obsessive characters are often effective in formal, public roles yet out of their depth in intimate, domestic ones. Although they are capable of loving attachments, they may not be able to express their tenderer selves without anxiety and shame; consequently, they may turn emotionally toned interactions into oppressively cognitive ones. In therapy and elsewhere, they may lapse into second-person locutions when describing emotions ("How did you feel when the earthquake hit?" "Well, you feel kind of powerless"). Not every human activity should be approached from the standpoint of rational analysis and problem solving. One man with whom I did an intake interview responded to my question about the quality of his sexual relationship with his wife with the somber assertion, "I get the job done."

Obsessionally organized people in the borderline and psychotic range may use isolation so relentlessly that they look schizoid. The prevalent misconception of the schizoid person as unfeeling may be based on observations of regressed obsessional people who have become wooden and robotic, so deep is the gulf between their thinking and feeling. Other more disturbed obsessional people border on paranoia; the distance between an extreme obsession and a delusion is not very great. I am told that in the era before antipsychotic medication, the only way to make a differential diagnosis between an extremely rigid, nonpsychotic obsessive compulsive person and a barely defended paranoid schizophrenic was to put the patient in question into a protected room and emphasize that now he or she would be safe and could relax. Thus invited to suspend obsessional defenses, a schizophrenic person would begin to talk about paranoid delusions, while an obsessive compulsive one would set about cleaning the room.

Behavioral Defenses against Drives, Affects, and Wishes

Undoing is the defining defense mechanism for the kind of compulsivity that is implicated in obsessive and compulsive symptoms and personality structure. Compulsive people undo by actions that have the unconscious meaning of atonement and/or magical protection. Deleterious compulsive behaviors like overdrinking, overeating, taking drugs, gambling, shoplifting, and sexualizing are more characteristic of people at the borderline and psychotic levels of compulsive organization, though they are not unknown in the neurotic range. Compulsivity differs from impulsivity in that a particular action is repeated over and over in a stylized and sometimes escalating way. Compulsive actions also differ from "acting out," strictly speaking, in that they are not so centrally driven by the need to master unprocessed past experiences by recreating them.*

Compulsive activity is familiar to all of us. Finishing the food on our plate when we are no longer hungry, cleaning the house when we should be studying for an exam, criticizing someone who offends us even though we know it will have no effect other than making an enemy, throwing "just one more" quarter into the slot machine. Whatever one's compulsive patterns, the disparity between what one feels impelled to do and what is reasonable to do can be glaring. Compulsive activities may be harmful or beneficial; what makes them compulsive is not their destructiveness but their drivenness. Florence Nightingale was probably compulsively helpful; Dana Carvey may be compulsively funny. People rarely come to treatment for their compulsivity if it works on their behalf, but they do come with related problems. Knowing that these patients are organized compulsively can aid therapists in helping them with whatever they *are* looking to do in therapy.

Compulsive actions often have the unconscious meaning of undoing a crime. Lady Macbeth's handwashing is a famous literary example of this dynamic, though in her case the crime was actually committed. In most instances, the compulsive person's crimes exist mainly in fantasy. One of my patients, a married oncologist who knew very well that AIDS was not transmitted by mouth-to-mouth contact, felt helplessly compelled to get tested repeatedly for HIV antibodies after she had kissed a man with whom she was tempted to have an affair. Even compulsions that are manifestly free of a sense of guilt can be found to have originated in guilt-inducing interactions; for example, most people who compulsively clean their plates were made to feel guilty as children about rejecting food when there is starvation in the world.

Compulsive behavior also betrays unconscious fantasies of omnipotent control. This dynamic is related to preoccupations with one's presumed crimes in that a determination to control, like the need to undo, derives from beliefs that originated before thoughts and deeds were differentiated. If I think my fantasies and urges are dangerous, that they are equivalent to powerful actions, I will try to restrain them with a comparably powerful counterforce. In prerational cognition (primary process thought), the self is the center of the world, and what happens

*As was true for the general meaning of masochism, most behavior that we consider pathological is by definition compulsive in a broad sense: The doer seems driven to act again and again in ways that prove useless or harmful. The schizoid person is compelled to avoid people, the paranoid to distrust, the psychopath to use, and so on. Only when an undoing dynamic is predominant is an action regarded as compulsive in the narrower sense of an obsessive compulsive dynamism or a compulsive personality organization.

to oneself is the result of one's own activity, not the chance twists of fate. The baseball player who performs a ritual before each game, the priest who gets anxious if he left something out of a prayer, the pregnant woman who keeps packing and repacking her suitcase for the hospital—all think at some level that they can control the uncontrollable if only they do the right thing.

Reaction Formation

Freud believed that the conscientiousness, fastidiousness, frugality, and diligence of obsessive compulsive people were reaction formations against wishes to be irresponsible, messy, profligate, and rebellious, and that one could discern in the overresponsible style of obsessive and compulsive patients a hint of the inclinations against which they had struggled. The incessant rationality of the obsessional person, for example, can be seen as a reaction formation against a superstitious, magical kind of thinking that obsessional defenses do not fully succeed in obscuring. The man who stubbornly insists on driving even though he is exhausted betrays the conviction that averting an accident depends on *his* being in charge of the car, not on a combination of an alert driver and some good fortune. In insisting on so much control, he is out of control in every significant way.

In Chapter 6 I talked about reaction formation as a defense against tolerating ambivalence. In working with obsessive and compulsive people, one is struck by their fixation on *both* sides of conflicts between cooperation and rebellion, initiative and sloth, cleanliness and slovenliness, order and disorder, thrift and improvidence, and so forth. Every compulsively organized person seems to have one messy drawer. Paragons of virtue may have a paradoxical island of corruption: The eminent theologian Paul Tillich had an extensive pornography collection; Martin Luther King Jr. was a wanton womanizer. People who try excessively hard to be upright and responsible may be struggling against more powerful temptations toward self-indulgence than most of us face; if this is so, then it should not surprise us when they are only partially able to counteract the impulses of which they are so afraid.

OBJECT RELATIONS IN OBSESSIVE AND COMPULSIVE PERSONALITIES

The parents and caregivers of people who develop in obsessive and compulsive directions are notorious for setting high standards of behavior and expecting early conformity to them. They tend to be strict and consistent in rewarding good behavior and punishing malfeasance. When they are basically loving, they produce emotionally advantaged children whose defenses lead them in directions that vindicate their parents' scrupulous devotion. The traditional American child-rearing style documented in McClelland's (1961) classic studies of achievement motivation tends to produce obsessive and compulsive people who expect a lot of themselves and have a good track record for achieving their goals.

When parents are unreasonably exacting, or prematurely demanding, or condemnatory not only of unacceptable behavior but also of accompanying feelings, thoughts, and fantasies, their children's obsessive and compulsive adaptations can take a problematic form. One man I worked with for several years had been raised in a stern midwestern Protestant family of deep religious conviction but shallow affectional capacity. His parents hoped he would become a minister and began working on him early to forego temptation and banish all thoughts of sin. This brand of pedagogy gave him no trouble—in fact, he found it easy to imagine assuming the morally elevated role into which they were so eager to cast him—until he reached puberty and found that sexual temptation was not nearly so abstract a danger as it had previously seemed. From then on, he overdosed with self-criticism, conducted incessant rationalistic ruminations about sexual morality, and launched heroic efforts to counteract erotic feelings that another boy would have simply learned to enjoy and master.

From an object relations point of view, what is notable about obsessive and compulsive people is the centrality of issues of *control* in their families of origin. While Freud depicted the anal phase as engendering a prototypical battle of wills, people with an object relations perspective emphasize that the parent who was unduly controlling about toilet training was probably equally controlling about oral- and oedipal-phase issues, and subsequent ones, for that matter. The mother who laid down the law in the bathroom is likely to have fed her child according to a schedule, demanded that naps be taken at particular times, inhibited many forms of spontaneous motor activity, prohibited masturbation, insisted on conventional sex-role behavior, punished loose talk, and so forth. The father who was forbidding enough to provoke regressions from oedipal to anal concerns was probably also reserved toward his infant, stern with his toddler, and authoritarian with his school-age child.

In old-fashioned obsessive compulsive-breeding families, control tended to be expressed in moralized, guilt-inducing terms, as in "I'm disappointed that you were not responsible enough to have fed your dog on time," or "I expect more cooperative behavior from a big girl like you," or "How would you like it if somebody else treated you that way?" Moralization was actively modeled. Parents explained their own actions on the basis of what was right ("I don't enjoy punishing you, but it's for your own good"). Productive behavior was associated with virtue, as in the "salvation through work" theology of Calvinism. Self-control and deferral of gratification were idealized.

There are still many families that operate this way, but post-Freudian, popularized ideas about the inhibiting effects of too moralistic an upbringing (combined with 20th-century dangers and cataclysms that suggest the wisdom of "getting it while you can" rather than postponing gratification) have changed child-rearing practices sufficiently that we now see fewer obsessive and compulsive people of the morally preoccupied type common in Freud's day. Many contemporary families that are organized around control issues foster obsessive and compulsive patterns through shaming rather than guilt-induction. Messages like "What will people think of you if you're overweight?" or "The other kids won't want to play with you if you behave like that," or "You'll never get into an Ivy League college if you don't do better," have, according to many clinicians and societal observers, become more common messages than communications stressing the primacy of individual conscience and the moral implications of one's behavior.

It is important to appreciate this change if one is working with more contemporary obsessive and compulsive psychopathologies such as eating disorders (not that anorexia and bulimia nervosa were unknown at the turn of the century, but they were almost certainly less prevalent). More traditional Freudian accounts of compulsion are insufficient in accounting for anorectic and bulimic compulsivity; theorists who have explored narcissistic object relations more thoroughly than Freud did have provided more clinically useful formulations (see Yarock, 1993). This caveat also applies to many instances of alcoholism, drug abuse, gambling, and other behavior disorders in which the background personality is not the moralistic obsessive compulsive of Freudian fame but the narcissistic perfectionist of more recent notoriety.

Guilt- and shame-inducing upbringings produce different kinds of superegos and different types of object relations. The traditional obsessive compulsive was more deeply motivated by guilt than by shame, although he or she was subject to feelings of shame when "out of control." Most early psychoanalytic writing on obsessive and compulsive dynamics concerns guilt-driven people, and what has come to be known as obsessive compulsive character structure—in the DSM and elsewhere—assumes that kind of psychology. It is thus critical for clinicians to distinguish between the traditional obsessive, compulsive, or obsessive compulsive person and the more narcissistically structured individual who has obsessive and compulsive defenses.

One other kind of family background has been noted in the formation of obsessive and compulsive personality, and as is typical in psychoanalytic observation, it is the polar opposite of the overcontrolling, moralistic variety. Some people feel so bereft of clear family standards, so unsupervised and casually ignored by the adults around them, that in order to push themselves to grow up they hold themselves to idealized criteria of behavior and feeling that they derive from the larger culture. These standards, since they are abstract and not modeled by people known personally to the unparented child, tend to be harsh and unbuffered by a humane sense of proportion. One of my patients, for example, whose father was a melancholy alcoholic and whose mother was overburdened and distracted, grew up in a house where nothing ever got done. The roof leaked, the weeds proliferated, the dishes sat in the sink. He was deeply ashamed of his parents' visible ineptitude, and he developed a powerful determination to be the opposite: organized, competent, in control. He became a very successful tax advisor, but a driven workaholic who lived in fear that he would betray himself as a fraud who was somehow in essence as ineffectual as his father and mother.

In the early psychoanalytic literature the phenomenon of the development of obsessive compulsive character in underparented children was noted with great interest, since it challenged Freud's model of superego formation, which postulated the presence of a strong and authoritative parent with whom the child identifies. Many analysts were finding that their patients with the harshest superegos had been laxly parented (cf. Beres, 1958). They concluded that having to model oneself after a parental image that one invents oneself, especially if one has an intense, aggressive temperament that is projected into that image, can create obsessive compulsive dynamics. Later, Kohut and other self psychologists made similar observations from the standpoint of their emphasis on idealization.

THE OBSESSIVE COMPULSIVE SELF

In keeping with the traditional use of the terms, I will limit this section to the self-concept and self-esteem issues that predominate in classical, guilt-based obsessive and compulsive personality structure. Material on more shame-based psychologies with obsessive and compulsive features can be found in Chapter 8. Obsessive and compulsive people are deeply concerned with issues of control and moral rectitude. They tend to define the latter in terms of the former; that is, they equate righteous behavior with keeping aggressive, lustful, and needy parts of the self under strict rein. They are apt to be seriously religious, hard-working, self-critical, and dependable. Their self-esteem comes from meeting the demands of internalized parental figures who hold them to a high standard of behavior and sometimes thought. They worry a lot, especially in situations in which they have to make a choice, and they can be easily paralyzed when the act of choosing has portentous implications.

This paralysis is one of the most unfortunate effects of the reluctance of obsessional people to make a choice that might turn out badly. Early analysts christened this phenomenon the "doubting mania." In the effort to keep all their options open, so that they can maintain (fantasied) control over all possible outcomes, they end up having no options. An obsessive compulsive acquaintance of mine, on becoming pregnant, lined up two different obstetricians who worked at two different medical centers with opposing philosophies about childbirth. All through her pregnancy she ruminated about which person and facility were preferable. When she went into labor, not having resolved this question, it took her so long to decide whether her condition warranted going to the hospital, and which hospital it should be, that she was suddenly in the later stages of giving birth and had to go to the nearest clinic and be delivered by the resident on duty. All her painstaking obsessing was rendered futile when reality finally enforced its own resolution of her ambivalence.

This is only one example of the tendency of obsessively structured people to postpone decision making until it is clear what the "perfect" (i.e., guilt and uncertainty-free) decision would be. It is common for them to come to therapy trying to resolve ambivalence over two boyfriends, two competing graduate programs, two contrasting job opportunities, and the like. The client's fear of making the "wrong" decision along with a tendency to cast the process of deciding in entirely rationalistic terms—lists of pros and cons are typical—often seduce the therapist into offering an opinion about which choice would be preferable, at which point the obsessional patient immediately responds with counterarguments. The well-known "Yes, but . . ." stance of this kind of person should be understood as, at least in part, an effort to avoid the guilt that inevitably comes with taking action. An unhappy outcome of this psychology is a tendency to postpone and procrastinate until external circumstances like the rejection of a suitor or the passing of a deadline determine one's direction. In standard neurotic fashion, then, the overzealousness to preserve one's autonomy serves eventually to destroy it.

People with a compulsive organization have the same problem with guilt and autonomy, but they solve it in the opposite direction: They jump into action before considering alternatives. Where the obsessive person postpones and procrastinates, the compulsive one speeds ahead. For compulsive people, certain situations have "demand characteristics" requiring certain behaviors. These are not always foolish or self-destructive (like knocking on wood every time one makes an optimistic prediction or jumping into bed every time a situation becomes sexually tinged, respectively); some individuals are compulsively helpful. Darley and Batson (1973), investigating altruistic behavior with a "Good Samaritan" experiment in which a shill who acted sick was put in the path of some theology students on the way to an exam, found that a subgroup of their subjects "couldn't leave the guy alone; they had to go the extra mile to help him" (Batson, personal communication, 1972).* Some drivers will risk their own safety and wreck their cars before hitting an animal, so automatic is their compulsion to preserve life.

The compulsion to act has the same effect on autonomy as the obsessional avoidance of acting. Instrumental thinking and expressive feeling are both circumvented lest the person notice that he or she is actually making a choice. Choice involves responsibility for one's actions, and responsibility involves tolerance of normal levels of both guilt and shame. Nonneurotic guilt is a natural reaction to exerting power, and a vulnerability to shame comes with the territory of taking deliberate action that can be seen by others. Both obsessive and compulsive people are so saturated with irrational guilt and shame that they cannot absorb any more of these feelings.

As mentioned earlier, obsessive people support their self-esteem by thinking; compulsive ones by doing. When circumstances make it hard for obsessive or compulsive individuals to feel good about themselves on the basis of what they are figuring out or accomplishing, respectively, they become depressed. Losing a job is a disaster for almost anybody, but it is catastrophic for a compulsive person because work is the primary source of his or her self-esteem. In the guilt-ridden type of obsessive compulsive client, depression is much more melancholic

*The main finding of this study, as of others designed by Darley and his colleagues, was that situational factors (e.g., whether one was in a hurry), not dispositional ones (e.g., measured personality traits), predicted helping behavior. But character is subtle, and *within the group of people who helped the shill*, there were some the researchers dubbed "superhelpers," who helped compulsively.

than narcissistic in nature (see Chapter 11), with an actively bad (uncontrolled, destructive) self-concept gaining ascendancy.

Obsessive and compulsive people fear their own hostile feelings and suffer inordinate self-criticism over both actual and purely mental aggression. Depending on the content of their family's messages, they may be equally nervous about giving in to lust, greed, vanity, sloth, envy, and the like. Rather than accepting such attitudes and basing their self-respect or self-condemnation solely on how they behave, they typically regard even *feeling* such impulses as reprehensible. Like moral masochists, with whom they share tendencies toward overconscientiousness and indignation, they may nurture a kind of private vanity about the stringency of their demands on themselves. They value self-control over most other virtues and emphasize attributes like discipline, order, reliability, loyalty, integrity, and perseverance. Their difficulties in suspending control diminish their capacities in areas like sexuality, play, humor, and spontaneity in general.

Finally, obsessive compulsive people are noted for avoidance of affect-laden wholes in favor of separably considered minutia (see Shapiro, 1965). People with obsessional psychologies hear all the words and none of the music. In an effort to bypass the overall import of any decision or perception, the appreciation of which might arouse guilt, they become fixed on specific details or implications ("What if . . ."). On the Rorschach test, obsessional subjects avoid whole percept responses and expound on the possible interpretations of small particulars of the inkblots. They cannot (unconsciously, will not) see the forest for the proverbial trees.

TRANSFERENCE AND COUNTERTRANSFERENCE WITH OBSESSIVE AND COMPULSIVE PATIENTS

Obsessive and compulsive people tend to be "good patients" (except toward the lower end of the developmental continuum, where they present formidable obstacles to therapy because of the rigidity of their isolation or the driving immediacy of their compulsions). They are serious, conscientious, honest, motivated, and hard-working. Nonetheless, their reputation for being difficult precedes them. It is typical for obsessional clients to experience the therapist as a devoted but demanding and judgmental parent, and to be consciously compliant and unconsciously oppositional. Despite all their dutiful cooperation, they convey an undertone of irritability and criticism. When a therapist comments on such feelings, they are usually denied. As Freud originally noted, obsessional patients tend to be subtly or overtly argumentative, controlling, critical, and resentful about parting with money. They wait impatiently for the therapist to speak and then interrupt before a sentence is completed. And at a conscious level, they are utterly innocent of their negativity.

Some years ago I treated a man for obsessions and compulsions of a type and intensity that Freud saw frequently. He was an engineering student from India, lost and homesick in an alien environment. In India, deference to authority is a powerfully reinforced norm, and in engineering, compulsivity is highly adaptive and rewarded. But even by the standards of these comparatively obsessive and compulsive reference groups his ruminations and rituals were excessive, and he wanted me to tell him definitively how to stop them. When I reframed the task as understanding the *feelings* behind his preoccupations, he was visibly dismayed. I suggested that he might be disappointed that my way of formulating his problem did not permit of a quick, authoritative solution. "Oh, no!" he insisted; he was sure I knew best, and he had only positive reactions to me.

The following week he came in asking how "scientific" the discipline of psychotherapy is. "Is it like physics or chemistry, an exact science?" he wanted to know. No, I replied, it is not so exact and has many aspects of an art. "I see," he pondered, frowning. I then asked if it troubled him that there is not more scientific accuracy in my field. "Oh, no!" he insisted, absentmindedly straightening up the papers on the end of my desk. Did the disorder in my office bother him? "Oh, no!" In fact, he added, it is probably evidence that I have a creative mind. He spent our third session educating me about how different things are in India, and wondering abstractedly about how a psychiatrist from his country might work with him. Did he sometimes wish I knew more about his culture, or that he could see an Indian therapist? "Oh, no!" He is very satisfied with me.

His was, by clinic policy, an eight-session treatment. By our last appointment, I had succeeded, mostly by gentle teasing, in getting him to admit to being occasionally a little irritated with me and with therapy (not angry, not even aggravated, but just slightly bothered, he carefully noted). I thought the treatment had been largely a failure, though I had not expected to accomplish much in eight meetings. But two years later he came back to tell me that he had thought a lot about feelings since he had seen me, particularly about his anger and sadness at being so far from his native country. As he had let in those emotions, his obsessions and compulsions had waned. In a manner typical of people in this clinical group, he had found a way to feel that he was in control of pursuing insights that came up in therapy, and this subjective autonomy was supporting his self-esteem.

The reader can probably infer that the countertransference with obsessional clients is an annoyed impatience, with wishes to shake them, to get them to be open about ordinary feelings, to give them a verbal enema or insist that they "shit or get off the pot." Their combination of excessive conscious submission and powerful unconscious defiance can be maddening. Therapists who have no personal inclination to regard affect as evidence of weakness or lack of discipline are mystified by the obsessional person's shame about it and resistance to admitting it. Sometimes, one can even feel one's rectal sphincter muscle tightening, in identification with the constricted emotional world of the patient (concordant), and in a physiological effort to contain one's retaliatory wish to "dump" on such an exasperating person (complementary).

The atmosphere of veiled criticism that an obsessive compulsive person emits can be discouraging and undermining. In addition, clinicians easily feel bored or distanced by the client's unremitting intellectualization. With one obsessive compulsive man I treated, I used to find myself having a vivid image that his head was alive and talking, but his body was a life-sized cardboard cut-out like the ones amusement parks provide for customers to put their heads through to be photographed.

Feelings of insignificance, boredom, and obliteration are not common during the treatment of obsessional clients, however (as they are with narcissistic patients who have obsessional defenses). There is something very object related about their unconscious devaluation, and something touching about their efforts to be "good" in such childlike ways as cooperating and deferring. Doubts about whether anything is being accomplished in therapy are typical for the practitioner as well as for the obsessive or compulsive client, especially before the latter is brave enough to express such worries directly to the therapist. But underneath all the obstinacy of the obsessional person is a capacity to appreciate the therapist's patient, noncondemnatory attitude, and as a result, an atmosphere of basic warmth is not hard to maintain.

THERAPEUTIC IMPLICATIONS OF THE DIAGNOSIS OF OBSESSIVE OR COMPULSIVE PERSONALITY

The first rule of practice with obsessive and compulsive people is ordinary kindness. They are used to being exasperating to others, for reasons they do not fully comprehend, and they are grateful for nonretaliatory responses to their irritating qualities. Appreciation for, and interpretation of, their vulnerability to shame is essential. Refusal to advise them, hurry them, and criticize them for the effects of their isolation, undoing, and reaction formation will foster more movement in therapy than more confronting measures. Countertransference-driven power struggles are common between therapists and obsessional clients; they produce temporary affective movement, but in the long run they only replicate early and detrimental object relations.

At the same time that one carefully avoids the therapeutic equivalent of becoming the demanding, controlling parent, one needs to keep relating warmly. The degree of therapist activity will depend on the patient—some obsessional people will not let the clinician get a word in edgewise until the last few minutes of a session, while others become disorganized and frightened if one remains quiet. Refusing to control should be distinguished from attitudes that will be felt as emotional disengagement. Remaining silent with a person who feels a pressure in silence is self-defeating, as is silence with a patient who feels abandoned when he or she is not addressed. Asking the patient's direction on how much the therapist should speak, like other respectful inquiries about what is helpful, may resolve the technical problem and provide the additional benefit of supporting the client's autonomy and sense of realistic control.

An exception to the rule of refusing to advise or control concerns people whose compulsions are outright dangerous. With self-destructive compulsivity, the therapist has two choices: Either tolerate anxiety about what the patient is doing until the slow integration of the therapy work reduces the compulsion to act, or, at the outset, make therapy contingent on the client's stopping the compulsive behavior. An example of the former would be hearing about one driven sexual affair after another while nonjudgmentally analyzing the dynamics involved, until the patient becomes unable to rationalize the defensive use of sexuality. An advantage of this position is its implicit encouragement of honesty (if one sets behavioral conditions for therapy, the patient will be tempted to hide it if he or she cheats). When the person's self-destructiveness is not life threatening, this choice is preferable.

Examples of the latter would include requiring that an addict go through a detoxification program before starting psychotherapy, insisting that a dangerously anorectic client first gain a given number of pounds in a hospital-supervised regime, or making therapy of an alcoholic person conditional on attendance at AA meetings. When undoing is automatic, the wishes, urges, and fantasied crimes being undone will not surface.* Moreover, by accepting compulsively self-harming people into analytic treatment unconditionally, the therapist may unwittingly contribute to their fantasies that therapy will operate magically, without their having at some point to exert self-control. This position is particularly advisable when the patient's compulsion involves substance abuse; doing therapy with someone whose mental processes are chemically altered is an exercise in futility.

The reader may wonder why anyone would want to go through psychotherapy if the compulsive behavior was under control. The answer is that people feel strongly the difference between being able to discipline a compulsion (by efforts of will or submission to authority) and not having one in the first place. Therapy with someone who has stopped behaving compulsively allows that person to master the issues that drove the compulsion, and to find internal serenity rather than a tenuous achievement of self-control. The alcoholic who feels no more need to drink is in a lot better shape than the one who, through constantly reinforced efforts of will, can manage to stay sober despite temptation (Levin, 1987).

The second important feature of good work with people in this diagnostic group, especially the more obsessional ones, is the avoidance of intellectualization. Interpretations that address the cognitive level of understanding, before affective responses have been disinhibited, will be counterproductive. We have all known people in psychoanalytic therapy who can discuss their dynamics in the tone of an auto mechanic detailing what is wrong with someone's motor, and who appear not a bit better for all this knowledge. It was experience with obsessive compulsive people that infused general analytic technique with all its familiar caveats about the dangers of premature interpretation (e.g., Strachey, 1934; Glover, 1955; Josephs, 1992) and the difference between intellectual and emotional insight (e.g., Richfield, 1954; Kris, 1956).

Because it can feel like a power struggle (to both parties) for the therapist to keep harping on the question "But how do you *feel*?" one way to bring a more affective dimension into the work is through imagery, symbolism, and artistic communication. Hammer (1990), in elaborating the consequences of how obsessional people use words

*Many compulsions are not responsive to treatment until the driven person encounters powerful negative consequences. Shoplifters and pedophiles tend to get serious about therapy only after they have been arrested; alcoholics and addicts often have to "bottom out" before getting help; cigarette smokers rarely try to stop before they get scared about their health. As long as one is "getting away with" compulsivity, there is little incentive to change.

more to fend off feeling than to express it, mentions the particular importance to this population of a more poetic style of speech, rich in analogy and metaphor. With extremely constricted patients, the combination of group therapy (where other clients tend to attack the isolative defense head-on) and individual treatment (where the therapist can help the person to process such experiences privately) has proven effective (Yalom, 1975).

A third component of good treatment with obsessionally and compulsively structured people is the practitioner's willingness to help them express their anger and criticism about therapy and the therapist. Usually one cannot do this right away, but one can pave the way for the patient's eventual acceptance of such feelings by preparatory comments such as, "It can be exasperating that the therapy process does not work as fast as we would both want it to. Don't be surprised if you find yourself having resentful thoughts about coming here or about me. If you noticed you were feeling dissatisfied with our work, would anything get in the way of your telling me that?" A frequent response to these ground-laying interventions is a protest that the client cannot imagine being actively dissatisfied and critical. The therapist's position that such a statement is very curious will begin the process of making ego alien the automatic process of isolation.

It is important to go beyond identification of affect to encouragement to enjoy it. Psychoanalytic therapy involves more than making the unconscious conscious; it requires changing the patient's conviction that what has been made conscious is shameful. Behind this susceptibility to shame lie pathogenic beliefs about sinfulness that propel both obsessive and compulsive mechanisms. That one could enjoy a sadistic fantasy, not just own up to it, or derive comfort from grieving, not just admit grudgingly that one is sad, is news to these clients. The sharing of the therapist's sense of humor may lighten the guilt and self-criticism that weigh so heavily on them.

"What good will it do to feel that?" is a frequent query of individuals with obsessive and compulsive psychologies. The answer is that harm is being done in not feeling it, and that emotions make one feel alive, energized, and fully human, even if they express attitudes that the patient has come to see as "not very nice." Especially with compulsive patients, it is useful to comment on their difficulty tolerating just *being*, rather than *doing*. It is no accident that 12-step programs, in their efforts to arrest self-destructive compulsivity, discovered the Serenity Prayer. Occasionally, one can appeal to the practical nature of obsessive and compulsive people when they are resisting the expression of feelings; for example, some scientifically minded patients find it helpful to know that crying rids the brain of certain chemicals associated with chronic mood disturbances. If these patients can rationalize expressiveness as being something other than pathetic self-indulgence, they may risk it sooner. But ultimately, the therapist's quiet dedication to emotional honesty, and the patient's growing experience that he or she will not be judged or controlled, will move the treatment toward a good outcome.

DIFFERENTIAL DIAGNOSIS

Ordinarily, obsessive and compulsive dynamics are easy to differentiate from other kinds of psychological organization. Assessing the operation of isolation and undoing is usually an uncomplicated matter; compulsive organization is particularly conspicuous, since the person's drivenness to act cannot be easily masked. Still, some kinds of confusion occur. Obsessive structure is sometimes hard to distinguish from schizoid psychology, especially at the lower-functioning end of the developmental continuum, and narcissistic personality organization with obsessive or compulsive overtones is frequently mistaken for obsessive and compulsive psychologies of the more "traditional" type.

Obsessive versus Narcissistic Personality

In Chapter 8 I discussed narcissistic versus obsessional character structure, with an emphasis on the damage done when an essentially narcissistic person is misunderstood as obsessive or compulsive, and when the therapist accordingly interprets in the areas of unconscious anger, fantasies of omnipotence, and guilt rather than subjective emptiness and fragile self-esteem. The damage is probably less serious when a mistake is made the other way, since all of us, whatever our character, can profit from therapies that focus on issues of self. Nevertheless, an old-fashioned, moralistic obsessive or compulsive person being treated by someone who construed him or her as narcissistic would be eventually distressed, demoralized, and even insulted by being seen as needy rather than conflicted.

Obsessive and compulsive people have a strong center of gravity psychologically; they are judgmental and self-critical. A therapist who communicates empathic acceptance of their subjective experience without evoking the deeper affects and beliefs that shape that experience is depriving such patients of any empathy worth its name. Sometimes interventions that a therapist conceives as mirroring are received by obsessive and compulsive clients as corrupting, in that the patient views the therapist as implicitly condoning aspects of the self that the patient sees as indefensible. Under these circumstances patients begin to doubt the moral credentials of the therapist. Analysis of the rationalistic and moralistic defenses of obsessive and compulsive clients should precede efforts to convey acceptance of the troublesome feelings these defenses have been erected to conceal.

Obsessive versus Schizoid Personality

In the symbiotic–psychotic range, a number of people who look schizoid may be in fact very regressed obsessional patients. The difference is that although a schizoid person withdraws from the outer world, he or she tends to be conscious of intense inner feelings and vivid fantasies. A withdrawn obsessional person uses isolation so completely that he or she may be subjectively "blank" or even stupid in appearance. The premorbid functioning of someone for whom this differential applies will give the therapist some clue as to whether to communicate to the patient that it is safe to express his or her inner experience, or to convey that it must be terrible to feel so cold and dead inside.

Obsessive Compulsive versus Organic Conditions

Psychopathology of organic origin cannot be covered here, but I should note the frequency with which inexperienced interviewers—whether or not they have had medical training—misconstrue behavior related to brain damage as obsessive compulsive. The perseverative thinking and repetitive actions typical of organic brain syndromes (Goldstein, 1959) can look like obsessiveness and compulsivity of a functional nature, but dynamically informed questioning will reveal that isolation of affect and undoing are not involved. A good history, with inquiries about possible fetal alcohol syndrome, complications at birth, illnesses with high fever (meningitis, encephalitis), head injury, and so forth may suggest an organic diagnosis, which may be confirmed by neurological examination.

Not all brain damage involves loss of intelligence. The practitioner should not assume that because a person is bright and competent, he or she could not suffer from organically based difficulties. This is a critical differential, since therapy to uncover unconscious dynamics in order to reduce a client's obsessive compulsive inflexibility is radically different from treatment that emphasizes, to the organically damaged person and to his or her family, the importance of maintaining order and predictability for the sake of the client's emotional security.

SUMMARY

I have discussed in this chapter people who preferentially think and/or act, in order to pursue emotional security, maintain self-esteem, and resolve internal conflicts. I reviewed classical conceptions of obsessive compulsive character structure, with emphasis on Freud's formulations about the centrality of anal-phase issues in its development. Defensive processes in obsessive and compulsive people (isolation and undoing, respectively, and reaction formation in both) suppress or distract from most affects, wishes, and drives, but unconscious guilt (over hostility) and conscious susceptibility to shame (over falling short of standards) are easily inferred. Family histories of people in this group are notable for either overcontrol or lack of control; contemporary object relations are formal, moralized, and somewhat juiceless, despite the basic capacity for attachment that obsessive compulsive people demonstrate. Perfectionism, ambivalence, and avoidance of guilt by either procrastination or impulsivity were addressed.

Transference and countertransference issues center around noticing and absorbing the patient's unconscious negativity. Therapeutic inferences include the importance of being unhurried, avoiding power struggles, discouraging intellectualization, inviting anger and criticism, and modeling the enjoyment of devalued feelings and fantasies. Obsessive and compulsive personalities were differentiated from narcissistically structured people with perfectionistic and compulsive defenses, from schizoid patients, and from those with organic brain syndromes.

SUGGESTIONS FOR FURTHER READING

Probably the most readable book on obsessionality is Salzman (1980). Nagera (1976) is comprehensive but a little advanced. Shapiro's (1965) study of the obsessional style remains a classic.

❖ 14 ❖
Hysterical (Histrionic) Personalities

Psychoanalysis began with the effort to understand hysteria and has repeatedly returned to that problem in every decade since the 1880s, when Freud first tackled it. Inspired by the work of the French psychiatrists Charcot, Janet, and Bernheim, who were investigating hysterical afflictions via hypnosis, Freud first began asking the kinds of questions that gave psychoanalytic theory its unique shape: How can someone know and not know at the same time? What accounts for forgetting important experiences? Does the body express what the mind cannot fathom? What would explain such sensational symptoms as full epileptic-like seizures in a person without epilepsy? Or blindness in someone optically normal? Or paralysis when nothing is wrong with the nerves?

At the time, hysterically ill women were being thrown out of physicians' offices and called names that were the 19th-century equivalents of "crock." Whatever Freud's mistakes about female psychology or sexual trauma, it is to his credit that he took these women seriously and paid them the respect of believing that by understanding their particular suffering, he would begin comprehending processes that operate in the emotionally healthy as well as in the emotionally disabled. This chapter is not about the dramatic disturbances that have been subsumed under the rubric of hysteria (conversion, amnesia, sudden and inexplicable attacks of anxiety, and many other disparate phenomena) but about a kind of personality structure that has been observed to accompany these conditions.

Hysterical (or, as per later editions of the DSM, histrionic) character is common in people without frequent or striking hysterical symptoms. As with obsessive compulsive people who lack obsessions and compulsions but who operate on the same principles that produce them, there are many of us who have never had hysterical outbreaks but whose subjective experience is colored by the dynamics and defenses that create them. Although this type of personality is seen more in women, hysterically organized men are not uncommon. In fact, Freud (e.g., 1897) regarded himself—with good reason—as somewhat hysterical, and one of his earliest publications (1886) was on hysteria in a man.

Analytically oriented therapists are accustomed to thinking of people with hysterical personality structure as in the neurotic range, since the defenses that mold their experience are considered more mature,* but borderline and psychotic-level hysterical people also exist. Elizabeth Zetzel (1968) observed some time ago the great distance between healthier and more deeply impaired individuals in this group. The phenomenon of *hysterical psychosis* has been known since antiquity (Veith, 1965, 1977) and across cultures (Linton, 1956). The absence from the DSM of this well-researched diagnosis (Hollender & Hirsch, 1964; Langness, 1967; Hirsch & Hollender, 1969; Richman & White, 1970) has arguably impoverished our approach to assessment and contributed to the overdiagnosis of schizophrenia when a trauma-related, hysteroid process should have been considered.†

People with hysterical personalities have high anxiety, high intensity, and high reactivity, especially interpersonally. They are warm, energetic, and intuitive "people people," attracted to situations of personal drama and risk. They may be so addicted to excitement that they go from crisis to crisis. Because of their anxiety level and the conflicts they suffer, their own emotionality may look superficial, artificial, and exaggerated to others, and their feelings may shift rapidly ("hysterical lability of affect"). Sarah Bernhardt may have had many hysterical features; the fictional Scarlett O'Hara had numerous qualities that a contemporary diagnostician would consider histrionic. People with hysterical character structures like high-visibility professions, such as acting, dancing, preaching, politics, and teaching.

*Paradoxically, starting with DSM-III the diagnosis of Histrionic Personality Disorder was reconceptualized toward the pathological end of the hysteroid continuum, indistinguishable from "Zetzel type 3 and 4" hysterical personalities (Zetzel, 1968) and the "infantile personality" of Kernberg (1975; also see Kernberg, 1984, 1992).

†Kernberg and others (see Kernberg, 1992) have used the term "hysterical" for higher-level patients, and "hysteroid," "pseudohysterical infantile," or "histrionic" to refer to borderline-to-psychotic ones.

DRIVE, AFFECT, AND TEMPERAMENT IN HYSTERIA

Many observers have suggested that hysterically organized people are by temperament intense, hypersensitive, and sociophilic. The kind of baby who kicks and screams when frustrated but shrieks with glee when entertained may well have the constitutional template for hysteria. Freud (e.g., 1931) suggested that powerful appetites may be characteristic of people who become hysterical, that they crave oral supplies, love, attention, and erotic closeness. They seek stimulation but get overwhelmed by too much of it, and they have trouble processing distressing experiences.

It has sometimes been suggested (e.g., Allen, 1977) that hysterical people are more dependent constitutionally on right-hemisphere brain functioning (Galin, 1974), in contrast to obsessively inclined individuals, who are inferred to be left-brain dominant. One basis for this speculation is the careful and seminal work of Shapiro (1965) on the hysterical cognitive style, some of which may be innate. Hysterically organized people differ strikingly from more obsessional ones in the quality of their mental operations; specifically, they are impressionistic, global, and imaginal. Some highly intelligent people with hysterical personality organization are remarkably creative; their integration of affective and sensory apperception with more linear, logical approaches to understanding produces a rich integration of intellectual and artistic sensibility.

Freud (1925a, 1932) and many later analysts (e.g., Marmor, 1953; Halleck, 1967; Hollender, 1971) suggested a dual fixation in hysteria, at oral and oedipal issues. An oversimplified account of this formulation follows: A sensitive and hungry little girl needs particularly responsive maternal care in infancy. She becomes disappointed with her mother, who fails to make her feel adequately safe, sated, and prized. As she approaches the oedipal phase, she achieves separation from the mother by devaluing her. She turns her intense love toward father, a most exciting object, especially because her unmet oral needs combine with later genital concerns to magnify oedipal dynamics. But how can she make a normal resolution of the oedipal conflict by identifying with and competing with her mother? She still needs her, and she has also devalued her.

This dilemma traps her at the oedipal level. As a result of her fixation, she continues to see males as strong and exciting, and females, herself included, as weak and insignificant. Because she regards power as inherently a male attribute, she looks up to men, but she also—unconsciously, for the most part—hates and envies them. She tries to increase her sense of adequacy and self-esteem by attaching to males, yet she also subtly punishes them for their assumed superiority. She uses her sexuality, the one kind of power she feels her gender affords, along with idealization and "feminine wiles"—the strategies of the subjectively weak—in order to access male strength. Because she uses sex defensively rather than expressively, and because she fears men and their abuses of power, she does not easily enjoy sexual intimacy with them and may suffer physical equivalents of fear and rejection, such as sexual pain or anesthesia, vaginismus, and failure of orgasm.

Freud's stress on penis envy as a universal female problem came out of his work with hysterically structured women. When he discovered that his patients symbolized male power in their dreams, fantasies, and symptoms with phallic images, he speculated that during their early years these women had equated powerlessness—their own and that of their mothers—with penislessness. In a patriarchal and increasingly complex urban culture where traditional feminine virtues carried little prestige, such a conclusion was probably easy for many young girls to draw. Freud (1932) stated:

> The castration complex of girls is . . . started by the sight of the genitals of the other sex. They at once notice the difference *and, it must be admitted, its significance too*. They feel seriously wronged, often declare that they want to "have something like it too," and fall victim to "envy for the penis," which will leave ineradicable traces on their development and the formation of their character. (p. 125; emphasis added)*

DEFENSIVE AND ADAPTIVE PROCESSES IN HYSTERIA

People with hysterical personalities use repression, sexualization, and regression. They act out in counterphobic ways, usually related to preoccupations with the fantasied power and danger of the opposite

*That Freud appreciated some negative consequences of patriarchy is implied in this quotation. In his life he encouraged women toward professional achievement and intellectual equality. He also hoped that by interpreting penis envy he would spur the revelation in his patients that men are not *in fact* superior—that a belief to that effect betrays an infantile fantasy that can be examined and discarded. Blame for the fact that ideas about penis envy were used by some subsequent therapists in the service of trying to keep women safely in an "appropriate" domestic sphere cannot justly be laid at Freud's door. See Young-Bruehl (1990) for a thoughtful commentary, with primary sources, on Freud's complex views on women.

sex. They also use dissociative defenses, broadly conceived, about which I will say more in the next chapter.

Freud regarded repression as the cardinal mental process in hysteria. Amnesia was a phenomenon of such singular fascination for him that it led to a whole theory about the structure of the mind and about how we can "forget" things that at some inaccessible level we also "know." Freud's first constructions of repression as an active *force* rather than an accidental lapse derived from his work with people who under hypnosis recalled and relived childhood traumas, often incestuous ones, and then lost their hysterical symptoms. In his earliest therapeutic attempts, first with hypnosis and then with nonhypnotic suggestion, he put all his energies into undoing repression, inviting his patients to relax and exhorting them to let their minds be open to recollection. He learned that when traumatic memories returned *with their original emotional power*, hysterical disabilities disappeared.*

Repressed memory and its associated affects became central objects of psychoanalytic study. Lifting repression became seen as a primary therapeutic task. Even now, most dynamically informed treatment seeks to unearth memories and to gain an understanding of the patient's actual background, though most analysts acknowledge that reconstruction of the past is always tentative, and essaying it resembles more the creation of a credible narrative than the retrieval of historical fact (Spence, 1982). Because of the vague, impressionistic nature of cognition in many hysterical people, the development of a linear and congruent account of their individual lives is especially therapeutic to them.

Eventually, Freud became convinced that some of the "memories" recovered by hysterical patients were actually fantasies, and his interest shifted from amnesia for trauma to the repression of wishes, fears, infantile theories, and painful affects.† He saw Victorian myths about the asexual nature of females as particularly inimical to psychological health, and he felt that women raised to repress their erotic strivings were at risk of hysteria because so compelling a biological force could only be deflected, not quelled. He began to see some maladies as

*Abreaction, the cathartic derepression of feelings that accompany trauma, has been rediscovered by students of multiple personality and dissociation. Their technical evolution has been remarkably like Freud's: Their early writings stressed abreactive work, while more recent articles have deemphasized and contextualized this in light of its potential to retraumatize a patient when other aspects of his or her functioning have not been addressed (see Chapter 15).

†Contrary to some popular impressions deriving from Masson's (1984) exposés, Freud did not promote the idea that all reports of early molestation were distortions. He did, however, eventually stress developmental processes over traumatic ones, and repression over dissociation, with mixed effects on subsequent therapeutic history.

conversions of impulse into bodily symptoms. A woman who, for instance, had been reared to regard sexual self-stimulation as depraved might lose feeling and movement in the hand with which she would be tempted to masturbate. This phenomenon, known as "glove paralysis" or "glove anesthesia" because only the hand was affected (which cannot be of neurological origin because any paralysis of the hand would involve the arm), was not uncommon in Freud's time, and it begged for an explanation.

It was symptoms like glove paralysis that inspired Freud to conceive of hysterical ailments as effecting a *primary gain* in the resolution of a conflict between a wish (e.g., to masturbate) and a prohibition (against masturbating), and also *secondary gains* in the form of concern and interest from others. The secondary gains compensated the afflicted person for the loss of sexual attention by the resulting nonerotic attention to his or her body and its disability. With the development of the structural theory, this dynamic was seen as a conflict between the id and the superego.

Freud also felt that such a solution was highly unstable, since sexual energy was being blocked up rather than expressed or sublimated, and he was inclined to interpret any outbreaks of sexualized interest as "the return of the repressed." Repression can be a very useful defense, but it is a brittle and undependable one when it is brought to bear against normal impulses that will continue to be stimulated and to exert a pressure for discharge. Freud's original formulation about the high degree of anxiety for which hysterical people are noted was that they were converting dammed-up sexual energy into diffuse nervousness (see Chapter 2).

I am dwelling on this formulation about hysterical symptoms because a comparable process can be inferred at a characterological level. People who repress erotic strivings and conflicts that seem dangerous or unacceptable tend to feel both sexually frustrated and vaguely anxious. Their normal wishes for closeness and love may become amplified, as if energized by unsatisfied sexual longing. They may be highly seductive (the return of the repressed) but unaware of the implied sexual invitation in their behavior. In fact, they are often shocked when their actions are construed as initiating a sexual connection. Moreover, if they proceed with such an encounter (as they sometimes do, both to placate the frightening sexualizing object and to assuage their guilt over the effects of their behavior), they generally do not enjoy it erotically.

In addition to these interacting processes of repression and sexualization, people with hysterical organization use *regression*. When insecure, fearful of rejection, or faced with a challenge that stimulates unconscious guilt and fear, they may become helpless and childlike in an attempt to fend off trouble by disarming potential rejecters and abusers. Like anyone in a state of high anxiety (cf. the "Stockholm syndrome" or the "Patty Hearst phenomenon," terms describing situations in which captive people become trusting toward their abductors or persecutors), hysterical personalities may be quite suggestible. In the high-functioning range they can be extremely charming when operating regressively; in the borderline and psychotic ranges histrionic patients may become physically ill, clingily dependent, or whiny. The regressive aspect of hysterical presentation was, until recently, so common in some female subcultures that playing dumb, giggling girlishly, and gushing over big, strong men were seen as normal. The 19th-century equivalent was the swoon.

Acting out in hysterical people is usually counterphobic: They approach what they unconsciously fear. Behaving seductively when they dread sex is only one example; they are also inclined to exhibit themselves when they are unconsciously ashamed of their bodies, to make themselves the center of attention when they are subjectively feeling inferior to others, to throw themselves into acts of bravery and heroism when they are unconsciously frightened of aggression, and to provoke authorities when they are intimidated by their power. The depiction of Histrionic Personality Disorder in the DSM-IV Draft Criteria (American Psychiatric Assocition, 1993) emphasizes the acting-out aspects of hysterical character to the exclusion of other equally important features. While counterphobic enactments are clearly the most striking of the purely behavioral phenomena associated with hysteria—and they are certainly the ones that get people's attention—the *meaning* of these behaviors is also important to the diagnosis, and the most pressing internal characteristic of the hysterical style is anxiety.

Because hysterically structured people have a surfeit of unconscious anxiety, guilt, and shame, and perhaps also because they are temperamentally intense and subject to overstimulation, they are easily overwhelmed. Experiences that are manageable for those with different psychologies may be traumatic to hysterical people. Consequently, they frequently use dissociative mechanisms to reduce the amount of affectively charged information that they must deal with all at once. Examples include the phenomenon that 19th-century French psychiatrists labeled *la belle indifférence*, a kind of strange minimization of the gravity of a situation or symptom; *fausse reconnaissance*, the conviction of remembering something that did not happen; *pseudologia fantastica*, the tendency to tell outrageous untruths while seeming, at least during the telling, to believe them; fugue states; body memories of traumatic events not recalled cognitively; dissociated behaviors such as binge eating or hysterical rages, and so forth.*

One of my patients, a highly successful professional woman in her 60s who had devoted a large portion of her career to educating people about safe sex, found herself during a conference going to bed with a man with whom she was not ready to have sex ("He wanted it, and somehow that felt like the final word"). It did not occur to her to ask him to use a condom. She dissociated both her capacity to say no and her awareness of the negative consequences of unprotected sex. The sources of her dissociation included a narcissistic father and unremitting childhood messages to the effect that the needs of the other person always come first.

OBJECT RELATIONS IN HYSTERIA

In the backgrounds of people of a hysterical bent, one almost always finds events and attitudes that assigned differential power and value to the different sexes. Common hysterogenic situations include families in which a little girl is painfully aware that one or both parents greatly favor her brother(s), or where she senses she was supposed to have been a boy. (Sometimes she is accurate; sometimes she erroneously deduces this theory from data such as her being the third of three daughters.) Or a young girl may notice that her father and the male members of the family have much more power than her mother, herself, and her sisters.

When positive attention is given to this child, it involves only superficial, external attributes like her appearance or nonthreatening, infantile ones like her innocence and cuteness. When negative attention is given to her brothers, their putative inadequacies are equated with femininity ("You throw like a *girl*!" or "You're not acting like someone who wears the pants in the family"). As she gets older and matures physically, she notices that her father pulls away from her and seems uncomfortable with her developing sexuality. She feels deeply rejected on the basis of her gender, yet she senses that femininity has a strange power over men (see Celani, 1976; Chodoff, 1978, 1982).

*In hysterical individuals, these mechanisms are secondary to the other defenses mentioned here, whereas in dissociative people they are primary. The two groups overlap considerably, and it is easy to confuse them. The diagnostic problem is complicated by the fact that diverse conditions have been lumped together under the label of hysteria. Freud and many subsequent analysts failed to distinguish between patients we would now clearly see as multiple personalities and those who were predominantly histrionic.

It has often been observed (e.g., Easser & Lesser, 1965; Herman, 1981) that the fathers of many histrionic women were both frightening and seductive. Men may easily underestimate how intimidating they are to their young female children; male bodies, faces, and voices are harsher than those of either little girls or mothers, and they take some getting used to. A father who is angry seems particularly formidable, perhaps especially to a sensitive female child. If a man also engages in tantrums, harsh criticism, erratic behavior, or especially incest, he may be terrifying. A doting father who also intimidates his little girl creates a kind of approach–avoidance conflict; he is an exciting but feared object. If he seems to dominate his wife, as in a patriarchal family, the effect is magnified. His daughter will learn that people of her own gender are less valued, especially once the days of delectable girlhood are gone, and that people of her father's gender must be approached with calculation. Mueller and Aniskiewitz (1986) emphasize the combination of maternal inadequacy and paternal narcissism in the etiology of hysterical personality:

> Whether the mother is resigned to a weak, ineffectual role or is threatened by the child and reacts competitively, the basic issue remains one of not having achieved a mature mutuality. . . . Similarly, whether the father's adequacy conflicts are expressed through a brittle, pseudomasculine exterior or directly in warm, sexual, or collusive ways with the daughter, he . . . reveals his own immaturity. . . . Despite variations in the manifest traits of the fathers, the common latent personality trends reflect a phallic–oedipal orientation. The fathers are self-centered and possessive, and view relationships as extensions of themselves. (pp. 15–17)

Thus, a frequent contributant to hysterical personality structure is the sense that one's sexual identity is problematic. Some little boys raised in matriarchies where their masculinity is denigrated (sometimes with scornful contrasts to hypothetical "real" men) develop in a hysterical direction, despite the advantages the larger culture has traditionally conferred on males. There is a small but identifiable subgroup of gay men, for example, who meet the DSM-IV criteria for histrionic personality, about whom such family dynamics have been reported (e.g., Friedman, 1988). The greater frequency of hysteria in females seems to me to be explicable by two facts: (1) men have more power than women in the larger culture, and no child fails to notice this; and (2) men do less of the primary care for infants, and their relative absence makes them more exciting, idealizable and "other" than women.

The outcome of an upbringing that magnifies the most simplistic gender stereotypes of the culture (men are powerful but narcissistic and dangerous; women are soft and warm but weak and helpless) is for a woman thus reared to seek security and self-esteem from attaching herself to males she sees as particularly powerful. She may use her sexuality to do this and then find she has no satisfactory sexual response to physical involvement with such a person. She may also, because his presumed power scares her, seek to evoke the more tender side of a male partner and then unconsciously devalue him for being less of a man (i.e., soft, feminine, weak). Some hysterically organized people, male as well as female, thus go through repetitive cycles of gender-specific overvaluation and devaluation, where power is sexualized but sexual satisfaction is curiously absent or ephemeral.

THE HYSTERICAL SELF

The main sense of self in hysteria is that of a small, fearful, and defective child coping as well as can be expected in a world dominated by powerful and alien others. Although people with hysterical personalities may come across as controlling and manipulative, their subjective state of mind is quite the opposite. The manipulation done by individuals with hysterical structure is, in marked contrast to the maneuvering of psychopathic people, quite secondary to their basic quest for safety and acceptance. Their orchestration of others involves efforts to achieve an island of security in a frightening world, to stabilize self-esteem, to master frightening possibilities by initiating them, to express unconscious hostility, or some combination of these motives. They do not seek pleasure from "getting over on" others.

For example, one of my patients, a graduate student in theater arts, a young woman who had grown up with a loving but capriciously explosive father, used to become infatuated with one after another man in authority and would knock herself out to be the favorite student of each. She would approach all her male teachers and coaches with subtle flattery and an attitude of awestruck discipleship, a demeanor she rationalized as going with the territory of being an acting student at the mercy of arbitrary men. Her seductiveness was hard for some of her mentors to ignore. When she began getting signals that they were attracted to her, she reacted with excitement (at feeling powerful and valued), exhilaration (at feeling attractive and desired), fear (of their translating their attraction into sexual demands), and guilt (for exerting her will over them and winning their forbidden erotic interest). Her manipulativeness was limited to men, and men in authority at that, and although powerfully driven, it was full of conflict.

Self-esteem in histrionic people is often dependent on their repetitively achieving the sense that they have as much status and power as people of the opposite gender (or, in the case of hysterically structured gay men, as much status and power as males who are seen as more masculine). Attachment to an idealized object—especially being seen with one—may create a kind of "derived" self-esteem (Ferenczi, 1913): "This powerful person is part of me." The autobiography of the rock groupie Pamela Des Barres (1987) suggests such a psychology. Sexual acting out may be fueled by the unconscious fantasy that to be penetrated by a powerful man is somehow to capture his strength.

Another way hysterically structured people attain self-esteem is through rescue operations. Via reversal, they may care for their internal frightened child by helping children at risk. Or they may handle their fear of authorities counterphobically and set out to change or heal present-day substitutes for a frightening–exciting childhood object. The phenomenon of sweet, warm, loving females falling in love with predatory, destructive males in the hope of "saving" them is bewildering but familiar to many parents, teachers, and friends of hysterical young women.

In the dream imagery of hysterical men and women one often finds symbols that represent possession of a secret uterus or penis, respectively. Women who are hysterically organized tend to see any power they have in their natural aggressiveness as representing their "masculine" side rather than as integrated with their gender identity. The inability to feel power in womanhood gives hysterically organized females an insoluble and self-perpetuating problem. As one of my clients put it, "When I feel strong, I feel like a man, not a strong woman."*

The perception that the other sex has the advantage creates an ostensible paradox in women with hysterical personality structure: Despite their unconscious sense that power is inherently masculine, their self-presentation is incontrovertibly feminine. Because they feel that the only potency in femaleness is sexual attractiveness, they may

*This kind of thinking—that maleness equates with activity and femaleness with passivity, and that therefore an assertive woman is by definition exercising her "masculine" side, or a tender man his "femininity"—was rife throughout the late 19th century and made its way into numerous psychoanalytic theories (e.g., Jung's [1954] archetypes of the animus and anima). Such ideas have some universality, as in the Chinese yin and yang, but the application of them to Western personality theory has always had problematic implications. A fascinating and talented hysterical woman who thought in these terms, with poignantly futile results, was the psychoanalyst Princess Marie Bonaparte (Bertin, 1982).

be overinvested in how they look and subject to a greater than average dread of aging. The tragicomic quality of the older hysterical woman was captured in the character of Blanche duBois in *A Streetcar Named Desire*. Any hysterically inclined client, male or female, should be encouraged to develop other areas besides attractiveness in which self-esteem may be sought and realized.

The tendency toward vanity and seductiveness in histrionic people, although constituting a narcissistic defense in that these attitudes function to achieve and maintain self-esteem, differs from behaviorally similar processes in individuals whose basic personality is narcissistic. Hysterically structured people are not internally empty and indifferent; they charm people because they fear intrusion, exploitation, and rejection. When these anxieties are not aroused, they are genuinely warm and caring. In healthier hysterical people, the loving aspects of the personality are conspicuously in conflict with the defensive and sometimes destructive ones. The aspiring actress described previously was painfully and guiltily aware of her complex effect on the men she worked so hard to beguile, and despite being able to dissociate the feeling most of the time, she felt guilt toward their wives.

The attention-seeking behavior of histrionic people has the unconscious meaning of attaining reassurance that they are acceptable—in particular that their gender is appreciated, in contrast to their childhood experiences. Hysterically organized individuals tend to feel unconsciously castrated; by showing off their bodies they may be converting a passive sense of physical inferiority into an active feeling of power in physicality. Their exhibitionism is thus counterdepressive.

Similar considerations apply to understanding the "shallow affect" associated with hysteria. It is true that when histrionic people express feelings, there is often a dramatized, inauthentic, exaggerated quality to what they say. This does not mean that they do not "really" have the emotions to which they are giving voice. Their superficiality and apparent playacting derive from their having extreme anxiety over what will happen if they have the temerity to express themselves to someone they see as powerful. Having been infantilized and devalued, they do not anticipate respectful attention to their feelings. They magnify their emotions in order to get past their anxiety and convince themselves and others of their right to self-expression; simultaneously, by communicating that they are not really serious, they preserve their option to retract or minimize what they are saying if it should turn out that this is another unsafe place to express oneself. Announcements such as "I was SOOOO furious!" accompanied by theatrically rolling eyes, invite an interviewer to see the emotion as not really there or as trivial. It is there, but it is drenched in conflict. Eventually, in an atmosphere of scrupulous respect, the histrionic person will be able to describe anger and other feelings in a credible and straightforward way, and to augment a reactive, impressionistic style with a proactive, analytic one.

TRANSFERENCE AND COUNTERTRANSFERENCE WITH HYSTERICAL PATIENTS

Transference was originally discovered with clients whose complaints were in the hysterical realm, and it is no accident that it became so visible there. Freud's whole conception of hysteria revolved around the observation that what is not consciously remembered remains active in the unconscious realm, finding expression in symptoms, enactments, and reexperiences of early scenarios. The present is misunderstood as containing the perceived dangers and insults of the past, partly because the hysterical person is too anxious to let contradictory information in.

In addition to these factors, histrionic people are strongly object related and emotionally expressive. They are more likely than other individuals to talk about their reactions to people in general and to the therapist in particular. Given the dynamics described above, the reader can probably see how the combination of a female hysterical patient and a male therapist would immediately evoke the client's central conflicts. Freud was initially quite exasperated to find that while he was trying to put himself across to his histrionic patients as a benevolent physician, they insisted on seeing him as a provocative male presence, with whom they would suffer, struggle, and sometimes fall in love (Freud, 1925b).

Because hysterical personality is a type of psychology in which gender-related issues dominate the patient's way of seeing the world, the nature of the initial transferences will differ as a function of the sex of both client and therapist. With male practitioners, female clients tend to be excited, intimidated, and defensively seductive. With female therapists, they are often subtly hostile and competitive. With both, they may seem somewhat childlike. Male hysterical patients are also psychologically organized around generalizations about sex differences, but their transferences will vary depending on whether their internal cosmology assigns greater power to maternal or paternal figures. Most hysterical clients are cooperative and appreciative of the therapist's interest. Borderline and psychotic-level hysteroid people are difficult to treat because they act out so destructively and feel so menaced by the treatment relationship (Lazare, 1971).

However, even high-functioning hysterical clients can have transferences of such intensity that they feel almost psychotic. Hot transferences are unnerving to both therapist and client, but they can be addressed effectively by interpretation. Therapists who are secure in their role will find them, as Freud did, not an obstacle to treatment but rather the means through which it heals. When histrionic patients are too afraid to admit to such passionate responses in the presence of the therapist, they may act out with objects who are transparent substitutes for him or her. A supervisee of mine named James began seeing a hysterical young woman whose father had alternated between traumatic intrusiveness and rejection; she had sequential affairs with men named Jim, Jamie, and Jay within the first several months of her treatment.

Occasionally the transference of a person with a hysterical character becomes painfully intense before he or she has sufficient trust in the therapist to bear it. Especially in the early months of treatment, histrionic patients may flee, sometimes with rationalizations and sometimes with conscious awareness that it is the strength of their attraction, or fear, or hatred—and the anxiety that it evokes—that is driving them away. Even though the frightening reactions generally coexist with warm feelings, they can be too upsetting to tolerate. I have worked with several women who became so upset by the hostility and devaluation they found themselves feeling in my presence that they could not keep coming to me. Similarly, several of my male colleagues have been fired by histrionic clients who became too obsessed with winning their therapist's love to benefit from therapy. In these cases, especially if the transference is somewhat ego alien, a change of therapists to someone who seems less like the original overstimulating or devalued object may work out well.

Countertransference with hysterical clients may include both defensive distancing and infantilization. The therapeutic dyad in which these potentials are most problematic is that of the male therapist, especially if his personality is at all narcissistic, and the female client. As I indicated earlier, it can be hard to attend respectfully to what feels like pseudoaffect in histrionic clients; the self-dramatizing quality of these chronically anxious patients invites ridicule. Most hysterically organized people are highly sensitive to interpersonal cues, however, and an attitude of patronizing amusement will be very injurious to them, even if they manage to keep the therapist's disrespect out of their awareness.

Before it was politically incorrect to talk openly and ego-syntonically about one's misogyny, it was common to hear (male) psychiatric residents condoling with each other man-to-man about their exasperating histrionic patients. "I've got this wacko hysteric—she bursts into tears every time I frown. And today she comes in with a skirt that barely reaches her thighs!" The female professionals within range of such conversations would exchange pained expressions and give silent thanks—or prayers—that they were not in treatment with someone who could talk like this about a person he hoped to help.

Related to this more condescending and hostile reaction to a histrionic woman is the temptation to treat her like a little girl. Again, since regression is a major weapon in the hysterical arsenal, this is to be expected. Still, it is surprising how many clinicians accept the hysterical invitation to act out omnipotence. The appeal of playing Big Daddy to a helpless and grateful young thing is evidently quite strong. I have known otherwise disciplined practitioners who, when treating a hysterically organized women, could not contain their impulse to give her advice, praise her, reassure her, and console her, despite the fact that the subtext in all these messages is that she is too weak to figure things out on her own, or to develop the capacity to give herself her own approval or reassurance or comfort.

Because regression in most histrionic people is defensive—that is, it protects them from feeling fears and guilts attendant upon taking adult responsibility—it should not be confused with genuine helplessness. Being afraid and being incompetent are not the same thing. The problem with being too commiserative and indulgent with a hysterical person, even if that stance lacks any hostile condescension, is that the client's diminished self-concept will be reinforced. An attitude of parental solicitude is as much of an insult as one of scorn for the patient's "manipulativeness."

Finally, I should mention countertransference temptations to respond to the patient's seductiveness. Again, this is a much greater danger to male than to female therapists, as has been demonstrated in every study to date about sexual abuse of clients (e.g., Pope, Tabachnick, & Keith-Spiegel, 1987). Women treating hysterical patients, even highly seductive heterosexual males, are protected by internalized social conventions that make the dyad of dependent male–authoritative female hard to erotize. The cultural acceptance of the phenomenon of the older or more powerful man's attraction to the younger or more needy woman, however, which has psychodynamic roots in male fears of female engulfment that are assuaged by this paradigm, leaves men much more vulnerable to sexual temptation in their therapeutic role. And we are only beginning to have a structure of ethics and consequences for sexual acting out that helps them with this.*

The implications of theory and the lessons of practice emphatically confirm that sexual acting out with patients has disastrous effects (Smith, 1984; Pope, 1987). What hysterical clients need, as opposed to what they may feel they need when their core conflicts are activated in treatment, is the experience of having powerful desires that are not exploited by the object on whom they rely. Trying and failing to seduce someone is profoundly transformative to histrionic people, because—often for the first time in their lives—they learn that an authority will put their welfare above the opportunity to use them, and that the direct exertion of their autonomy is more effective than defensive, sexualized distortions of it.†

THERAPEUTIC IMPLICATIONS OF THE DIAGNOSIS OF HYSTERIA

Standard psychoanalytic treatment was invented for people with hysterical personality structure, and it is still the treatment of choice. By standard treatment, I mean that the therapist is relatively quiet and nondirective, interprets process rather than content, deals with defenses rather than what is being defended against, and limits interpretation mostly to addressing resistances as they appear in the transference. As David Allen (1977) notes:

> Hysterical patients make contact immediately, and it is a reparative contact they seek. . . . For the beginning therapist, such patients give the clearest and most accessible evidence of transference. . . . The crux of the treatment of the hysterical personality *is* the transference. If we give wrong interpretations, we can correct them

*The doctoral dissertation of my former student Sharon Greenfield (1991) involved interviews with practitioners treating women whose prior therapist had acted out with them sexually. She found that while the female interviewees saw the prior male therapist as an exploitive narcissist or psychopath, the male ones expressed some sympathy and understanding of how a man subject to the seductive pressure of a patient could have lost his professional moorings.

†In the early 1970s, when so many experiments in the obliteration of boundaries were going on, one sometimes heard apparently sincere people contending that it could be therapeutic for patients to have their sexuality so concretely appreciated by their therapist. It is of interest that this argument was never heard in circumstances in which the patient was elderly or obese or physically unattractive.

> in the light of later information. If we miss opportunities to interpret, they will occur again and again. But if we mishandle the transference, the treatment is in trouble. *Mishandling of the transference or failing to establish a therapeutic alliance is almost the only vital mistake*, and it is exceedingly difficult to repair. (p. 291)

One must first establish a cordial working alliance and spell out the responsibilities of both parties to the therapy contract— a swift and easy process with healthier hysterical clients because of their basic relatedness. Then, by a nonintrusive but warm demeanor, along with a judicious avoidance of self-disclosure, the therapist allows the transference to flourish. Once the patient's issues surface in the treatment relationship, the therapist can tactfully interpret feelings, fantasies, frustrations, wishes, and fears as they appear directly in the consulting room.

It is critical that the therapist allow the hysterical client to come to his or her own understandings. A rush to interpret will only intimidate someone with hysterical sensibilities, reminding him or her once again of the superior power and insight of others. Comments with any trace of the attitude "I know you better than you know yourself" may, in the imagery that often dominates the internal representational world of the hysterical person, feel castrating or penetrating to the client. Raising gentle questions, remarking casually when the patient seems stuck, and continually bringing him or her back to what is being felt, and how that is understood, comprise the main features of effective technique.

With neurotic-level hysterical people, the therapist may have the experience of sitting back and watching the patient make him- or herself well. It is important to rein in one's narcissistic needs to be valued for making a contribution; the best contribution one can make to a histrionic person is confidence in the patient's capacity to figure things out and make responsible adult decisions. One should attend not only to the elicitation of feelings but to the integration of thinking and feeling. Allen (1977) observes:

> An essential part of craftsmanship in therapy is to communicate within the cognitive style of the patient with full respect for the

---

The alleged behavior of Jules Masserman, whose patronizing attitude toward histrionic patients always saturated his writings, represents a logical extreme in narcissistic exploitation of hysterical dynamics. According to Noel (1992), he progressed from mild paternalism to unwarranted sodium amytal treatment to the rape of patients while they were drugged.

> patient's feelings and values. The hysterical thinking style is not inferior as far as it goes, but the hysterical style needs the complementary advantages of detailed, linear "left-hemisphere thinking" as well. In a sense, the hysteric does need to learn how to think and what to connect in thinking, just as the obsessive compulsive needs to learn how to feel and what to connect in feeling. (p. 324)

More disturbed hysterical clients require much more active and educative work. In the first interview, besides tolerating and naming their crippling anxiety, one should predict any temptations that may imperil the treatment. For example: "I know that right now you are determined to work these problems out in therapy. But we can see that in your life so far when your anxiety has gotten too high, you have escaped into an exciting love affair [or gotten sick, or gone into a rage and left—whatever is the pattern]. That is bound to happen here. Do you think you can stick with our work over the long haul?" Lower-functioning hysterical clients should be told to expect powerful and negative reactions to the therapist, and urged to come in and talk about them. In general, approaches that apply to borderline patients across the typological spectrum are useful with more disturbed hysterical people, with special attention to their transference reactions.

DIFFERENTIAL DIAGNOSIS

The main conditions with which hysterical personality organization can be confused, on the basis of its manifest characteristics, are psychopathy and narcissism. In addition, some imprecision exists, as it did in Freud's day, between the diagnoses of hysterical and dissociative psychology. Finally, also as in the time of Freud and earlier, some people with undiagnosed physiological conditions are misunderstood as having a hysterical personality disorder.

Hysterical versus Psychopathic Personality

Many writers, over many decades (e.g., Kraepelin, 1915; Rosanoff, 1938; Vaillant, 1975; Chodoff, 1982; Lilienfield, Van Valkenburg, Larntz, & Akiskal, 1986; Meloy, 1988), have noted connections between psychopathy and hysteria. Anecdotal evidence suggests that there is an affinity between the two psychologies; specifically, some histrionic women, especially in the borderline range, are attracted to sociopathic men. Meloy (1988) mentions the familiar phenomenon of the convicted murderer who gets inundated with letters from female sympathizers looking to come to his defense and/or to become his lover.

Qualities seen as hysterical in women are often construed as psychopathic in men. A study by Richard Warner (1978), in which a fictional case vignette was given to mental health professionals, found that identical descriptions of sensational, flirtatious, excitable behavior attributed to either a man or a women yielded assessments of antisocial or hysterical personality, respectively, depending on the gender of the patient portrayed. Warner concluded that hysteria and sociopathy are essentially the same. And yet every experienced clinician has seen at least a few women who were unquestionably psychopathic rather than hysterical, and a few men who were clearly histrionic and not antisocial. If these categories were just gendered versions of the same psychology, that would not be so. (Also, Warner's vignettes featured behaviors that make differential diagnosis difficult.) A more reasonable view of his findings is that because of the greater frequency of sociopathy in men and of hysteria in women, most of his diagnosticians engaged in the research task with an explanatory "set" that was not sufficiently counteracted to change their expectancies.*

Confusion of hysteria with sociopathy is likelier toward the more disturbed end of the hysterical continuum; in the borderline and psychotic ranges, many people have aspects of both psychologies. But a determination of which dynamic predominates is critical to the formation of an alliance and to the ultimate success of therapy. Hysterical individuals are intensely object related, conflicted, and frightened, and a therapeutic relationship with them depends on the clinician's appreciation of their fear. Psychopathic people equate fear with weakness, and they disdain therapists who mirror their trepidation. Hysterical and antisocial people both behave dramatically, but the defensive theatricality of the histrionic person is absent in sociopathy. Demonstrating one's power as a therapist will engage a psychopathic person positively yet will intimidate or infantilize a hysterical client.

*Another example of the influence of explanatory sets on research findings is Rosenhan's (1973) study in which students entered hospitals complaining they heard voices but otherwise giving honest accounts of themselves. Most were diagnosed schizophrenic, a finding that putatively exposed psychiatric pathologizing. Yet when a therapist sees a patient claiming to hear voices (a "first-rank symptom" of schizophrenia), the assumption that he or she is in serious trouble is more reasonable than alternative conjectures—such as that he or she is a mildly depressed but imaginative person, or a malingerer, or a researcher's plant. See also Slavney (1990).

Hysterical versus Narcissistic Personality

As I have noted, hysterical people use narcissistic defenses. Both hysterical and narcissistic individuals have basic self-esteem defects, deep shame, and compensatory needs for attention and reassurance; both idealize and devalue. But the sources of these similarities differ. First, for the hysterical person, self-esteem problems are usually related to gender identification or to particular conflicts, while with narcissistic people they are diffuse. Second, people who are hysterically organized are basically warm and caring; their exploitive qualities arise only when their core dilemmas and fears are activated. Third, hysterical people idealize and devalue in specific, often gender-related ways; their idealization frequently has its origins in counterphobia ("This wonderful man would not hurt me"), and their devaluation has a reactive, aggressive quality. In contrast, narcissistic people habitually rank all others in terms of better and worse, without the press of powerful, object-directed affects. Kernberg (1982) has commented on how a hysterical and a narcissistic woman may both have unsatisfactory intimate relationships, but the former tends to pick bad objects whom she has counterphobically idealized, while the latter picks adequate objects whom she then devalues.

Implications of this differential for treatment are substantial, though too complex to cover except with the overall observation that basically hysterical people do very well with standard analytic treatment, whereas narcissistic ones need therapeutic efforts adapted to the primacy of their efforts to maintain self-cohesion and a positively valued self-concept.

Hysterical versus Dissociative Personality

Hysterical and dissociative psychologies are closely related. Because it is much more common for a dissociative person to be presumed to be hysterical than vice versa, I will discuss the distinctions between these two conditions in the next chapter.*

*It will not be surprising if, as professional consciousness of dissociation and trauma continues to be raised, misunderstandings go in the opposite direction in the near future. Even now, some patients are eager to find evidence of the incest and sexual trauma that create dissociation, in preference to exploring the internal conflicts that manifest as hysteria.

Hysterical versus Physiological Conditions

Although it is much less common now than in the heyday of American pop Freudianism to attribute any baffling physical symptom to unconscious conflict, a final word should be said about not overlooking the possibility of physical origins of mysterious ailments. Symptoms of some systemic illnesses—multiple sclerosis, for example—are frequently assumed to be of hysterical origin, as are many "female complaints" that frustrate physicians. In England in recent years, there was an outbreak of what was widely diagnosed as "gardener's hysteria" in members of a group of horticulturists who had visited the United States; eventually it was discovered that they had gathered examples of American fall foliage on the trip, including a lot of brilliantly red poison ivy. More consequentially, George Gershwin probably would have lived well beyond 38 if his therapist had not interpreted the symptoms of his brain tumor as psychogenic rather than organic.

Because histrionic people regress when they are anxious, and have off-putting ways of expressing their complaints, a physical illness in a person with hysterical tendencies is at risk of not being thoroughly investigated. It is more than simply scrupulous and prudent to pursue the possibility of an organic problem in a histrionic person; it also sends a therapeutic message to a scared human being whose basic dignity has not always been respected.

SUMMARY

Hysterical personality has been described in the context of evolving analytic conceptualizations that include aspects of drive (intense and affectionate basic temperament, with oral and oedipal struggles aggravated by gender-related disappointments), ego (impressionistic cognitive style; defenses of repression, sexualization, regression, acting out, dissociation), object relations (inadequate parenting that includes narcissistic and seductive messages, replicated in later relationships dominated by the repetition compulsion), and self (self-image as small, defective, and endangered, and self-esteem burdened by conflicts over sexualized expressions of power).

Transference–countertransference experiences were said to include strong competitive and erotized reactions, depending on the sexual orientation and gender of client and therapist, as well as regressive trends that invite contempt or indulgence rather than respect. The danger of therapist sexualization was addressed. Treatment recommendations include the careful maintenance of professional boundaries, a warm and empathic attitude, and an economy of interpretation guided by traditional psychoanalytic technique. Hysterical character was contrasted with psychopathic, narcissistic, and dissociative personality, and a final caveat was offered about investigating possible physiological causes of presumptively hysterical symptoms.

SUGGESTIONS FOR FURTHER READING

I am partial to Horowitz's (1977) anthology and also to the work of Mueller and Aniskiewitz (1986), whose tone lacks the condescension so common in writing on hysteria by male therapists. Again, Shapiro's (1965) essay on the hysterical cognitive style is superior, and Veith's (1965) historical review is both illuminating and entertaining.

15
Dissociative Personalities

In this chapter, I shall diverge somewhat from representing mainstream psychodynamic personality diagnosis, since to my knowledge, this is the first psychoanalytic textbook in which dissociative personality is included as simply one other possible type of character structure. In this century, until approximately the 1980s, multiple personality disorder and related psychologies based on dissociation were considered rare enough to preclude their incorporation into schemata of personality types and disorders. It has become abundantly clear, however, that many people dissociate frequently, and that some do it so regularly that dissociation can be said to be their prime mechanism for dealing with stress. If multiple personality disorder were not "a pathology of hiddenness" (Gutheil, in Kluft, 1985), where the patient is often unaware of having alter personalities, and where trust is so problematic that even those parts of the self that know about the dissociation are reluctant to divulge their secret, we would have known long ago how to begin identifying and helping dissociative clients.

In fact, some people did know long ago. A regrettable side effect of Freud's ultimate emphasis on maturational issues rather than traumatic ones, and on repression rather than dissociation, is that they distracted us from some fine scholarship on dissociation that was available at the end of the 19th century. Pierre Janet (1890), for example, explained many hysterical symptoms by reference to dissociative processes, explicitly disputing Freud's preference for repression as a primary explanatory principle. In America, William James and Alfred Binet were both seriously interested in dissociation. Morton Prince (1906) published his detailed case of the dissociative "Miss Beauchamps" around the same time that *The Interpretation of Dreams* (Freud, 1900) was beginning to be noticed, and the eventual impact of the latter virtually eclipsed that of the former. Colin Ross (1989b) and Frank Putnam (1989) have each written texts that cover the fascinating history of the phenomenon and the motley etiological speculations that have surrounded it.

Therapists experienced with dissociative clients regard multiplicity not as a bizarre aberration but as the understandable adaptation of a particular kind of person to a particular kind of history—specifically, as a chronic posttraumatic stress syndrome of childhood origin (cf. D. Spiegel, 1984). In this respect dissociative personality is not qualitatively different from any other kind of character structure or pathology. Because of the extensively documented differences among the dissociated selves of someone with multiple personality disorder, the condition has been widely sensationalized.* These differences (which may include subjective age, sexual identity and preference, systemic illnesses, allergies, eyeglass prescriptions, EEG readings, handwriting, handedness, addictions, and language facility) are so impressive that lay people consider multiple personality disorder the most exotic mental illness they have ever heard of. So do many therapists. No other documented disorder has inspired comparable arguments about whether it exists at all independent of iatrogenesis.

Yet considered in context, multiple personality is not so incomprehensible. Research on dissociative states and hypnosis (people who dissociate are actually entering spontaneous hypnotic trances) has revealed some remarkable capacities of the human organism and has raised absorbing questions about consciousness, brain functioning, integrative and disintegrative mental processes, and latent potential. Still, clinicians know that each of their dissociative patients is in most respects an ordinary human being—a *single* person with the *subjective experience* of different selves†—one whose suffering is only too real.

The first carefully documented case of multiple personality in

*As this book goes to press, there is talk of renaming Multiple Personality Disorder in the DSM-IV as Dissociative Identity Disorder. Some have wondered whether the label "multiple personality" has sensationalized the condition by implicitly reifying the alter personalities. I shall use both terms interchangeably in this chapter.

†Phenomena associated with dissociation certainly strain credulity, and yet who is to say that people with multiple personality disorder are any more peculiar than people who starve themselves to death on the basis of a false conviction that they are fat, or people who believe that influencing machines control their actions, or people who will not leave their homes because some nameless fear immobilizes them. It may be the talent—the achievement of so many different albeit dissociated skills—more than the disability of dissociative individuals that invites the skepticism with which their symptoms are often greeted.

In my view, recent philosophical efforts to grapple with multiple personality disorder have leaned toward a category mistake to the effect that there are *actually* different personalities involved, not one person with the subjective sense of multiplicity. A notable exception is the work of Braude (1991).

recent decades (Thigpen & Cleckley, 1957; Sizemore & Pittillo, 1977; Sizemore, 1989) was Eve (of *The Three Faces of . . .*), the pseudonym of Christine Costner Sizemore. Sizemore, now a fully integrated woman of impressive energy and achievement, is a good exemplar of a high-functioning dissociative person. It is notable that the first sufferer of characterological dissociation to "come out" to a therapist in this era was someone with considerable basic trust, ego strength, and object constancy. More disturbed dissociative people, even when they suspect their multiplicity, are much too afraid of mistreatment to let a naive therapist in on their troubled inner life—especially early in treatment.* Josef Breuer's famous patient "Anna O" (Bertha Pappenheim), a person who influenced psychoanalytic history in incalculable ways, is another example of a high-functioning multiple personality. Breuer and Freud (1883–1885) regarded her dissociation as only one aspect of her hysterical illness, but most contemporary diagnosticians would consider her primarily dissociative rather than hysterical. Consider the following description:

> Two entirely distinct states of consciousness were present which alternated very frequently and without warning and which became more and more differentiated in the course of her illness. In one of these states she recognized her surroundings; she was melancholy and anxious, but relatively normal. In the other state she hallucinated and was "naughty"—that is to say, she was abusive, used to throw the cushions at people. . . . [I]f something had been moved in the room or someone had entered or left it (during her other state of consciousness) she would complain of having "lost" some time and would remark upon the gap in her train of conscious thoughts. . . . At moments when her mind was quite clear she would complain . . . of having two selves, a real one and an evil one which forced her to behave badly. (p. 24)

This remarkable woman went on, after her abortive treatment with Breuer, to be a devoted and highly effective social worker (Karpe, 1961).

In dramatic contrast to Christine Sizemore and Bertha Pappen-

*Currently, sufferers of dissociation encounter enough information about multiple personality disorder—from television talk shows, newspapers, magazines, biographies, and acquaintance with other dissociators in incest-survivor and 12-step groups—to suspect their diagnosis. But before the 1980s, individual dissociative people knew only that they were "crazy" in a way that defied description. They consequently harbored a terror of being found out and locked up for life in some snake pit. A woman of 60 whom I treat for multiple personality disorder says that the deinstitutionalization of mental patients in the 1970s contributed to her developing the courage to admit to her hallucinatory experiences and "lost time."

heim, in the borderline and psychotic ranges of the developmental spectrum are the ruthlessly self-destructive and "polyfragmented" patients, who dissociate so automatically and chaotically that they experience themselves as having hundreds of "personalities," most of which consist of limited attributes that address some current issue. Truddi Chase (1987), who has attained some notoriety in the popular media, may be in this category, though it is arguable that if her therapist were less invested in publicizing her dissociated condition, she might not look so splintered. Many dissociative people in the psychotic range may be in jails rather than mental hospitals; alter personalities who rape and kill, often in delusional states of mind, are possible outcomes of the traumatic abuse that creates multiplicity. It is reasonable to suppose that others with psychotic-level dissociative structure belong to cults* that structure and normalize dissociative experiences, sometimes to the benefit of their dissociative members and sometimes to the drastic harm of everyone involved.

An interesting mutual ambivalence exists between the psychoanalytic community and the therapists who have led the recent movement to gain and disseminate knowledge of dissociation. On the one hand, analytic practitioners are much more appreciative of the power of organized unconscious forces than are therapists of most other stripes; consequently, the idea of traumatically created, out-of-consciousness alter personalities does not require from them a leap of imagination. Moreover, they tend to work with clients over many years, during which time the covert consciousnesses of a dissociative person may build up the courage to expose parts of the self for which the host personality is amnestic.† Thus, analysts and analytic therapists are more likely than other professionals to have worked with people

*It is beyond the scope of this chapter to address the currently raging debate on the prevalence of ritual and cult abuse, but perhaps I should state my own bias. I have seen enough evidence for the existence of sadistic subcultures, satanic and otherwise, to believe, along with many colleagues who treat dissociative patients, that contemporary Western cultures contain numerous underground groups and sects that operate like factories for dissociation. For every destructive cult that has been identified—the most notorious of recent years being David Koresh's Branch Davidians—there may be several that operate in complete secrecy. In an era that has seen the crimes of the Nazis, the Ku Klux Klan, the Mafia, and more isolated groups like the Manson family, we cannot afford to ignore any evidence that evil is being propagated in organized ways.

†Richard Kluft, a pioneer in diagnosing and treating dissociation, is a psychoanalyst. A long-time collaborator of his told me that one of his early cases of multiplicity was a high-functioning women in classical analysis whose treatment had gone on for several years. Suddenly she jumped up, pointed at the couch, and announced, "*She* may believe in this analysis crap, but *I don't!*" In a triumph of seat-of-the-pants judgment, Kluft replied, "Back on the couch. You're in analysis, too."

who have revealed their multiplicity, and they are also more likely to have taken it seriously.

On the other hand, analytic practitioners have inherited the explanatory preferences of Freud, who eventually put less emphasis on trauma and molestation than on fantasy and its interaction with developmental challenges. Also, and curiously, Freud had little to say about multiple personality disorder, a condition that was recognized in his day by several of the psychiatrists he revered.* And his blind spots here did contribute to a tendency in some of his adherents to regard reports of incest and molestation as fantasy. Intriguingly, Freud's original "seduction theory" ran aground on a problem that is once again surfacing in evaluating the reports of victims of sexual abuse: Trauma distorts perception and creates a basis for later confusions of fact and fantasy.

In addition to habits of thought that derive from Freudian assumptions, people trained in the psychodynamic tradition have sometimes misapplied concepts from object relations theory that seem to account for the switches in consciousness that signal the emergence of alter personalities. Specifically, they have been more inclined than other mental health professionals to interpret such switches not as alterations in consciousness but as evidence of the primitive defense of splitting. As a result, they have often failed to ask questions that would discriminate between splitting and dissociation.

Some therapists who have distinguished themselves by their commitment to learning and teaching about multiplicity have thus found it hard to forgive Freud and Freudians for minimizing both the prevalence and the destructiveness of the sexual abuse of children. Some also lament the influence of thinkers like Kernberg, on the grounds that they have confused dissociation with splitting and have thereby misdiagnosed many people with dissociative personalities as borderline or schizophrenic—a mistake that can cost a dissociative patient years of misguided treatment. Specialists in dissociation (e.g., C. A. Ross, 1989b) rightly complain that legions of desperate people have been misunderstood and even retraumatized over many years by unnecessary medical procedures (e.g., major tranquilizers, electroshock). Critics of exponents of dissociation counter that when one is looking for them, one can find a multiple under every rock (cf. D. Ross,

*Freud knew of the phenomenon of multiple personality but probably believed he had never encountered a case of it. In *The Ego and the Id* (1923), in the course of discussing object-identification, he made the offhand comment, "perhaps the secret of the cases of what is described as 'multiple personality' is that the different identifications seize hold of consciousness in turn" (pp. 30–31).

1992). Fads in psychopathology are not unknown, especially in hysterically related conditions where suggestibility may play a large role.*

I am commenting on all this because the reader who pursues knowledge of dissociation will still find, even though Dissociative Identity Disorder and other dissociative conditions have attained respectability by inclusion in the later editions of the DSM, a certain polemicism infiltrating the work of explicators and critics of dissociative concepts. This is to be expected when there has been a paradigm shift (Kuhn, 1970; R. J. Loewenstein, 1988; R. J. Loewenstein & Ross, 1992) in any field. I recommend that whatever the reader's bias, he or she try to comprehend the phenomenon of dissociation with an "experience-near" sensibility; that is, from the standpoint of empathy with the internal experience of the person who feels and behaves like a composite of many different selves.

DRIVE, AFFECT, AND TEMPERAMENT IN DISSOCIATIVE CONDITIONS

People who use dissociation as their primary defense mechanism are essentially virtuosos in self-hypnosis. Movement into an altered state of consciousness when one is distressed is not possible for everybody; you have to have the talent. Just as people differ in their basic levels of hypnotizability (R. Spiegel & D. Spiegel, 1978), they differ in their capacities for autohypnosis. In order to become a multiple personality, one has to have the constitutional potential to enter a hypnotic state; otherwise, trauma may be handled in other ways (e.g., repression, acting out, flights into addiction).

*The iatrogenic hypothesis has never been empirically substantiated (Braun, 1984; Kluft, 1989; C. A. Ross, 1989a), and there is not one documented case of iatrogenic multiple personality disorder in the literature. It may be true, however, that a public tone can be set that encourages people to express posttraumatic reactions by one psychological means rather than another. In my view, the "choice" of symptom—amnesia versus bulimia versus conversion, for example—is of far less importance than the fact that the creation of *any* disabling symptom evidences a person's suffering. With the exception of criminals who hope to cop an insanity plea, people do not elect dissociation for the secondary gain; it is too disturbing a way to live.

Lately, I have seen several patients who wrongly thought they might be multiple—a remarkable change from a few years ago, when telling a person with textbook multiple personality disorder that he or she was dissociative would provoke grave alarm. Although the organizing defenses of these would-be multiples turned out not to be dissociative, all were in serious psychological difficulty and needed professional help. Their pain was real even if their understanding of its nature was flawed.

Some evidence suggests that the kind of person who dissociates is innately more resourceful and interpersonally sensitive than the norm. A child with a complex, rich inner life (imaginary friends, fantasy identities, internal dramas, and a penchant for imaginative play) may be more able to retreat to a secret world when terrorized than a less gifted youngster. Anecdotal reports suggest that people with dissociative personality are as a group brighter and more creative than average.* Such observations may be artifactual; the kind of dissociative person who *comes for help* may not represent the whole dissociative spectrum. It used to be thought that Eve and Sybil (Schrieber, 1973) were paradigmatic multiples, but their respective, hysteroid presentations are now seen as typical of only a small percentage of those who dissociate (Kluft, 1991).

To my knowledge, no drive constructs have been put forward to account for dissociative character, probably because by the time the mental health community gave concentrated attention to dissociation, the hegemony of psychoanalytic drive theory was over. With respect to affect, however, the picture is clear: Dissociative people have been overwhelmed with it and have gotten virtually no help processing it. Primordial terror and horror are foremost among the emotions that provoke dissociation in any traumatic situation; rage, excitement, shame, and guilt may also be involved. The more numerous and conflicting the emotional states activated, the harder it is to assimilate an experience without dissociation. Bodily states that may instigate trance include insufferable pain and confusing sexual arousal. While it may be possible to become a multiple personality in the absence of early sexual trauma and abuse by caregivers (e.g., via repeated catastrophes in the context of war or persecution), empirical studies have established this relationship in 97 to 98% of diagnosed cases (Braun & Sacks, 1985; Putnam, 1989).

DEFENSIVE AND ADAPTIVE PROCESSES IN DISSOCIATIVE CONDITIONS

Dissociative defenses are like any others in that they begin as the best possible adaptation of an immature organism to a particular situation,

*One of my pet (unprovable) speculations is that Marilyn Monroe was dissociative. Her magnetism, genuineness, and dramatic talent fit the profile, as do her traumatic history, her problems with time, and other eccentricities. Ralph Greenson's misconstrual of her as schizophrenic and his emotional overinvolvement in her therapy—shamefully misunderstood and burlesqued in Spoto's (1993) biography—is also consistent with such an assessment.

then become automatic and hence maladaptive in later circumstances. Some people with dissociative personalities in adulthood have simply kept on dissociating ever since the time of their original traumas; others, once the abusive practices ceased, have achieved for significant periods either a tenuous cooperation of alter personalities or the consistent domination of their subjective world by one part of the self (the "host personality").

One common clinical presentation is the person whose flagrant dissociation stopped when he or she left the family in which it originated, only to surface again when a son or daughter reached the age at which the parent was first abused. (This identificatory connection is usually completely out of consciousness.) Another frequent trigger for dissociation in an adult whose autohypnotic tendencies have been dormant is an encounter with some circumstance that unconsciously reminds him or her of childhood trauma. One woman in my practice suffered a household fall that injured her in the same places where she had been mutilated during childhood ritual abuse, and for the first time in years she suddenly became someone else. In taking a careful history, one often finds many minor instances of dissociation throughout the patient's adult life, but what usually brings him or her to treatment is some dramatic and disabling dissociative reaction (losing significant amounts of time, being told of things one cannot remember, and so forth). It is phenomena like these that prompted Kluft (1987) to talk about "windows of diagnosability" in dissociative conditions.

Dissociation is an oddly invisible defense. When one alter or system of alters is running things smoothly, no one outside the patient can see the dissociative process. Many therapists believe they have never treated a multiple personality, because they expect such a client to announce his or her multiplicity, or to generate a dramatically alien alter. Sometimes this happens (in fact, it happens more and more as the topic of dissociation is demystified), but more commonly, indications of multiplicity are subtle. Frequently, only one alter personality goes to therapy.* Even when a fairly identifiable alter personality emerges in treatment (e.g., a frightened child), an unenlightened therapist will tend to read the change in the patient in nondissociative terms (e.g., as a passing regressive phenomenon).

*A psychologist I supervised treated a dissociative woman who had gone for 5 years to a rational–emotive therapist. Because she liked him and appreciated his interest, yet suspected he would debunk the phenomenon of multiple personality, she generated a rational–emotive alter personality who came to treatment regularly and seemed to be making splendid progress.

My first experience with a dissociative client—knowingly, that is—was at one remove. In the early 1970s, a close friend and colleague in my department was conferring with me about treating a student who had exposed her multiplicity in the second year of her therapy with him. I found his accounts of her behavior riveting. *Sybil* had just been published, and I remember thinking that this client must be one of only a dozen or so extant multiples. Then he mentioned that she was in a course that I taught and, with her permission, told me her name. I was stunned. I would never have guessed that this young woman was dissociative; from the outside, the shifts that indicated "switching" looked like minor changes of mood. Since I knew from my friend how painfully she struggled with amnesia, it was an unforgettable lesson in how opaque the condition is to observers, even credulous ones. I began to wonder how many other hidden dissociators there might be.

Accurate appraisal of the demographics of dissociation is hampered by its invisibility. I have sometimes consulted with spouses of people with dissociative psychologies, who, despite full awareness of their partner's diagnosis, have made comments like, "But yesterday, she said the *opposite*!" Cerebral knowledge that one was talking to a different alter yesterday pales against the data provided by one's senses: *I was speaking to the same physical person on both days*. If intimate partners of people with admitted, diagnosed multiple personality disorder miss signs of dissociation, it is not hard to see how uninitiated professionals can be even blinder. People who dissociate learn to "cover" for their lapses. They develop techniques of evasion and fabrication in childhood, as they find themselves repeatedly accused of "lying" about things they do not remember. Because they have suffered horrific abuse at the hands of people who were supposed to protect them, they do not trust authorities, and they do not come to treatment with the expectation that full disclosure is in their interest.

The estimation of how many of us are centrally dissociative also depends on how dissociation is defined. In addition to "classic" multiple personality, there is the condition currently called "DDNOS" (Dissociative Disorder Not Otherwise Specified), in which alter personalities exist but do not take executive control of the body. There are also other dissociative phenomena such as depersonalization—after depression and anxiety the third most commonly reported psychiatric symptom (Cattell & Cattell, 1974; Steinberg, 1991)—that presumably can be frequent and longstanding enough to be considered characterological.

Bennett Braun (1988) has suggested a useful conceptualization that has come to be known by the acronym BASK (Behavior, Affect, Sensation, Knowledge). With it, Braun has elevated the concept of dissociation to the status of a superordinate category rather than, as Freud conceived it, a more peripheral defense. His model subsumes many processes that often occur together but have not always been seen as related. According to Braun, one can dissociate *behavior*, as in a paralysis or a trance-driven self-mutilation; or *affect*, as in acting with *la belle indifférence* or the memory of trauma without feeling; or *sensation*, as in conversion anesthesias and "body memories" of abuse; or *knowledge*, as in fugue states and amnesia. The BASK model regards repression as a subsidiary of dissociation and puts a number of phenomena that have previously been regarded as hysterical into the dissociative domain. It also links to historical trauma many issues that have tended to be seen as solely expressing intrapsychic conflict. Therapists working with characterologically dissociative patients find his formulation very useful clinically; those working with people other than multiples find that it sensitizes them to the dissociative processes that occur in everyone.

OBJECT RELATIONS IN DISSOCIATIVE CONDITIONS

The outstanding feature of the childhood relationships of someone who becomes characterologically dissociative is abuse, usually including but not limited to sexual abuse. The parents of people with multiple personality disorder are frequently themselves dissociative, either directly, as a result of their own traumatic histories, or indirectly, via alcoholism or drug addiction. Because the parents often have amnesia for what they do—whether it is psychogenic amnesia or substance abuse-related blackouts—they both traumatize their children and fail to help them understand what has happened to them. Sometimes they are involved in cults preoccupied with torture, the witnessing of torture, and blood sacrifice.

Many have wondered whether multiple personality is in fact more common now than it was generations ago, or whether the current explosion in diagnosing it derives entirely from our increased capacity to identify it. It is not impossible that severe child abuse has been on the rise over the past decades and that a greater portion of the total human population has resulting dissociative problems. Sociological factors that might contribute to more child abuse include the nature of modern warfare (in which whole civilizations rather than small groups of warriors are traumatized, and more people may reenact their horror with their children); destabilization of families; increases in addiction, including the spread of drugs to previously abstemious middle-class groups (as the Lisa Steinberg case illustrated, an intoxicated parent will do things that he or she would not even conceive of doing sober); the increase in violent imagery in the media (such that dissociative defenses are more often stimulated in a susceptible person); and the mobility, anonymity, and privacy of contemporary life (I have no idea how my next-door neighbors treat their kids, and I have no personal influence on their behavior).

On the other hand, children have been traumatized since antiquity, and when one treats a patient for dissociative problems, one frequently finds that that person's parent was also sexually abused, as was the parent's parent, and so on. Stephanie Coontz's (1992) indictment of nostalgia in sociological theorizing should give pause to anyone inclined to postulate easier times for children in prior generations. All we can say with certainty is that currently more people are talking about their childhood abuse and seeking help for its dissociative legacy.

Kluft (1984) has derived from extensive clinical data and systematic research a four-factor theory of the etiology of multiple personality disorder and severe dissociation. First, the individual is talented hypnotically. Second, he or she is severely traumatized. Third, the patient's dissociative responses are shaped by particular childhood influences; that is, dissociation is adaptive and to some extent rewarded by the family. Fourth, there is no comfort during and after traumatic episodes. I have already talked some about Kluft's first three prerequisites; the last is equally critical, and it never fails to move therapists. No one seems ever to have held the dissociative child, or wiped away a tear, or explained an upsetting experience. Typically, emotional responses to trauma were punished by more abuse ("Now I'll *really* give you something to cry about!"). There is often a kind of systemic family collusion to deny feeling, to forget pain, to act as if the horrors of the preceding night were all imaginary.*

One fascinating aspect of multiple personality disorder is how lovable most dissociative people are—at least those who get into treatment. Despite all the devastations to their basic emotional security and all the corruptions of parental care that one would expect to have destroyed the capacity to attach, it is almost universally

*Given how memory can be distorted by both trauma and trance, a question is frequently raised as to how accurate are the abuse histories remembered in therapy by dissociative clients. Clinical experience suggests that while specific details of abuse may be confabulated, the fact of trauma is certain. In spite of the vagaries of memory and the elusiveness one would expect from childhood abusers and witnesses, efforts to get independent corroboration of the recollections of abuse victims have substantiated their claims at an astonishing rate of over 80% (Coons & Milstein, 1986; Herman & Schatzow, 1987).

reported that dissociative patients evoke deep feelings of concern and tenderness. Although they often get involved with abusive people (via the repetition compulsion, as in masochism), they also attract some generous, understanding friends. In the histories of dissociative people, there is often one person after another—a childhood friend who stayed in touch for years, a nurse who felt this patient was different from the "other" schizophrenics on the ward, a beloved teacher, an indulgent cop—who saw something special in the dissociator and tried to act as a force for good.

The reader may recall that I have sequenced these typological chapters according to degree of object relatedness. Even more than the hysterical person, the dissociative patient is object-seeking, hungry for relationship, and appreciative of care.* I have not seen any explanation for this widely acknowledged phenomenon in the literature on dissociation, but perhaps when one is systematically abused by a parent, one feels perversely important to the persecutor and therefore confirmed in one's basic value to others. Whatever the reasons, people with multiple personality disorder tend to attach powerfully and with hope.

THE DISSOCIATIVE SELF

The most striking feature of the self of someone with multiple personality disorder is, of course, that it has been fractured into numerous split-off partial selves, each of which performs certain functions.† These selves typically include the host personality (the one most often in evidence, usually the seeker of treatment, who tends to be anxious, dysthymic, and overwhelmed), infant and child components, internal persecutors, victims, protectors and helpers, and special-purpose alters (see Putnam [1989] for a more complete list). The host may know all, some, or none of the alters, and each alter may likewise know all, some, or none (T. Tudor, personal communication, July 19, 1993).

*Many psychopathic people have had abusive childhoods, with the opposite outcome. Perhaps they lack some constitutional advantage, or perhaps when abuse is chaotic and negligent (as opposed to deliberate, ritualized, or done in an altered state), a child feels hated, discarded, and defensively predatory. Or perhaps, as a dissociative patient of mine who read a first draft of this chapter pointed out, only those multiples who have had an early good object have enough experience of love to come to treatment expecting help.

†Where abuse starts in early infancy, it is more accurate to say that a self was prevented from integrating in the first place.

It can be hard for the inexperienced or naturally skeptical person to appreciate how discrete and "real" the alters can seem, both to the dissociative individual and to knowledgeable others. One evening I picked up my telephone just when my answering machine was beginning to record and found myself talking to a petulant child, an alter personality of one of my patients. She was calling to tell me about an early trauma whose existence I had suspected and to ask why the host personality needed to know about it. The next day when I told my client about the tape, she asked to hear it. We attended together to my conversation with this dissociated aspect of herself, after which she was amused to note that as she listened, she was not feeling at all identified with the childish voice recounting her own history but was instead feeling sympathy with me, the voice of parental reason (she was a mother), trying to persuade a peevish little girl that I knew what was good for her.

Running through all the identities of a dissociative person, like the themes in a complex musical composition, are certain core beliefs engendered by childhood abuse. Colin Ross, discussing the "cognitive map" of multiple personality disorder, summarizes these core beliefs as follows:

1. Different parts of the self are separate selves.
2. The victim is responsible for the abuse.
3. It is wrong to show anger (or frustration, defiance, a critical attitude . . .).
4. The past is present.
5. The primary personality can't handle the memories.
6. I love my parents but she hates them.
7. The primary personality must be punished.
8. I can't trust myself or others. (Ross, 1989b, p. 126)

Ross (1989b) then dissects each of these convictions, exposing its component beliefs and inevitable extrapolations. For example:

2. *The victim is responsible for the abuse.*
    a. I must have been bad otherwise it wouldn't have happened.
    b. If I had been perfect, it wouldn't have happened.
    c. I deserve to be punished for being angry.
    d. If I were perfect, I would not get angry.
    e. I never feel angry—she is the angry one.
    f. She deserves to be punished for allowing the abuse to happen.
    g. She deserves to be punished for showing anger. (p. 127)

Recent literature on multiple personality disorder contains

extensive information on how to access alter personalities, and how to reduce amnestic barriers so that the alter personalities may eventually become integrated into one person with all the memories, feelings, and assets that were previously sequestered and inaccessible. A critical fact for the therapist to keep in mind is that "everyone" is the patient.* Even the most unsavory persecutory personality is a valuable, potentially adaptive part of the person.† Even when alters are not in evidence, one should assume they are listening and address their concerns by "talking through" the available personality (Putnam, 1989).

TRANSFERENCE AND COUNTERTRANSFERENCE WITH DISSOCIATIVE PATIENTS

The most impressive feature of transference in dissociative clients is that there is so much of it. A person who has been severely mistreated lives in constant readiness to see the abuser in anyone on whom he or she comes to depend. Especially when child alter personalities are in ascendance, the present can feel so much like the past that hallucinatory convictions (e.g., the therapist is about to rape me, to torture me, to desert me) are not uncommon. These psychotic transferences do not indicate characterological psychosis, though diagnosticians untrained in dissociative phenomena have frequently made that inference. Rather, they are posttraumatic perceptions, sensations, and affects that were severed from awareness at the time of the original abuse and that remain unintegrated into the client's personal historical narrative. They can perhaps be best conceptualized as conditioned emotional responses to a class of stimuli associated with abuse.

A common sequence with people who have undiagnosed dissociative psychologies is for the therapist to feel a vague and benign positive transference from the host personality, who is treated as the whole patient for several weeks, months, or years, followed by a sudden

*Some early therapies of dissociative patients, including that of Eve, came to grief when the therapist advocated discarding or "killing off" troublesome alters. Dissociative people worry that this is a therapist's goal—even when explicitly reassured, as they should be, that no part of them will be sacrificed.

†People who have not worked closely with dissociative patients can be unsettled by the tendency of dissociation-savvy practitioners to join in the patient's habit of reifying dissociated parts, but to do anything else is unempathic and incongruent with one's affective experience. In fact, treatment feels a lot like doing family therapy with one person, and as in well-conducted family work, the system, not a particular favored member, is the client.

treatment crisis driven by the patient's emerging recollection of trauma and its activation of alter personalities, somatic memories, or reenactments of abuse. Such developments can be deeply disturbing and can invite counterphobic responses from the naive practitioner who assumes a schizophrenic break. The histories of dissociative patients are littered with referrals for electroshock, unwarranted pharmacological treatment (including major tranquilizers, which may aggravate dissociation), invasive medical procedures, and infantilizing "management" approaches. But for a therapist who can see what has really happened, this crisis signals the beginning of a truly reparative collaboration.

Because transference inundates dissociative patients, it is valuable for the therapist to be somewhat more "real" than he or she may customarily behave. Many clinicians find that they do this naturally—albeit with guilt if their training emphasized an invariant, "orthodox" technique. Nondissociative people of neurotic-level character structure are so grounded in reality that for their underlying projections to become evident, the therapist must be neutral. Transferences become analyzable because the client discovers a tendency to make attributions in the absence of evidence, and he or she discovers that the sources of such assumptions are historical. In contrast, dissociative people (even at the neurotic level) tend to assume that current reality is only a distraction from a more ominous *real* reality: exploitation, abandonment, torment. To explore a dissociative person's transference, the therapist must first establish that he or she is someone different from the expected abuser—someone respectful, devoted, modest, and scrupulously professional. The dissociative person's world is so infused with unexamined transferences that only the active contradiction of them permits their eventual analysis.

As mentioned previously, dissociative patients induce intense responses of love, care, and wishes to rescue. Their suffering is so profound and undeserved, their responsiveness to simple consideration so touching, that one yearns to put them on one's lap (especially the child alters) or take them home. But however effectively they evoke this reaction, they are also petrified by any violation of normal boundaries between therapists and clients; it smacks of incest. Pioneers in the rediscovery of multiplicity in the second half of the twentieth century had a tendency toward excessive nurturance: Cornelia Wilbur was very motherly toward Sybil, and David Caul could not avoid some overinvolvement with Billy Milligan (Keyes, 1982). In the autobiographical book *The Flock* (Casey, 1991), the recovered patient describes being treated as a surrogate child by a therapist and her husband; the therapist, whose notes accompany the client's account, later comments, "I will never regret 'adopting' Joan . . . but I am pleased to find that I can give multiples what they need without leaving the office" (p. 290).

Like their intrepid predecessors, most clinicians seeing their first dissociative client tend to overextend themselves. Patients with multiple personality disorder are notoriously hard to contain; at the end of each session they may linger and chat, evidently seeking a few extra shreds of moral support in facing the horrors that therapy has unearthed.* Even experienced practitioners report that sessions with their dissociative clients tend to creep past the time boundary. Being warmer and more real than one usually is, while at the same time being fastidiously observant of limits, gets easier with practice. And when one inevitably blunders, some alter will usually be happy to provide corrective instruction.

One rather amusing countertransference to dissociative people is dissociation. Like other psychologies, dissociation is catching. Not only is it easy to get into trance states while working with an autohypnotist, one also gets oddly forgetful. When I began to work with my first multiple (or "index patient," as people in dissociative studies like to say), I enrolled in the International Society for the Study of Multiple Personality and Dissociation twice, having forgotten that I had already joined.

THERAPEUTIC IMPLICATIONS OF THE DIAGNOSIS OF A DISSOCIATIVE CONDITION

Most novice therapists are intimidated by the prospect of working with someone with multiple personality disorder, and at the time I am writing this, many psychotherapy training programs still consider such patients too complex and challenging for a beginner. This is unfortunate. There is a range of dissociative pathology, and treatment should vary accordingly. A dissociative person at a neurotic level is usually easy to treat; borderline and psychotic-level cases of multiple personality present more challenges but are not any more difficult than people with other kinds of character structure in those ranges.†

*Putnam (1989) suggests 90-minute sessions, possibly in part because of this phenomenon. But most experts find the ordinary 45- or 50-minute meeting adequate for dissociative clients, with possible exceptions for extended intakes or scheduled abreactions.

†It is true, though, that people whose training program imposes time limits on clinical work should not take on someone with significant dissociative tendencies. Attachment–abandonment sequences retraumatize dissociative people, in conspicuous opposition to the Hippocratic principle "Do no harm."

Putnam (1989) rightly stresses that there is nothing fancy, no special wizardry, required to conduct good therapy with a dissociative client. With an empathic sensibility and ordinary training, one can expect to do a good job. Ross (1989b) describes the work as "extended short-term therapy," meaning that a here-and-now focus on dissociative reactions, over the long term, is the treatment of choice. One need not graduate from an analytic institute to do such work. The problem with the dissociative conditions has always been more at the diagnostic level; when people with multiple personality disorder are misunderstood as generically borderline or schizophrenic or bipolar or psychopathic, their prognosis is indeed dubious. Not only do they feel misunderstood (often in ways they cannot articulate) and hence distrustful, they are also refractory to treatment because large parts of the self are not participating in it. Once the diagnosis is clear and the patient understands the therapist's approach, psychotherapy will usually progress.

I have already mentioned some of the special aspects of technique with dissociative patients. In distilling the essence of effective therapy with this population, I could not do better than Kluft (1991), who has derived the following principles:

> 1. MPD [multiple personality disorder] is a condition that was created by broken boundaries. Therefore, a successful treatment will have a secure treatment frame and firm, consistent boundaries.
>
> 2. MPD is a condition of subjective dyscontrol and passively endured assaults and changes. Therefore, there must be a focus on mastery and the patient's active participation. . . .
>
> 3. MPD is a condition of involuntariness. Its sufferers did not elect to be traumatized and find their symptoms are often beyond their control. Therefore, the therapy must be based on a strong therapeutic alliance, and efforts to establish this must be undertaken throughout the process.
>
> 4. MPD is a condition of buried traumata and sequestered affect. Therefore, what has been hidden away must be uncovered, and what feeling has been buried must be abreacted.
>
> 5. MPD is a condition of perceived separateness and conflict among the alters. Therefore, the therapy must emphasize their collaboration, cooperation, empathy, and identification. . . .
>
> 6. MPD is a condition of hypnotic alternate realities. Therefore, the therapist's communications must be clear and straight. . . .
>
> 7. MPD is a condition related to the inconsistency of important others. Therefore, the therapist must be evenhanded to all the alters, avoiding "playing favorites" or dramatically altering his or her behavior toward the different personalities. The

therapist's consistency across all of the alters is one of the most powerful assaults on the patient's dissociative defenses.

8. MPD is a condition of shattered security, self-esteem, and future orientation. Therefore, the therapy must make efforts to restore morale and inculcate realistic hope.

9. MPD is a condition stemming from overwhelming experiences. Therefore, the pacing of the therapy is essential. Most treatment failures occur when the pace of the therapy outstrips the patient's capacity to tolerate the material. . . . [I]f one cannot get into the difficult material one planned to address in the first third of the session, to work on it in the second, and process it and restabilize the patient in the third [one should not approach] the material, lest the patient leave the session in an overwhelmed state . . . .

10. MPD is a condition that results from the irresponsibility of others. Therefore, the therapist must be very responsible, and hold the patient to a high standard of responsibility once the therapist is confident that the patient, across alters, actually grasps what reasonable responsibility entails.

11. MPD is a condition that often results because people who could have protected a child did nothing. The therapist can anticipate that technical neutrality will be interpreted as uncaring and rejecting and is best served by taking a warmer stance that allows for a latitude of affective expression.

12. MPD is a condition in which the patient has developed many cognitive errors. The therapy must address and correct them on an ongoing basis. (pp. 177–178)

It also helps to know a little hypnosis. Since dissociative people by definition go into trance states spontaneously all the time, it is not possible to work with them *without* hypnosis—either they are doing it alone, or you and they are doing it cooperatively. A therapist who can help the patient learn how to get the hypnotic process under control and use it autonomously and therapeutically rather than traumatically and defensively is providing a critical service. Trance-inducing techniques are extremely easy to use with this population of hypnotic prodigies. These techniques are especially effective in building a sense of safety, containing surplus anxiety, and handling emergencies.

I say this as someone who came to hypnosis kicking and screaming. My colleague Jeffrey Rutstein calls this the "If-it-wasn't-good-enough-for-Freud-it-isn't-good-enough-for-me!" reaction. My resistance to learning hypnotic techniques came from my misgivings about any intervention I regarded as authoritarian; I did not want to tell someone he or she was getting sleepy if that was actually my directive rather than the client's natural experience. This prejudice remitted when I learned to hypnotize in an egalitarian, collaborative way (having the patient direct me as to induction images and other particulars), and when I saw how much calmer it made my dissociative clients in managing the emotional maelstrom created by going in and out of traumatic memories. For therapists who have no background in it, a weekend workshop in hypnosis is enough to provide adequate skill for work with most dissociative clients. The training also helps one to appreciate the full range of dissociative phenomena.

Occasionally, other deviations from standard treatment may be called for. Tudor (1989) has recommended "field trips," in which the therapist and patient visit the scene of early traumas in order to establish the reality of what happened there. Readers of *Sybil* may remember how critical it was to her recovery to find physical evidence of her early abuse. Whether exceptional practices should occur more with dissociative patients than with others is moot. I have sometimes attended the wedding of a nondissociative client, or accepted a gift, or walked around the block with a person whose anxiety was too high that day to stay on the couch—even in the most classical treatment there may arise a compelling therapeutic reason, usually involving disconfirmation of specific pathogenic beliefs, to suspend ordinary arrangements. As with any "parameter" (Eissler, 1953), the therapist should behave anomalously only with a clear therapeutic rationale, and should look with the client at his or her reactions to the atypical activity. Since dissociative people are even more concerned than others about boundary infractions, attention to their responses to departures from standard operating procedure is particularly critical.

Finally, I want to underscore Kluft's comments about pacing. With dissociative patients even more than with others, the practitioner is wise to remember the old psychoanalytic chestnut "The slower you go, the faster you get there" (that is, assuming you have the diagnosis right; otherwise, a lot of time is being wasted treating the alter who comes for therapy as the only patient). Now that multiplicity has been rediscovered, some hospitals and clinics are experimenting with ways to cut down on treatment time. But as with any problem that inheres in character, shortcuts are contraindicated. With dissociative people, they are not only futile (trust takes a long time to build, and premature pressure on the patient actually prolongs distrust), they may make things dramatically worse. We have no business, especially in the name of mental health, retraumatizing someone who has already had more than an ordinary share of injury.

DIFFERENTIAL DIAGNOSIS

In this chapter the differential diagnosis section will be more thorough than usual because so much of the misunderstanding and mistreatment of dissociative patients derives from diagnostic errors. I was never taught to "rule out" dissociation, and it is my impression that psychotherapy training programs are only beginning to teach people how to distinguish dissociative pathology from other kinds of problems. As a case in point, when I was in training, I was taught that if a patient reported hearing voices, he or she was presumptively psychotic, organically or functionally, with the best bet being some variety of schizophrenia. I was not instructed to ask whether the voices seemed to be inside or outside the person's head. This rudimentary way of discriminating posttraumatic hallucinatory states from psychotic decompensation was not even known in the 1970s, and despite the impressive research that has since then established its value (see C. A. Ross, 1989b, Kluft, 1991), it is still taught only rarely.

Fortunately, things are changing very fast in the dissociative realm. Although recent research (Coons, Bowman, & Milstein, 1988) into the mental health backgrounds of people with multiple personality disorder disclosed that an average of 7 *years* intrudes between the patient's initial application for treatment and his or her eventual accurate diagnosis, this lag seems already to be shrinking. Yet it is still true that one of the factors that should alert a diagnostician to the possible existence of a dissociative identity problem is the presence of several prior, serious, and/or mutually exclusive diagnostic labels in the treatment history of a patient.

I cannot stress enough that most people with dissociative psychologies do not come to therapy announcing that their problem is dissociation. The condition must be inferred. Data suggesting the possibility of a dissociative process include a known history of trauma; a family background of severe alcoholism or drug abuse; a personal background of unexplained serious accidents; amnesia for the elementary-school years; a pattern of self-destructive behavior for which the patient can offer no rationale; complaints of "lost time," blank spells, or time distortion; headaches (common during switching); referral to the self in the third person or the first person plural; eye-rolling and trance-like behaviors; voices or noises in the head; and previous treatment failures.

Dissociative problems range from mild depersonalization to polyfragmented multiple personality disorder. Although this chapter is about characterological dissociation, many of us have occasional dissociative symptoms, and neither they nor entrenched dissociative personality patterns can be addressed by a therapist who is not open to seeing them. There now exist two excellent screening devices for dissociation, the Dissociation Experiences Scale (E. M. Bernstein & Putnam, 1986) and the Structured Clinical Interview for DSM-IV Dissociative Disorders (SCID-D; Steinberg, 1993), that augur well for both diagnosis and future research.

Dissociative Conditions versus the Functional Psychoses

Because dissociative patients in crisis or under stress show most of Schneider's "first-rank" symptoms of schizophrenia (see Hoenig, 1983), they are easily construed as schizophrenic.* If an observer regards dissociative switching as lability of mood, the client may be seen as schizoaffective or bipolar at the psychotic level. The main ways in which dissociative people differ from those with functional psychoses involve their premorbid personalities and their object relatedness: Genuinely schizophrenic people have a deadened, flat quality and do not tend to draw the therapist into an intense attachment. Their withdrawal from reality and relatedness tends to have started in their teens and progressed insidiously toward a more complete isolation in adulthood. Manic–depressive and schizoaffective people have shifts of mood but no disorders of memory, and in the manic state they are much more grandiose than the agitated dissociative person.

Complicating the diagnostic challenge is the fact that dissociative symptoms can coexist with schizophrenia and with the affective psychoses. To assess whether dissociation is a major part of a psychotic picture when voices are reported, one should ask to speak with "the part of you that is saying these things." If dissociation predominates, an alter will often answer back. The first time one does this it feels

*Many have wondered recently whether some of the more spectacular cures of "schizophrenia" (e.g., Sechehaye, 1951a, 1951b; Green, 1964) might have involved patients whose primary dynamic was actually dissociative. If this is so, and if most empirical investigations of schizophrenia have included dissociative subjects along with genuinely schizophrenic ones, we need to redo much of that research. This comment is *not* made in support of the position that in contrast to dissociative disorders, "real" schizophrenia is incurable; still, there is little doubt that dissociatively based hallucinations, delusions, and disorders of thinking remit much faster, and carry a better eventual prognosis, than similar symptoms that express an underlying psychotic disorganization.

ludicrous, but after that it seems a rather prosaic intervention. The neophyte dissociation-evaluator should remember that the worst that can happen is for the patient to stare blankly and ascribe the request to some weird professional rite of intake.

Dissociative versus Borderline Conditions

The diagnoses of borderline and dissociative conditions are not mutually exclusive. To be consistent about psychoanalytic concepts of character organization, we would have to assume that a dissociative person can be organized at a psychotic, borderline, or neurotic level, and fortunately for the point of view represented in this book, contemporary research in dissociation supports such an assumption. Referring to the DSM-III-R definitions of Multiple Personality Disorder and Borderline Personality Disorder, Kluft (1991) reports that:

> of treatment-adherent patients who appear to have both MPD and BPD [borderline personality disorder], one-third rapidly ceased to show BPD features once they settled into treatment, one-third lost their apparent BPD as their MPD resolved, and one-third retained BPD features even after integration. (p. 175)

Presumably, once patients in this last group had stopped dissociating, their borderline status could be addressed in further expressive therapy.

Even though some dissociative patients are rightly regarded as in the borderline range, where separation–individuation issues prevail, it is also common for neurotic-level people with multiple personality or chronic dissociative responses to be misunderstood as generically borderline. Dissociation resembles splitting, and switches to alter personalities can be easily mistaken for changes in ego states. The important questions to ask here are sensitive to the presence or absence of amnesia. Their phrasing is critical, since traumatized people do not trust in the benevolence of authorities and offer certain information only if it is expressly welcomed. Saying "Last Monday you were furious at me and thought I was worthless, but today you're saying I'm wonderful" will evoke defensiveness in either a dissociative or a generically borderline person. But "Do you happen to remember that you were feeling quite different about me last Monday?" may distinguish borderline from dissociative shifts. The dissociative person has been given permission by the phrasing of the question to admit that he or she has forgotten everything about the Monday session, while the one with borderline dynamics is free to say, "Yeah, so what?"

Dissociative versus Hysterical Conditions

As mentioned previously, there is considerable overlap between hysterical and dissociative psychologies; many of us have both. Conversion symptoms are common in people with multiple personality disorder; hysterical people dissociate in many small ways. The basic temperament of people who become more dissociative and people who become more histrionic is probably similar, but the childhood mistreatment of the former is profound. Some individuals with hysterical personalities, especially at the neurotic level, have suffered no abuse to speak of, while no one with diagnosable dissociative identity disorder, even at the neurotic level, has escaped severe trauma. In anyone with pronounced hysterical symptoms, one should assess for dissociation.

The therapeutic ramifications of this differential revolve around the importance with hysterical people of interpreting their recurrent impulses, fantasies, and unconscious strivings, in contrast with an emphasis with dissociative patients on remembering and abreacting a traumatic history. If one does the former with a basically dissociative client, one will reinforce denial, increase guilt, and fail to deal with the pain that a terrible history has created. If one does the latter with a histrionic client, one may prevent the flowering of the sense of agency that comes from acknowledging internal dynamics and redirecting one's energies in directions that are genuinely satisfying.

Dissociative versus Psychopathic Conditions

As mentioned in Chapter 7, many antisocial people have dissociative defenses. Discriminating between a sociopathic person with a dissociative streak and a dissociative person with a sociopathic alter is a maddeningly difficult enterprise—mostly because by the time this question is asked, so many legal consequences hinge on it. A person apprehended for a serious crime may have a huge stake in convincing a judge or jury of multiplicity; less commonly, a persecutory alter may be trying to punish the host personality by getting the self assessed as antisocial. It is prudent to assume psychopathy when someone has powerful reasons to malinger. Several recent books in the "true-crime" genre (e.g., Weissberg, 1992) have explored the mind-bending complications that have arisen in cases when a suspect has claimed to be a multiple.

If we do become adept at reliably differentiating essentially dissociative from essentially psychopathic people, even when there is significant secondary gain to the patient in presenting as one or the other, the consequences for the criminal justice system could be substantial. Since dissociative people (except the most polyfragmented) have a good prognosis, there would be significant crime-preventive value in giving intensive therapy to perpetrators discovered to have multiple personality disorder. Clinicians can resolve dissociation more expeditiously than they can modify antisocial patterns; under conditions of limited resources, people working in jails or with the probation system could concentrate on those clients most receptive to their help.

SUMMARY

In this chapter I have discussed the history of the concept of dissociation and its intriguing characterological variant, multiple personality disorder. In accounting for individual development of dissociation as a core process, I mentioned constitutional talent for self-hypnosis, often coexisting with high intelligence, creativity, and sociophilia. These factors may predispose a person to respond to trauma with a dissociative defense invisible to outsiders. Braun's BASK model of dissociation was discussed as an alternative to Freudian concepts of defense. Object relations of dissociative people were explained as rooted in traumatic childhood abuse, undiluted by help in processing such injuries emotionally. The self of someone with a dissociative identity was depicted not only as fragmented but also as permeated by paralyzing fears and self-blaming cognitions.

The power of transference and countertransference reactions with dissociative patients was emphasized, especially as they provoke rescue fantasies and overinvolvement in the therapist. Treatment implications of this diagnosis included a stress on nurturing the sense of basic safety and cooperation in the therapeutic relationship, promoting recall and emotional comprehension of dissociated experiences, maintaining consistency toward all personalities, being "real" and warm while adhering strictly to professional boundaries, analyzing pathogenic beliefs, using hypnosis adjunctively, and respecting the client's need to take time to tolerate abreaction and integration. Dissociative dynamics were differentiated from schizophrenic and bipolar psychoses, generically borderline conditions, and hysterical and psychopathic personality organizations.

SUGGESTIONS FOR FURTHER READING

Putnam (1989) and C. A. Ross (1989b) have each written excellent basic texts on the diagnosis and treatment of dissociative conditions.

Psychoanalytically friendly readers should not be put off by Ross's somewhat cranky attitude toward analysts; his expertise is vast. The most concise, state-of-the-art article on multiple personality disorder and dissociation that I know of is Kluft's (1991) summary. The chapters in Kluft and Fine's (1993) edited anthology on multiple personality disorder are almost uniformly readable and of the highest quality.

Appendix: Suggested Diagnostic Interview Format

DEMOGRAPHIC DATA

Name, age, sex, ethnic and racial background, religious orientation, relationship status, parental status, level of education attained, employment status, previous experience with psychotherapy, source of referral, informants other than client.

CURRENT PROBLEMS AND THEIR ONSET

Chief complaints, and the patient's ideas about their origins; history of these problems; any medications being taken for them; why therapy is being sought *now*.

PERSONAL HISTORY

Where born, reared, number of children in family and client's place among them, major moves. Parents and siblings: Get objective data (whether alive, cause and time of death if not; age, health, occupation) and subjective data (personality, nature of relationship with patient). Psychological problems in family (diagnosed psychopathology and other conditions; e.g., alcoholism).

Infancy and Toddlerhood

Whether patient was wanted; family conditions after birth; anything unusual in developmental milestones; any early problems (eating, bowel control, talking, locomoting; bedwetting, night terrors, sleepwalking, nailbiting, etc.); earliest memories; family stories or jokes about the client.

Latency

Separation problems, social problems, academic problems, behavioral problems, cruelty to animals; illnesses, losses, moves, or family stresses at this time; sexual or physical abuse.

Adolescence

Age of puberty, any physical problems with sexual maturation, family preparation for sexuality, first sexual experiences, sexual preference, masturbation fantasies; school experience, academically and socially; patterns of self-destructiveness (eating disorders, drug use, questionable sexual judgment, excessive risk-taking, suicidal impulses, antisocial patterns); illnesses, losses, moves or family stresses at this time.

Adulthood

Work history; relationship history; adequacy of current intimate relationship; relationship to children; hobbies, talents, pleasures, areas of pride and satisfaction.

CURRENT PRESENTATION (MENTAL STATUS)

General appearance, affective state, mood, quality of speech, soundness of reality testing, estimated intelligence, adequacy of memory, assessed reliability of information. Pursue further investigation into any of these areas that suggest problems; e.g., if mood is depressed, assess suicide.

Dreams: Are they remembered? Any recurrent? Example of a recent dream.

Substance use, prescribed and otherwise, including alcohol.

CONCLUDING TOPICS

Ask the patient if he or she can think of any other important information that has not been asked about.

Ask whether the patient is comfortable with you and whether he or she has anything to ask.

INFERENCES

Major recurring themes; areas of fixation and conflict; favored defenses; inferred unconscious fantasies, wishes and fears; central identifications, counteridentifications, unmourned losses; self-cohesion and self-esteem.

References

Abraham, K. (1924). A short study of the development of the libido, viewed in light of mental disorders. In *Selected papers on psycho-analysis* (pp. 418–501). London: Hogarth Press, 1927.

Abraham, K. (1935). The history of a swindler. *Psychoanalytic Quarterly*, *4*, 570–587.

Abrahamsen, D. (1985). *Confessions of Son of Sam*. New York: Columbia University Press.

Adler, A. (1927). *Understanding human nature*. Garden City, NY: Garden City Publishing.

Adler, G. (1972). Hospital management of borderline patients and its relationship to psychotherapy. In P. Hartcollis (Ed.), *Borderline personality disorders: The concept, the syndrome, the patient* (pp. 307–323). New York: International Universities Press.

Adler, G. (1973). Hospital treatment of borderline patients. *American Journal of Psychiatry*, *130*, 32–36.

Adler, G. (1985). *Borderline psychopathology and its treatment*. New York: Jason Aronson.

Adler, G., & Buie, D. (1979). The psychotherapeutic approach to aloneness in the borderline patient. In J. LeBoit & A. Capponi (Eds.), *Advances in psychotherapy of the borderline patient* (pp. 433–448). New York: Jason Aronson.

Adorno, T. W., Frenkl-Brunswick, E., Levinson, D. J., & Sanford, R. N. (1950). *The authoritarian personality*. New York: Harper.

Aichhorn, A. (1936). *Wayward youth*. London: Putnam.

Akhtar, S. (1992). *Broken structures: Severe personality disorders and their treatment*. Northvale, NJ: Jason Aronson.

Akiskal, H. S. (1984). Characterologic manifestations of affective disorders: Toward a new conceptualization. *Integrative Psychiatry*, *2*, 83–88.

Allen, D. W. (1977). Basic treatment issues. In M. J. Horowitz (Ed.), *Hysterical personality* (pp. 283–328). New York: Jason Aronson.

Altschul, S. (Ed.). (1988). *Childhood bereavement and its aftermath*. Madison, CT: International Universities Press.

American Psychiatric Association. (1968). *Diagnostic and statistical manual of mental disorders* (2nd ed.). Washington, DC: Author.

American Psychiatric Association. (1980). *Diagnostic and statistical manual of mental disorders* (3rd ed.). Washington, DC: Author.

American Psychiatric Association. (1987). *Diagnostic and statistical manual of mental disorders* (3rd ed., rev.). Washington, DC: Author.

American Psychiatric Association. (1993, March 1). *DSM-IV draft criteria*. Washington, DC: Author.

Arieti, S. (1955). *Interpretation of schizophrenia*. New York: Brunner/Mazel.

Arieti, S. (1961). Introductory notes on the psychoanalytic therapy of schizophrenics. In A. Burton (Ed.), *Psychotherapy of the psychoses* (pp. 68–89). New York: Basic Books.

Arieti, S. (1974). *Interpretation of schizophrenia* (2nd ed.). New York: Basic Books.

Arlow, J. A., & Brenner, C. (1964). *Psychoanalytic concepts and the structural theory*. New York: International Universities Press.

Aronson, M. L. (1964). A study of the Freudian theory of paranoia by means of the Rorschach Test. In C. F. Reed, I. E. Alexander, & S. S. Tomkins (Eds.), *Psychopathology: A source book* (pp. 370–387). New York: Wiley.

Ashe, S. S. (1985). The masochistic personality. In R. Michels & J. Cavenar (Eds.), *Psychiatry 1* (pp. 1–9). Philadelphia: Lippincott.

Bach, S. (1985). *Narcissistic states and the therapeutic process*. New York: Jason Aronson.

Bak, R. C. (1946). Masochism in paranoia. *Psychoanalytic Quarterly*, *15*, 285–301.

Balint, M. (1945). Friendly expanses—Horrid empty spaces. *International Journal of Psycho-Analysis*, *36*, 225–241.

Balint, M. (1960). Primary narcissism and primary love. *Psychoanalytic Quarterly*, *29*, 6–43.

Balint, M. (1968). *The basic fault: Therapeutic aspects of regression*. London: Tavistock.

Bateson, G., Jackson, D. D., Haley, J., & Weakland, J. (1956). Toward a theory of schizophrenia. *Behavioral Science*, *1*, 251–264.

Baumeister, R. F. (1989). *Masochism and the self*. Hillsdale, NJ: Lawrence Erlbaum.

Bellak, L., & Small, L. (1978). *Emergency psychotherapy and brief psychotherapy*. New York: Grune & Stratton.

Beres, D. (1958). Vicissitudes of superego formation and superego precursors in childhood. *Psychoanalytic Study of the Child*, *13*, 324–335.

Bergler, E. (1949). *The basic neurosis*. New York: Grune & Stratton.

Bergman, P., & Escalona, S. K. (1949). Unusual sensitivities in very young children. *Psychoanalytic Study of the Child, 3/4*, 333–352.

Bergmann, M. S. (1985). Reflections on the psychological and social functions of remembering the Holocaust. *Psychoanalytic Inquiry*, *5*, 9–20.

Bergmann, M. S. (1987). *The anatomy of loving: The story of man's quest to know what love is*. New York: Columbia University Press.

Berliner, B. (1958). The role of object relations in moral masochism. *Psychoanalytic Quarterly*, *27*, 38–56.

Bernstein, D. (1993). *Female identity conflict in clinical practice*. Northvale, NJ: Jason Aronson.

Bernstein, E. M., & Putnam, F. W. (1986). Development, reliability, and validity of a dissociation scale. *Journal of Mental and Nervous Disease*, *174*, 727–735.

Bernstein, I. (1983). Masochistic psychology and feminine development. *Journal of the American Psychoanalytic Association*, *31*, 467–486.

Bertin, C. (1982). *Marie Bonaparte: A life*. New York: Quarter Books.

Bettelheim, B. (1960). *The informed heart: Autonomy in a mass age*. Glencoe, IL: The Free Press.

Bettelheim, B. (1983). *Freud and man's soul*. New York: Knopf.

Bibring, E. (1953). The mechanism of depression. In P. Greenacre (Ed.), *Affective disorders* (pp. 13–48). New York: International Universities Press.

Bion, W. R. (1959). *Experiences in groups*. New York: Basic Books.

Bion, W. R. (1967). *Second thoughts*. New York: Jason Aronson.

Biondi, R., & Hecox, W. (1992). *The Dracula killer: The true story of California's vampire killer*. New York: Pocket Books.

Blanck, G., & Blanck, R. (1974). *Ego psychology: Theory and practice*. New York: Columbia University Press.

Blanck, G., & Blanck, R. (1979). *Ego psychology II: Psychoanalytic developmental psychology*. New York: Columbia University Press.

Blanck, G., & Blanck, R. (1986). *Beyond ego psychology: Developmental object relations theory*. New York: Columbia University Press.

Blanck, R., & Blanck, G. (1968). *Marriage and personal development*. New York: Columbia University Press.

Blatt, S. J. (1974). Levels of object representation in anaclitic and introjective depression. *Psychoanalytic Study of the Child*, *24*, 107–157.

Blatt, S. J., & Bers, S. (1993). The sense of self in depression: A psychoanalytic perspective. In Z. V. Segal & S. J. Blatt (Eds.), *The self in emotional distress: Cognitive and psychodynamic perspectives* (pp. 171–210). New York: Guilford Press.

Bleuler, E. (1911). *Dementia praecox or the group of schizophrenias* (J. Zinkin, Trans.). New York: International Universities Press, 1950.

Bleuler, M. (1977). *The schizophrenic disorders* (S. M. Clemens, Trans.). New Haven: Yale University Press.

Bollas, C. (1987). Loving hate. In *The shadow of the object* (pp. 117–134). New York: Columbia University Press.

Bornstein, B. (1949). The analysis of a phobic child: Some problems of theory and technique in child analysis. *Psychoanalytic Study of the Child, 3/4,* 181–226.

Bowlby, J. (1969). *Attachment and loss: Vol. I. Attachment.* New York: Basic Books.

Bowlby, J. (1973). *Attachment and loss: Vol. II. Separation: Anxiety and anger.* New York: Basic Books.

Braude, S. E. (1991). *First person plural: Multiple personality and the philosophy of mind.* New York: Routledge, Chapman & Hall.

Braun, B. G. (1984). Hypnosis creates multiple personality: Myth or reality? *International Journal of Clinical Hypnosis, 32,* 191–197.

Braun, B. G. (1988). The BASK (behavior, affect, sensation, knowledge) model of dissociation. *Dissociation, 1,* 4–23.

Braun, B. G., & Sacks, R. G. (1985). The development of multiple personality disorder: Predisposing, precipitating, and perpetuating factors. In R. P. Kluft (Ed.), *Childhood antecedents of multiple personality* (pp. 37–64). Washington, DC: American Psychiatric Press.

Brazelton, T. B. (1962). Observations of the neonate. *Journal of the American Academy of Child Psychiatry, 1,* 38–58.

Brazelton, T. B. (1980, May). *New knowledge about the infant from current research: Implications for psychoanalysis.* Paper presented at the meeting of the American Psychoanalytic Association, San Francisco.

Brazelton, T. B. (1982). Joint regulation of neonate-parent behavior. In E. Tronick (Ed.), *Social interchange in infancy.* Baltimore: University Park Press.

Brenman, M. (1952). On teasing and being teased and the problems of "moral masochism." *Psychoanalytic Study of the Child, 7,* 264–285.

Brenner, C. (1955). *An elementary textbook of psychoanalysis.* New York: International Universities Press.

Brenner, C. (1959). The masochistic character. *Journal of the American Psychoanalytic Association, 7,* 197–226.

Brenner, C. (1982). The calamities of childhood. In *The mind in conflict* (pp. 93–106). New York: International Universities Press.

Breuer, J., & Freud, S. (1893–1895). Studies in hysteria. *Standard Edition, 2,* 21–47.

Brody, S., & Siegel, M. (1992). *The evolution of character: Birth to eighteen years. A longitudinal study.* New York: International Universities Press.

Brown, R. (1965). *Social psychology.* New York: The Free Press.

Buckley, P. (Ed.). (1988). *Essential papers on psychosis.* New York: New York University Press.

Bursten, B. (1973a). *The manipulator: A psychoanalytic view.* New Haven: Yale University Press.

Bursten, B. (1973b). Some narcissistic personality types. *International Journal of Psycho-Analysis, 54,* 287–300.

Cameron, N. (1959). Paranoid conditions and paranoia. In S. Arieti (Ed.), *American handbook of psychiatry* (Vol. 1, pp. 508–539). New York: Basic Books.

Capote, T. (1965). *In cold blood.* New York: Random House.

Casey, J. F. (1991). *The flock: The autobiography of a multiple personality* (with L. Wilson). New York: Knopf.

Cath, S. H. (1986). Fathering from infancy to old age: A selective overview of recent psychoanalytic contributions. *Psychoanalytic Review, 74,* 469–479.

Cattell, J. P., & Cattell, J. S. (1974). Depersonalization: Psychological and social perspectives. In S. Arieti (Ed.), *American handbook of psychiatry* (pp. 767–799). New York: Basic Books.

Celani, D. (1976). An interpersonal approach to hysteria. *American Journal of Psychiatry, 133,* 1414–1418.

Chase, T. (1987). *When Rabbit howls.* New York: Jove.

Chasseguet-Smirgel, J. (1971). *Female sexuality: New psychoanalytic views.* Ann Arbor: University of Michigan Press.

Chasseguet-Smirgel, J. (1984). *Creativity and perversion.* London: Free Association.

Chasseguet-Smirgel, J. (1985). *The ego ideal: A psychoanalytic essay on the malady of the idea.* New York: Norton.

Chess, S., Rutter, M., Thomas, A., & Birch, H. G. (1963). Interaction of temperament and the environment in the production of behavioral disturbances in children. *American Journal of Psychiatry, 120,* 142–147.

Chess, S., Thomas, A., & Birch, H. G. (1967). Behavior problems revisited: Findings of an anteretrospective study. *Journal of the American Academy of Child Psychiatry,* 6, 321–331.

Chessick, R. D. (1969). *How psychotherapy heals: The process of intensive psychotherapy.* New York: Jason Aronson.

Chessick, R. D. (1985). *Psychology of the self and the treatment of narcissism.* Northvale, NJ: Jason Aronson.

Chodoff, P. (1978). Psychotherapy of the hysterical personality disorder. *Journal of the American Academy of Psychoanalysis,* 6, 496–510.

Chodoff, P. (1982). The hysterical personality disorder: A psychotherapeutic approach. In A. Roy (Ed.), *Hysteria* (pp. 277–285). New York: Wiley.

Chodorow, N. J. (1978). *The reproduction of mothering: Psychoanalysis and the sociology of gender.* Berkeley: University of California Press.

Chodorow, N. J. (1989). *Feminism and psychoanalytic theory.* New Haven: Yale University Press.

Cleckley, H. (1941). *The mask of sanity: An attempt to clarify some issues about the so-called psychopathic personality.* St. Louis: Mosby.

Cohen, M. B., Baker, G., Cohen, R. A., Fromm-Reichmann, F., & Weigert, E. (1954). An intensive study of twelve cases of manic–depressive psychosis. *Psychiatry, 17,* 103–137.

Colby, K. (1951). *A primer for psychotherapists.* New York: Ronald.

Coleman, M., & Nelson, B. (1957). Paradigmatic psychotherapy in borderline treatment. *Psychoanalysis, 5,* 28–44.

Coons, P. M., Bowman, E. S., & Milstein, V. (1988). Multiple personality disorder: A clinical investigation of 50 cases. *Journal of Nervous and Mental Disease, 176,* 519–527.

Coons, P. M., & Milstein, V. (1986). Psychosexual disturbances in multiple personality. *Journal of Nervous and Mental Disease, 174*, 106–110.

Coontz, S. (1992). *The way we never were: American families and the nostalgia gap*. New York: Basic Books.

Cooper, A. M. (1988). The narcissistic–masochistic character. In R. A. Glick & D. I. Meyers (Eds.), *Masochism: Current psychoanalytic perspectives* (pp. 189–204). Hillsdale, NJ: The Analytic Press.

Darley, J., & Batson, C. D. (1973). From Jerusalem to Jericho: A study of situational and dispositional variables in helping behavior. *Journal of Personality and Social Psychology, 27*, 100–108.

Davanloo, H. (1978). *Basic principles and techniques in short-term dynamic psychotherapy*. New York: Spectrum.

Davanloo, H. (1980). *Short-term dynamic psychotherapy*. New York: Jason Aronson.

de Monchy, R. (1950). Masochism as a pathological and as a normal phenomenon in the human mind. *International Journal of Psycho-Analysis, 31*, 95–97.

Deri, S. (1968). Interpretation and language. In E. Hammer (Ed.), *The use of interpretation in treatment*. New York: Grune & Stratton.

Des Barres, P. (1987). *I'm with the band: Confessions of a groupie*. New York: Morrow.

Deutsch, H. (1942). Some forms of emotional disturbance and their relationship to schizophrenia. *Psychoanalytic Quarterly, 11*, 301–321.

Deutsch, H. (1944). *The psychology of women: A psychoanalytic interpretation: Vol. 1. Girlhood.* New York: Grune & Stratton.

Deutsch, H. (1955). The impostor: Contribution to ego psychology of a type of psychopath. *Psychoanalytic Quarterly, 24*, 483–503.

Diamond, M. J. (1993, April). *Fathers and sons: Psychoanalytic perspectives on "good-enough" fathering throughout the life cycle*. Paper presented at the Spring Meeting of the Division of Psychoanalysis (39) of the American Psychological Association, New York.

Dinnerstein, D. (1976). *The mermaid and the minotaur*. New York: Harper & Row.

Dorpat, T. (1982). An object-relations perspective on masochism. In P. L. Giovacchini & L. B. Boyer (Eds.), *Technical factors in the treatment of severely disturbed patients* (pp. 490–513). New York: Jason Aronson.

Easser, B. R., & Lesser, S. (1965). The hysterical personality: A reevaluation. *Psychoanalytic Quarterly, 34*, 390–405.

Edelstein, M. G. (1981). *Trauma, trance, and transformation: A clinical guide to hypnotherapy*. New York: Brunner/Mazel.

Ehrenberg, D. B. (1992). *The intimate edge: Extending the reach of psychoanalytic interaction*. New York: Norton.

Eigen, M. (1986). *The psychotic core*. New York: Jason Aronson.

Eissler, K. R. (1953). The effects of the structure of the ego on psychoanalytic technique. *Journal of the American Psychoanalytic Association, 1*, 104–143.

Ekstein, R., & Wallerstein, R. S. (1958; rev. ed., 1971). *The teaching and learning of psychotherapy*. Madison, CT: International Universities Press.

Ellis, A. (1961). The treatment of a psychopath with rational emotive psychotherapy. In *Reason and emotion in psychotherapy* (pp. 288–299). New York: Lyle Stewart.

Erikson, E. H. (1950). *Childhood and society*. New York: Norton.

Erikson, E. H. (1968). *Identity: Youth and crisis*. New York: Norton.

Escalona, S. K. (1968). *The roots of individuality: Normal patterns of development in infancy*. Chicago: Aldine.

Fairbairn, W. R. D. (1941). A revised psychopathology of the psychoses and psychoneuroses. *International Journal of Psycho-Analysis*, *22*, 250–279.

Fairbairn, W. R. D. (1954). *An object-relations theory of the personality*. New York: Basic Books.

Fast, I. (1990). Aspects of early gender development: Toward a reformulation. *Psychoanalytic Psychology*, *7* (Suppl.), 105–107.

Federn, P. (1952). *Ego psychology and the psychoses*. New York: Basic Books.

Fenichel, O. (1928). On "isolation." In *The collected papers of Otto Fenichel, first series* (pp. 147–152). New York: Norton.

Fenichel, O. (1941). *Problems of psychoanalytic technique*. Albany, NY: Psychoanalytic Quarterly.

Fenichel, O. (1945). *The psychoanalytic theory of neurosis*. New York: Norton.

Ferenczi, S. (1913). Stages in the development of a sense of reality. In *First contributions to psycho-analysis* (pp. 213–239). New York: Brunner/Mazel, 1980.

Ferenczi, S. (1925). Psychoanalysis of sexual habits. *Further contributions to the theory and technique of psycho-analysis* (pp. 259–297). New York: Brunner/Mazel, 1980.

Finell, J. (1986). The merits and problems with the concept of projective identification. *Psychoanalytic Review*, *73*, 103–120.

Fisher, S. (1970). *Body experience in fantasy and behavior*. New York: Appleton-Century-Crofts.

Fisher, S., & Greenberg, R. P. (1985). *The scientific credibility of Freud's theories and therapy*. New York: Columbia University Press.

Fogelman, E. (1988). Intergenerational group therapy: Child survivors of the Holocaust and offspring of survivors. *Psychoanalytic Review*, *75*, 619–640.

Fogelman, E., & Savran, B. (1979). Therapeutic groups for children of Holocaust survivors. *International Journal of Group Psychotherapy*, *29*, 211–235.

Fonda, H. (1981). *My life. As told to Howard Teichmann*. New York: New American Library.

Forster, E. M. (1921). *Howard's End*. New York: Vintage.

Fraiberg, S. (1959). *The magic years: Understanding and handling the problems of early childhood*. New York: Charles Scribner's Sons.

Frances, A., & Cooper, A. M. (1981). Descriptive and dynamic psychiatry: A perspective on DSM-III. *American Journal of Psychiatry*, *138*, 1198–1202.

Frank, J. D., Margolin, J., Nash, H. T., Stone, A. R., Varon, E., & Ascher, E.

(1952). Two behavior patterns in therapeutic groups and their apparent motivation. *Human Relations*, *5*, 289–317.
Freud, A. (1936). *The ego and the mechanisms of defense*. New York: International Universities Press, 1966.
Freud, S. (1886). Observation of a severe case of hemianaesthesia in a hysterical male. *Standard Edition*, *1*, 23–31.
Freud, S. (1897). Letter to Wilhelm Fliess. *Standard Edition*, *1*, 259.
Freud, S. (1900). The interpretation of dreams. *Standard Edition*, *4*.
Freud, S. (1901). The psychopathology of everyday life. *Standard Edition*, *6*.
Freud, S. (1905). Three essays on the theory of sexuality. *Standard Edition*, *7*, 135–243.
Freud, S. (1908). Character and anal eroticism. *Standard Edition*, *9*, 169–175.
Freud, S. (1909). Notes upon a case of obsessional neurosis. *Standard Edition*, *10*, 151–320.
Freud, S. (1911). Psycho-analytic notes on an autobiographic account of a case of paranoia (dementia paranoides). *Standard Edition*, *13*, 1–162.
Freud, S. (1912). The dynamics of transference. *Standard Edition*, *12*, 97–108.
Freud, S. (1913). The disposition to obsessional neurosis. *Standard Edition*, *12*, 311–326.
Freud, S. (1914a). Remembering, repeating and working through (Further recommendations on the technique of psycho-analysis II). *Standard Edition*, *12*, 147–156.
Freud, S. (1914b). On narcissism: An introduction. *Standard Edition*, *14*, 67–102.
Freud, S. (1915a). Instincts and their vicissitudes. *Standard Edition*, *14*, 111–140.
Freud, S. (1915b). Repression. *Standard Edition*, *14*, 147.
Freud, S. (1916). Some character types met with in psychoanalytic work. *Standard Edition*, *14*, 311–333.
Freud, S. (1917a). Mourning and melancholia. *Standard Edition*, *14*, 243–258.
Freud, S. (1917b). On transformations of instinct as exemplified in anal erotism. *Standard Edition*, *17*, 125–133.
Freud, S. (1918). From the history of an infantile neurosis. *Standard Edition*, *17*, 7–122.
Freud, S. (1919). A child is being beaten: A contribution to the study of the origin of sexual perversions. *Standard Edition*, *17*, 179–204.
Freud, S. (1920). Beyond the pleasure principle. *Standard Edition*, *18*, 7–64.
Freud, S. (1923). The ego and the id. *Standard Edition*, *19*, 13–59.
Freud, S. (1924). The economic problem in masochism. *Standard Edition*, *19*, 159–170.
Freud, S. (1925a). Some psychical consequences of the anatomical distinction between the sexes. *Standard Edition*, *19*, 248–258.
Freud, S. (1925b). Autobiographical study. *Standard Edition*, *20*, 32–76.
Freud, S. (1931). Libidinal types. *Standard Edition*, *21*, 215–222.
Freud, S. (1932). Femininity. *Standard Edition*, *22*, 112–135.

Freud, S. (1937). Analysis terminable and interminable. *Standard Edition, 22,* 216–253.
Freud, S. (1938). An outline of psycho-analysis. *Standard Edition, 23,* 144–207.
Friedenberg, E. Z. (1959). *The vanishing adolescent.* Boston: Beacon.
Friedman, R. C. (1988). *Male homosexuality: A contemporary psychoanalytic perspective.* New Haven: Yale University Press.
Fromm, E. (1947). *Man for himself: An inquiry into the psychology of ethics.* New York: Rinehart.
Fromm-Reichmann, F. (1950). *Principles of intensive psychotherapy.* Chicago: University of Chicago Press.
Frosch, J. (1964). The psychotic character: Clinical psychiatric considerations. *Psychoanalytic Quarterly, 38,* 91–96.
Furman, E. (1982). Mothers have to be there to be left. *Psychoanalytic Study of the Child, 37,* 15–28.
Gabbard, G. O. (1990). *Psychodynamic psychiatry in clinical practice.* Washington, DC: American Psychiatric Press.
Gaddis, T., & Long, J. (1970). *Killer: A journal of murder.* New York: Macmillan.
Galenson, E. (1988). The precursors of masochism: Protomasochism. In R. A. Glick & D. I. Meyers (Eds.), *Masochism: Current psychoanalytic perspectives* (pp. 189–204). Hillsdale, NJ: The Analytic Press.
Galin, D. (1974). Implications for psychiatry of left and right cerebral specialization. *Archives of General Psychiatry, 31,* 572–583.
Gardiner, M. (1971). *The wolf-man: By the wolf-man.* New York: Basic Books.
Gardner, M. R. (1991). The art of psychoanalysis: On oscillation and other matters. *Journal of the American Psychoanalytic Association, 39,* 851–870.
Gay, P. (1968). *Weimar culture.* New York: Harper & Row.
Gay, P. (1988). *Freud: A life for our time.* New York: Norton.
Gaylin, W. (Ed.). (1983). *Psychodynamic understanding of depression: The meaning of despair.* New York: Jason Aronson.
Gill, M. M. (1983). The interpersonal paradigm and the degree of the therapist's involvement. *Contemporary Psychoanalysis, 19,* 200–237.
Gill, M. M, Newman, R., & Redlich, F. C. (1954). *The initial interview in psychiatric practice.* New York: International Universities Press.
Gilligan, C. (1982). *In a different voice: Psychological theory and women's development.* Cambridge, MA: Harvard University Press.
Giovacchini, P. L. (1979). *The treatment of primitive mental states.* New York: Jason Aronson.
Giovacchini, P. L. (1986). *Developmental disorders: The transitional space in mental breakdown and creative imagination.* Northvale, NJ: Jason Aronson.
Giovacchini, P. L., & Boyer, L. B. (Eds.). (1982). *Technical factors in the treatment of the severely disturbed patient.* New York: Jason Aronson.
Glick, R. A., & Meyers, D. I. (1988). *Masochism: Current psychoanalytic perspectives.* Hillsdale, NJ: The Analytic Press.

Glover, E. (1955). *The technique of psycho-analysis*. New York: International Universities Press.

Goldberg, A. (1990a). Disorders of continuity. *Psychoanalytic Psychology, 7,* 13–28.

Goldberg, A. (1990b). *The prisonhouse of psychoanalysis*. New York: The Analytic Press.

Goldstein, K. (1959). Functional disturbances in brain damage. In S. Arieti (Ed.), *American handbook of psychiatry* (Vol. 1, pp. 770–794). New York: Basic Books.

Gottesman, I. (1991). *Schizophrenia genesis: The origins of madness*. New York: W. H. Freeman.

Green, H. (1964). *I never promised you a rose garden*. New York: Holt, Rinehart & Winston.

Greenacre, P. (1958). The impostor. *Psychoanalytic Quarterly, 27,* 359–382.

Greenberg, J. R., & Mitchell, S. A. (1983). *Object relations in psychoanalytic theory*. Cambridge, MA: Harvard University Press.

Greenfield, S. (1991). Experiences of subsequent therapists with female patients sexually involved with a prior male therapist. Unpublished doctoral dissertation. Graduate School of Applied and Professional Psychology, Rutgers University. *Dissertation Abstracts International, 52,* 3905B.

Greenson, R. R. (1967). *The technique and practice of psychoanalysis*. New York: International Universities Press.

Greenspan, S. I. (1981). *Clinical infant reports: Number 1: Psychopathology and adaptation in infancy and early childhood: Principles of clinical diagnosis and preventive intervention*. New York: International Universities Press.

Greenwald, H. (1958). *The call girl: A sociological and psychoanalytic study*. New York: Ballantine Books.

Greenwald, H. (1974). Treatment of the psychopath. In H. Greenwald (Ed.), *Active psychotherapy* (pp. 363–377). New York: Jason Aronson.

Grinker, R. R., Werble, B., & Drye, R. C. (1968). *The borderline syndrome: A behavioral study of ego functions*. New York: Basic Books.

Grossman, W. (1986). Notes on masochism: A discussion of the history and development of a psychoanalytic concept. *Psychoanalytic Quarterly, 55,* 379–413.

Groth, A. N. (1979). *Men who rape: The psychology of the offender*. New York: Plenum.

Grotstein, J. (1982). Newer perspectives in object relations theory. *Contemporary Psychoanalysis, 18,* 43–91.

Grünbaum, A. (1979). Is Freudian psychoanalysis pseudo-scientific by Karl Popper's criterion of demarcation. *American Philosophical Quarterly, 16,* 131–141.

Grunberger, B. (1979). *Narcissism: Psychoanalytic essays* (J. Diamanti, Trans.). New York: International Universities Press.

Gunderson, J. G. (1984). *Borderline personality disorder*. Washington, DC: American Psychiatric Press.

Gunderson, J. G., & Singer, M. T. (1975). Defining borderline patients: An overview. *American Journal of Psychiatry, 133*, 1–10.

Guntrip, H. (1952). The schizoid personality and the external world. In *Schizoid phenomena, object relations and the self* (pp. 17–48). New York: International Universities Press, 1969.

Guntrip, H. (1961). The schizoid problem, regression, and the struggle to preserve an ego. In *Schizoid phenomena, object relations and the self* (pp. 49–86). New York: International Universities Press, 1969.

Guntrip, H. (1969). *Schizoid phenomena, object relations and the self*. New York: International Universities Press.

Guntrip, H. (1971). *Psychoanalytic theory, therapy, and the self: A basic guide to the human personality in Freud, Erikson, Klein, Sullivan, Fairbairn, Hartmann, Jacobson, and Winnicott*. New York: Basic Books.

Hall, C. S. (1954). *A primer on Freudian psychology*. New York: Octagon Books (reprinted 1990).

Halleck, S. L. (1967). Hysterical personality traits— psychological, social, and iatrogenic determinants. *Archives of General Psychiatry, 16*, 750–759.

Hammer, E. (1968). *The use of interpretation in treatment*. New York: Grune & Stratton.

Hammer, E. (1990). *Reaching the affect: Style in the psychodynamic therapies*. New York: Jason Aronson.

Hare, R. (1970). *Psychopathy: Theory and research*. New York: Wiley.

Harris, D. (1982). *Dreams die hard: Three men's journey through the sixties*. New York: St. Martin's/Marek.

Hartcollis, P. (Ed.). (1977). *Borderline personality disorders: The concept, the syndrome, the patient*. New York: International Universities Press.

Hartmann, H. (1958). *Ego psychology and the problem of adaptation*. New York: International Universities Press.

Hedges, L. E. (1983). *Listening perspectives in psychotherapy*. New York: Jason Aronson.

Hendin, H. (1975). *The age of sensation: A psychoanalytic exploration*. New York: Norton.

Herman, J. L. (1981). *Father–daughter incest*. Cambridge, MA: Harvard University Press.

Herman, J. L. (1992). *Trauma and recovery: The aftermath of violence—from domestic abuse to political terror*. New York: Basic Books.

Herman, J. L., & Schatzow, E. (1987). Recovery and verification of memories of childhood sexual abuse. *Psychoanalytic Psychology, 4*, 1–14.

Herzog, J. (1980). Sleep disturbance and father hunger in 18–to 28–month-old boys: The Erlkönig syndrome. *Psychoanalytic Study of the Child, 35*, 219–236.

Hirsch, S. J., & Hollender, M. H. (1969). Hysterical psychoses: Clarification of the concept. *American Journal of Psychiatry, 125*, 909.

Hoch, P. H., & Polatin, P. (1949). Pseudoneurotic forms of schizophrenia. *Psychoanalytic Quarterly*, *23*, 248–276.

Hoenig, J. (1983). The concept of schizophrenia: Kraepelin–Bleuler–Schneider. *British Journal of Psychiatry*, *142*, 547–556.

Hollender, M. H. (1971). Hysterical personality. *Comments on Contemporary Psychiatry*, *1*, 17–24.

Hollender, M., & Hirsch, S. (1964). Hysterical psychosis. *American Journal of Psychiatry*, *120*, 1066–1074.

Horner, A. J. (1979). *Object relations and the developing ego in therapy*. New York: Jason Aronson.

Horner, A. J. (1990). *The primacy of structure: Psychotherapy of underlying character pathology*. Northvale, NJ: Jason Aronson.

Horner, A. J. (1991). *Psychoanalytic object relations therapy*. Northvale, NJ: Jason Aronson.

Horney, K. (1926). The flight from womanhood: The masculinity-complex in women as viewed by men and women. *International Journal of Psycho-Analysis*, *7*, 324–339.

Horney, K. (1939). *New ways in psycho-analysis*. New York: Norton.

Horowitz, M. J. (Ed). (1977). *Hysterical personality*. New York: Jason Aronson.

Hughes, J. M. (1989). *Reshaping the psychoanalytic domain: The work of Melanie Klein, W. R. D. Fairbairn, and D. W. Winnicott*. Berkeley, CA: University of California Press.

Isaacs, K. (1990). Affect and the fundamental nature of neurosis. *Psychoanalytic Psychology*, *7*, 259–284.

Jacobs, T. J. (1991). *The use of the self: Countertransference and communication in the analytic situation*. Madison, CT: International Universities Press.

Jacobson, E. (1964). *The self and the object world*. New York: International Universities Press.

Jacobson, E. (1967). *Psychotic conflict and reality*. London: Hogarth Press.

Jacobson, E. (1971). *Depression: Comparative studies of normal, neurotic, and psychotic conditions*. New York: International Universities Press.

Janet, P. (1890). *The major symptoms of hysteria*. New York: Macmillan.

Jaspers, K. (1963). *General psychopathology* (J. Hoenig & M. W. Hamilton, Trans.). Chicago: University of Chicago Press.

Johnson, A. (1949). Sanctions for superego lacunae of adolescents. In K. R. Eissler (Ed.), *Searchlights on delinquency* (pp. 225–245). New York: International Universities Press.

Jones, E. (1913). The God complex: The belief that one is God, and the resulting character traits. In *Essays in applied psycho-analysis* (Vol. 2, pp. 244–265). London: Hogarth Press, 1951.

Josephs, L. (1992). *Character structure and the organization of the self*. New York: Columbia University Press.

Jung, C. G. (1945). The relations between the ego and the unconscious. In H. Read, M. Fordham, & G. Adler (Eds.), *The collected works of* C. G. *Jung* (Bollinger Series 20, Vol. 7, pp. 120–239). Princeton, NJ: Princeton University Press, 1953.

Jung, C. G. (1954). Concerning the archetypes, with special reference to the *anima* concept. In H. Read, M. Fordham, G. Adler, & W. McGuire (Eds.), *The collected works of* C. G. *Jung* (Bollinger Series 20, Vol. 9, pp. 54–72). Princeton, NJ: Princeton University Press, 1959.

Kahn, H. (1962). *Thinking about the unthinkable.* New York: Horizon.

Kalafat, J. (1984). Training community psychologists for crisis intervention. *American Journal of Community Psychology, 12,* 241–251.

Karasu, T. B. (1990). *Psychotherapy for depression.* Northvale, NJ: Jason Aronson.

Karon, B. P. (1989). On the formation of delusions. *Psychoanalytic Psychology, 6,* 169–185.

Karon, B. P. (1992). The fear of understanding schizophrenia. *Psychoanalytic Psychology, 9,* 191–211.

Karon, B. P., & VandenBos, G. R. (1981). *Psychotherapy of schizophrenia: The treatment of choice.* New York: Jason Aronson.

Karpe, R. (1961). The rescue complex in Anna O's final identity. *Psychoanalytic Quarterly, 30,* 1–27.

Kasanin, J. S. (Ed.). (1944). *Language and thought in schizophrenia.* New York: Norton.

Kasanin, J. S., & Rosen, Z. A. (1933). Clinical variables in schizoid personalities. *Archives of Neurology and Psychiatry, 30,* 538–553.

Katan, M. (1953). Mania and the pleasure principle: Primary and secondary symptoms. In P. Greenacre (Ed.), *Affective disorders* (pp. 140–209). New York: International Universities Press.

Kernberg, O. F. (1970). Factors in the psychoanalytic treatment of narcissistic personalities. *Journal of the American Psychoanalytic Association, 18,* 51–85.

Kernberg, O. F. (1975). *Borderline conditions and pathological narcissism.* New York: Jason Aronson.

Kernberg, O. F. (1976). *Object relations theory and clinical psychoanalysis.* New York: Jason Aronson.

Kernberg, O. F. (1981). Some issues in the theory of hospital treatment. *Nordisk Tidsskrift for Loegeforen, 14,* 837–842.

Kernberg, O. F. (1982, August). Conference on treating borderline and narcissistic patients. Eastham, MA.

Kernberg, O. F. (1984). *Severe personality disorders: Psychotherapeutic strategies.* New Haven: Yale University Press.

Kernberg, O. F. (1988). Clinical dimensions of masochism. *Journal of the American Psychoanalytic Association, 36,* 1005–1029.

Kernberg, O. F. (1989). An ego psychology object relations theory of the structure and treatment of pathologic narcissism: An overview. *Psychiatric Clinics of North America, 12,* 723–729.

Kernberg, O. F. (1991). Aggression and love in the relationship of the couple. *Journal of the American Psychoanalytic Association, 39,* 45–70.

Kernberg, O. F. (1992). *Aggression in personality disorders and perversions.* New Haven: Yale University Press.

Kernberg, O. F., Selzer, M. A., Koenigsberg, H. W., Carr, A. C., &

Appelbaum, A. H. (1989). *Psychodynamic psychotherapy of borderline patients*. New York: Basic Books.

Keyes, D. (1982). *The minds of Billy Milligan*. New York: Bantam.

Khan, M. M. R. (1963). The concept of cumulative trauma. *Psychoanalytic Study of the Child, 18*, 286–306.

Khan, M. M. R. (1974). *The privacy of the self*. New York: International Universities Press.

Klein, M. (1932). *The psycho-analysis of children*. London: Hogarth Press.

Klein, M. (1935). A contribution to the psychogenesis of manic–depressive states. In *Love, guilt and reparation and other works 1921–1945* (pp. 262–289). New York: The Free Press, 1975.

Klein, M. (1937). Love, guilt and reparation. In *Love, guilt and reparation and other works 1921–1945* (pp. 306–343). New York: The Free Press, 1975.

Klein, M. (1940). Mourning and its relation to manic–depressive states. In *Love, guilt and reparation and other works 1921–1945* (pp. 311–338). New York: The Free Press, 1975.

Klein, M. (1945). The oedipus complex in light of early anxieties. In *Love, guilt and reparation and other works 1921–1945* (pp. 370–419). New York: The Free Press, 1975.

Klein, M. (1946). Notes on some schizoid mechanisms. *International Journal of Psycho-Analysis, 27*, 99–110.

Klein, M. (1957). Envy and gratitude. In *Envy and gratitude and other works 1946–1963* (pp. 176–235). New York: The Free Press, 1975.

Kluft, R. P. (1984). Treatment of multiple personality disorder: A study of 33 cases. *Psychiatric Clinics of North America, 7*, 9–29.

Kluft, R. P. (Ed.). (1985). *Childhood antecedents of multiple personality*. Washington, DC: American Psychiatric Press.

Kluft, R. P. (1987). Making the diagnosis of multiple personality disorder. In F. F. Flach (Ed.), *Diagnostics and psychopathology*, (pp. 201–225). New York: Norton.

Kluft, R. P. (1989). Dissociation: The David Caul Memorial Symposium symposium papers: Iatrogenesis and MPD. *Dissociation*, 2, 66–104.

Kluft, R. P. (1991). Multiple personality disorder. In A. Tasman & S. M. Goldfinger (Eds.), *American Psychiatric Press review of psychiatry* (Vol. 10, pp. 161–188). Washington, DC: American Psychiatric Press.

Kluft, R. P., & Fine, C. G. (Eds.). (1993). *Clinical perspectives on multiple personality disorder*. Washington, DC: American Psychiatric Press.

Knight, R. (1953). Borderline states in psychoanalytic psychiatry and psychology. *Bulletin of the Menninger Clinic, 17*, 1–12.

Kohut, H. (1968). The psychoanalytic treatment of narcissistic personality disorders. *Psychoanalytic Study of the Child, 23*, 86–113.

Kohut, H. (1971). *The analysis of the self: A systematic approach to the psychoanalytic treatment of narcissistic personality disorders*. New York: International Universities Press.

Kohut, H. (1977). *The restoration of the self*. New York: International Universities Press.

Kohut, H. (1984). *How does analysis cure?* (A. Goldberg, Ed., with P. Stepansky). Chicago: University of Chicago Press.

Kohut, H., & Wolf, E. S. (1978). The disorders of the self and their treatment—an outline. *International Journal of Psycho-Analysis*, 59, 413–425.

Kraepelin, E. (1913). *Lectures on clinical psychiatry*. London: Bailliere, Tindall, & Cox.

Kraepelin, E. (1915). *Psychiatrie: Ein lehrbuch* (8th ed.). Leipzig: Barth.

Kraepelin, E. (1919). *Dementia praecox and paraphrenia* (R. M. Barclay, Trans.). Huntington, NY: Robert E. Krieger, 1971.

Krafft-Ebing, R. (1900). *Psychopathia sexualis* (F. J. Rebman, Trans.). New York: Physicians and Surgeons Book Company, 1935.

Kretschmer, E. (1925). *Physique and character* (J. H. Sprott, Trans.). New York: Harcourt, Brace & World.

Kris, E. (1956). On some vicissitudes of insight in psychoanalysis. *International Journal of Psycho-Analysis*, *37*, 445–455.

Kuhn, T. S. (1970). *The structure of scientific revolutions* (2nd rev. ed.). Chicago: University of Chicago Press.

Kupperman, J. (1991). *Character*. New York: Oxford University Press.

Lachmann, F., & Beebe, B. (1989). Oneness fantasies revisited. *Psychoanalytic Psychology*, 6, 137–149.

Laing, R. D. (1965). *The divided self: An existential study in sanity and madness*. Baltimore: Penguin.

Langness, L. L. (1967). Hysterical psychosis—the cross-cultural evidence. *American Journal of Psychiatry*, *124*, 143–151.

Langs, R. J. (1973). *The technique of psychoanalytic psychotherapy: The initial contact, theoretical framework, understanding the patient's communications, the therapist's interventions* (Vol. 1). New York: Jason Aronson.

LaPlanche, J., & Pontalis, J. B. (1973). *The language of psychoanalysis*. New York: Norton.

Lasch, C. (1978). *The culture of narcissism: American life in an age of diminishing expectations*. New York: Norton.

Lasch, C. (1984). *The minimal self: Psychic survival in troubled times*. New York: Norton.

Laughlin, H. P. (1956). *The neuroses in clinical practice*. Philadelphia: Saunders.

Laughlin, H. P. (1967). *The neuroses*. New York: Appleton-Century-Crofts.

Laughlin, H. P. (1970; 2nd ed., 1979). *The ego and its defenses*. New York: Jason Aronson.

Lax, R. F. (1977). The role of internalization in the development of certain aspects of female masochism: Ego psychological considerations. *International Journal of Psycho-Analysis*, 58, 289–300.

Lax, R. F. (Ed.) (1989). *Essential papers on character neurosis and treatment*. New York: New York University Press.

Lazare, A. (1971). The hysterical character in psychoanalytic theory: Evolution and confusion. *Archives of General Psychiatry*, 25, 131–137.

Levenson, E. A. (1972). *The fallacy of understanding: An inquiry into the changing structure of psychoanalysis*. New York: Basic Books.

Levin, J. D. (1987). *Treatment of alcoholism and other addictions: A self-psychology approach*. Northvale, NJ: Jason Aronson.

Lewis, H. B. (1971). *Shame and guilt in neurosis*. New York: International Universities Press.

Lichtenberg, J. (Ed.). (1992). Perspectives on multiple personality disorder. *Psychoanalytic Inquiry, 12*(1).

Lidz, T. (1973). *The origin and treatment of schizophrenic disorders*. New York: Basic Books.

Lidz, T., & Fleck, S. (1965). Family studies and a theory of schizophrenia. In T. Lidz, S. Fleck, & A. R. Cornelison (Eds.), *Schizophrenia and the family*. New York: International Universities Press.

Lifton, R. J. (1968). *Death in life: Survivors of Hiroshima*. New York: Random House.

Lilienfeld, S. O., Van Valkenburg, C., Larntz, K., & Akiskal, H. S. (1986). The relationship of histrionic personality disorder to antisocial personality disorder and somatization disorders. *American Journal of Psychiatry, 142*, 718–722.

Lindner, R. (1955). The jet-propelled couch. In *The fifty-minute hour: A collection of true psychoanalytic tales* (pp. 221–293). New York: Jason Aronson, 1982.

Linton, R. (1956). *Culture and mental disorders*. Springfield, IL: Charles C. Thomas.

Lion, J. R. (1978). Outpatient treatment of psychopaths. In W. Reid (Ed.), *The psychopath: A comprehensive study of antisocial disorders and behaviors* (pp. 286–300). New York: Brunner/Mazel.

Lion, J. R. (Ed.). (1986). *Personality disorders: Diagnosis and management* (2nd ed.). Malabar, FL: Robert E. Krieger.

Litman, R. E., & Farberow, N. L. (1970). Emergency evaluation of suicidal potential. In E. S. Schneiderman, N. L. Farberow, & R. E. Litman (Eds.), *The psychology of suicide* (pp. 259–272). New York: Science House.

Little, M. I. (1981). *Transference neurosis and transference psychosis: Toward basic unity*. New York: Jason Aronson.

Little, M. I. (1990). *Psychotic anxieties and containment: A personal record of an analysis with Winnicott*. Northvale, NJ: Jason Aronson.

Livingston, M. S. (1991). *Near and far: Closeness and distance in psychotherapy*. New York: Rivercross.

Loeb, J., & Mednick, S. A. (1977). *A prospective study of predictors of criminality: Three electrodermal response patterns*. In S. A. Mednick & K. O. Christiansen (Eds.), *Biosocial bases of criminal behavior* (pp. 245–254). New York: Gardner.

Loewald, H. W. (1957). On the therapeutic action of psychoanalysis. In *Papers on psychoanalysis* (pp. 221–256). New Haven: Yale University Press, 1980.

Loewenstein, R. M. (1951). The problem of interpretation. *Psychoanalytic Quarterly*, *20*, 1–14.

Loewenstein, R. M. (1955). A contribution to the psychoanalytic theory of masochism. *Journal of the American Psychoanalytic Association*, *5*, 197–234.

Loewenstein, R. J. (1988). The spectrum of phenomenology in multiple personality disorder: Implications for diagnosis and treatment. In B. G. Braun (Ed.), *Proceedings of the Fifth National Conference on Multiple Personality Disorder/ Dissociative States* (p. 7). Chicago: Rush University.

Loewenstein, R. J., & Ross, D. R. (1992). Multiple personality and psychoanalysis: An introduction. *Psychoanalytic Inquiry*, *12*, 3–48.

Lothane, Z. (1992). *In defense of Schreber: Soul murder and psychiatry*. Hillsdale, NJ: The Analytic Press.

Lovinger, R. J. (1984). *Working with religious issues in therapy*. New York: Jason Aronson.

Lykken, D. (1957). A study of anxiety in the sociopathic personality. *Journal of Abnormal and Social Psychology*, *55*, 6–10.

Lynd, H. M. (1958). *On shame and the search for identity*. New York: Harcourt, Brace & World.

MacKinnon, R. A., & Michels, R. (1971). *The psychiatric interview in clinical practice*. Philadelphia: Saunders.

Maheu, R., & Hack, R. (1992). *Next to Hughes*. New York: Harper Collins.

Mahler, M. S. (1968). *On human symbiosis and the vicissitudes of individuation*. New York: International Universities Press.

Mahler, M. S. (1971). A study of the separation–individuation process and its possible application to borderline phenomena in the psychoanalytic situation. *Psychoanalytic Study of the Child*, *26*, 403–424.

Mahler, M. S. (1972a). On the first three subphases of the separation–individuation process. *International Journal of Psycho-Analysis*, *53*, 333–338.

Mahler, M. S. (1972b). Rapprochement subphase of the separation–individuation process. *Psychoanalytic Quarterly*, *41*, 487–506.

Mahler, M. S., Pine, F., & Bergman, A. (1975). *The psychological birth of the human infant*. New York: Basic Books.

Main, T. F. (1957). The ailment. *British Journal of Medical Psychology*, *30*, 129–145.

Malan, D. H. (1963). *A study of brief psychotherapy*. New York: Plenum.

Mandelbaum, A. (1977). The family treatment of the borderline patient. In P. Hartcollis (Ed.), *Borderline personality disorders: The concept, the syndrome, the patient* (pp. 423–438). New York: International Universities Press.

Mann, J. (1973). *Time-limited psychotherapy*. Cambridge, MA: Harvard University Press.

Marmor, J. (1953). Orality in the hysterical personality. *Journal of the American Psychiatric Association*, *1*, 656–671.

Masling, J. (Ed.). (1986). *Empirical studies of psychoanalytic theories* (Vol. 2). Hillsdale, NJ: The Analytic Press.

Masson, J. M. (1984). *The assault on truth: Freud's suppression of the seduction theory*. New York: Farrar, Straus, & Giroux.

Masterson, J. F. (1972). *Treatment of the borderline adolescent: A developmental approach*. New York: Wiley-Interscience.

Masterson, J. F. (1976). *Psychotherapy of the borderline adult: A developmental approach*. New York: Brunner/Mazel.

McClelland, D. C. (1961). *The achieving society*. Princeton, NJ: Van Nostrand.

McDougall, J. (1980). *Plea for a measure of abnormality*. New York: International Universities Press.

McDougall, J. (1989). *Theaters of the body: A psychoanalytic approach to psychosomatic illness*. New York: Norton.

McGoldrick, M. (1982). Irish families. In M. McGoldrick, J. K. Pearce, & J. Giordano (Eds.), *Ethnicity and family therapy* (pp. 310–339). New York: Guilford Press.

McWilliams, N. (1979). Treatment of the young borderline patient: Fostering individuation against the odds. *Psychoanalytic Review*, 66, 339–357.

McWilliams, N. (1984). The psychology of the altruist. *Psychoanalytic Psychology*, *1*, 193–213.

McWilliams, N. (1986). Patients for life: The case for devotion. *The Psychotherapy Patient*, 3, 55–69.

McWilliams, N. (1991). Mothering and fathering processes in the psychoanalytic art. *Psychoanalytic Review*, *78*, 526–545.

McWilliams, N., & Lependorf, S. (1990). Narcissistic pathology of everyday life: The denial of remorse and gratitude. *Journal of Contemporary Psychoanalysis*, 26, 430–451.

McWilliams, N., & Stein, J. (1987). Women's groups led by women: The management of devaluing transferences. *International Journal of Group Psychotherapy*, *37*, 139–153.

Mednick, S. A., Gabrielli, W., & Hutchings, B. (1984). Genetic influences in criminal convictions: Evidence from an adoption cohort. *Science*, *224*, 891–894.

Meissner, W. W. (1978). *The paranoid process*. New York: Jason Aronson.

Meissner, W. W. (1979). Narcissistic personalities and borderline conditions: A differential diagnosis. *Annual Review of Psychoanalysis*, *7*, 171–202.

Meissner, W. W. (1984). *The borderline spectrum: Differential diagnosis and developmental issues*. New York: Jason Aronson.

Meissner, W. W. (1988). *Treatment of patients in the borderline spectrum*. Northvale, NJ: Jason Aronson.

Meissner, W. W. (1991). *What is effective in psychoanalytic therapy: A move from interpretation to relation*. Northvale, NJ: Jason Aronson.

Meloy, J. R. (1988). *The psychopathic mind: Origins, dynamics, and treatment*. Northvale, NJ: Jason Aronson.

Menaker, E. (1942). The masochistic factor in the psychoanalytic situation. *Psychoanalytic Quarterly*, *11*, 171–186.

Menaker, E. (1953). Masochism—A defense reaction of the ego. *Psychoanalytic Quarterly*, *22*, 205–220.

Menaker, E. (1982). *Otto Rank: A rediscovered legacy*. New York: Columbia University Press.

Menninger, K. (1963). *The vital balance: The life process in mental health and illness* (with M. Mayman & P. Pruyser). New York: Viking.

Michaud, S., & Aynesworth, H. (1983). *The only living witness*. New York: New American Library.

Milgram, S. (1963). Behavioral study of obedience. *Journal of Abnormal and Social Psychology, 67*, 371–378.

Miller, A. (1975). *Prisoners of childhood: The drama of the gifted child and the search for the true self*. New York: Basic Books.

Miller, J. B. (Ed.). (1973). *Psychoanalysis and women: Contributions to new theory and therapy*. New York: Brunner/Mazel.

Miller, J. B. (1984). The development of women's sense of self. In J. V. Jordan, A. G. Kaplan, J. B. Miller, I. P. Stiver, & J. L. Surrey (Eds.), *Women's growth in connection: Writings for the Stone Center* (pp. 11–26). New York: Guilford Press.

Mischler, E., & Waxler, N. (Eds.). (1968). *Family processes and schizophrenia*. New York: Jason Aronson.

Modell, A. H. (1975). A narcissistic defense against affects and the illusion of self-sufficiency. *International Journal of Psycho-Analysis, 56*, 275–282.

Modell, A. H. (1976). The "holding environment" and the therapeutic action of psychoanalysis. *Journal of the American Psychoanalytic Association, 24*, 285–308.

Money, J. (1980). *Love and lovesickness: The science of sex, gender difference, and pair bonding*. Baltimore: Johns Hopkins University Press.

Money, J. (1988). *Gay, straight, and in-between: The sexology of erotic orientation*. New York: Oxford University Press.

Morrison, A. P. (1983). Shame, the ideal self, and narcissism. *Contemporary Psychoanalysis, 19*, 295–318.

Morrison, A. P. (Ed.). (1986). *Essential papers on narcissism*. New York: New York University Press.

Morrison, A. P. (1989). *Shame: The underside of narcissism*. Hillsdale, NJ: The Analytic Press.

Mowrer, O. H. (1950). *Learning theory and personality dynamics*. New York: Ronald.

Mueller, W. J., & Aniskiewitz, A. S. (1986). *Psychotherapeutic intervention in hysterical disorders*. Northvale, NJ: Jason Aronson.

Mullahy, P. (1970). *Psychoanalysis and interpersonal psychiatry: The contributions of Harry Stack Sullivan*. New York: Science House.

Murray, H. A., & members of the Harvard Psychological Clinic (1938). *Explorations in personality*. New York: Oxford University Press.

Myerson, P. G. (1991). *Childhood dialogues and the lifting of repression: Character structure and psychoanalytic technique*. New Haven: Yale University Press.

Nagera, H. (1976). *Obsessional neuroses: Developmental pathology*. New York: Jason Aronson.

Nannarello, J. J. (1953). "Schizoid." *Journal of Nervous and Mental Diseases, 118*, 242.

Nemiah, J. C. (1973). *Foundations of psychopathology*. New York: Jason Aronson.

Niederland, W. (1959). Schreber: Father and son. *Psychoanalytic Quarterly, 28*, 151–169.

Noblin, C. D., Timmons, E. O., & Kael, H. C. (1966). Differential effects of positive and negative verbal reinforcement on psychoanalytic character types. *Journal of Personality and Social Psychology, 4*, 224–228.

Noel, B. (1992). *You must be dreaming* (with K. Watterson). New York: Poseidon Press.

Nunberg, H. (1955). *Principles of psycho-analysis*. New York: International Universities Press.

Nydes, J. (1963). The paranoid–masochistic character. *Psychoanalytic Review, 50*, 215–251.

Ogden, T. H. (1982). *Projective identification: Psychotherapeutic technique*. New York: Jason Aronson.

Ovesey, L. (1955). Pseudohomosexuality, the paranoid mechanism and paranoia. *Psychiatry, 18*, 163–173.

Panken, S. (1973). *The joy of suffering: Psychoanalytic theory and therapy of masochism*. New York: Jason Aronson.

Paolino, T. J. Jr. (1981). *Psychoanalytic psychotherapy: Theory, technique, therapeutic relationship and treatability*. New York: Brunner/Mazel.

Peralta, V., Cuesta, M. J., & de Leon, J. (1991). Premorbid personality and positive and negative symptoms in schizophrenia. *Acta Psychiatrica Scandinavica, 84*, 336–339.

Piaget, J. (1937). *The construction of reality in the child*. New York: Basic Books.

Pine, F. (1985). *Developmental theory and clinical process*. New Haven: Yale University Press.

Pine, F. (1990). *Drive, ego, object, and self: A synthesis for clinical work*. New York: Basic Books.

Pope, K. S. (1987). Preventing therapist–patient sexual intimacy: Therapy for a therapist at risk. *Professional Psychology: Research and Practice, 18*, 624–628.

Pope, K. S., Tabachnick, B. G., & Keith-Spiegel, P. (1987). Ethics of practice: The beliefs and behaviors of psychologists as therapists. *American Psychologist, 42*, 993–1006.

Prichard, J. C. (1835). *Treatise on insanity*. London: Sherwood Gilbert & Piper.

Prince, M. (1906). *The dissociation of a personality: A biographical study in abnormal personality*. New York: Longman, Green.

Putnam, F. W. (1989). *Diagnosis and treatment of multiple personality disorder*. New York: The Guilford Press.

Racker, H. (1968). *Transference and countertransference*. New York: International Universities Press.

Rado, S. (1928). The problem of melancholia. *International Journal of Psycho-Analysis*, 9, 420–438.

Rank, O. (1929). *The trauma of birth*. Harper & Row, 1973.

Rank, O. (1945). *Will therapy and truth and reality*. New York: Knopf.

Rasmussen, A. (1988). Chronically and severely battered women: A psychodiagnostic investigation. Unpublished doctoral dissertation. Graduate School of Applied and Professional Psychology, Rutgers University. *Dissertation Abstracts International*, 50, 2634B.

Rawn, M. L. (1991). The working alliance: Current concepts and controversies. *Psychoanalytic Review*, 78, 379–389.

A Recovering Patient. (1986). "Can we talk?" The schizophrenic patient in psychotherapy. *American Journal of Psychiatry*, 143, 68–70.

Redl, R., & Wineman, D. (1951). *Children who hate*. New York: The Free Press.

Reich, A. (1960). Pathological forms of self-esteem regulation. *Psychoanalytic Study of the Child*, 15, 215–231.

Reich, W. (1933). *Character analysis*. New York: Farrar, Straus, and Giroux, 1972.

Reik, T. (1941). *Masochism in modern man*. New York: Farrar, Straus.

Reik, T. (1948). *Listening with the third ear*. New York: Grove.

Ressler, R. K., & Schactman, T. (1992). *Whoever fights monsters: My twenty years of hunting serial killers for the FBI*. New York: St. Martin's.

Rhodes, J. (1980). *The Hitler movement: A modern millenarian revolution*. Stanford, CA: Hoover Institution Press.

Rice, J., Reich, T., Andreason, N. C., Endicott, J., Van Eerdewegh, M., Fishman, R., Hirschfeld, R. M., & Klerman, G. L. (1987). The familial transmission of bipolar illness. *Archives of General Psychiatry*, 44, 441–447.

Richfield, J. (1954). An analysis of the concept of insight. *Psychoanalytic Quarterly*, 23, 390–408.

Richman, J., & White, H. (1970). A family view of hysterical psychosis. *American Journal of Psychiatry*, 127, 280–285.

Rinsley, D. B. (1982). *Borderline and other self disorders: A developmental and object-relations perspective*. New York: Jason Aronson.

Robbins, A., with contributors. (1980). *Expressive therapy*. New York: Human Sciences Press.

Robbins, A. (1988). The interface of the real and transference relationships in the treatment of schizoid phenomena. *Psychoanalytic Review*, 75, 393–417.

Robbins, A. (1989). *The psychoaesthetic experience: An approach to depth-oriented treatment*. New York: Human Sciences Press.

Robbins, A. (1991, April). Unpublished comments. Symposium at the Spring Meeting of the Division of Psychoanalysis (39) of the American Psychological Association, Chicago.

Rockland, L. H. (1992). *Supportive therapy: A psychodynamic approach*. New York: Basic Books.

Rogers, C. R. (1951). *Client-centered therapy: Its current practice, implications, and theory*. Boston: Houghton Mifflin.

Rogers, C. R. (1961). *On becoming a person.* Boston: Houghton Mifflin.

Roland, A. (1981). Induced emotional reactions and attitudes in the psychoanalyst as transference and in actuality. *Psychoanalytic Review, 68,* 45–74.

Roland, A. (1988). *In search of self in India and Japan: Toward a cross-cultural psychology.* Princeton, NJ: Princeton University Press.

Rosanoff, A. J. (1938). *Manual of psychiatry and mental hygiene.* New York: Wiley.

Rosenfeld, H. (1947). Analysis of a schizophrenic state with depersonalization. *International Journal of Psycho-Analysis, 28,* 130–139.

Rosenhan, D. L. (1973). On being sane in insane places. *Science, 179,* 250–258.

Rosenwald, G. C. (1972). Effectiveness of defenses against anal impulse arousal. *Journal of Consulting and Clinical Psychology, 39,* 292–298.

Ross, C. A. (1989a). Effects of hypnosis on the features of multiple personality disorder. *American Journal of Clinical Hypnosis, 32,* 99–106.

Ross, C. A. (1989b). *Multiple personality disorder: Diagnosis, clinical features, and treatment.* New York: Wiley.

Ross, D. R. (1992). Discussion: An agnostic viewpoint on multiple personality disorder. *Psychoanalytic Inquiry, 12,* 124–138.

Rosse, I. C. (1890). Clinical evidences of borderland insanity. *Journal of Nervous and Mental Diseases, 17,* 669–683.

Rowe, C. E., & MacIsaac, D. S. (1989). *Empathic attunement: The "technique" of psychoanalytic self psychology.* Northvale, NJ: Jason Aronson.

Salzman, L. (1960a). Masochism and psychopathy as adaptive behavior. *Journal of Individual Psychology, 16,* 182–188.

Salzman, L. (1960b). Paranoid state: Theory and therapy. *Archives of General Psychiatry, 2,* 679–693.

Salzman, L. (1962). *Developments in psychoanalysis.* New York: Grune & Stratton.

Salzman, L. (1980). *Treatment of the obsessive personality.* New York: Jason Aronson.

Sampson, H. (1983, May). *Pathogenic beliefs and unconscious guilt in the therapeutic process: Clinical observation and research evidence.* Paper presented at Symposium on Narcissism, Masochism, and the Sense of Guilt in Relation to the Therapeutic Process. Letterman General Hospital, San Francisco.

Sandler, J. (1976). Countertransference and role-responsiveness. *International Review of Psycho-Analysis, 3,* 43–47.

Sandler, J. (1987). *Projection, identification, and projective identification.* Madison, CT: International Universities Press.

Sass, L. A. (1992). *Madness and modernism: Insanity in the light of modern art, literature, and thought.* New York: Basic Books.

Schafer, R. (1968). *Aspects of internalization.* New York: International Universities Press.

Schafer, R. (1983). *The analytic attitude.* New York: Basic Books.

Schafer, R. (1984). The pursuit of failure and the idealization of unhappiness. *American Psychologist, 39*, 398–405.

Scharff, J. S. (1992). *Projective and introjective identification and the use of the therapist's self*. New York: Jason Aronson.

Schneider, K. (1950). Psychoanalytic therapy with the borderline adult: Some principles concerning technique. In J. Masterson (Ed.), *New perspectives on psychotherapy of the borderline adult* (pp. 41–65). New York: Brunner/Mazel.

Schneider, K. (1959). *Clinical psychopathology* (5th ed.; M. W. Hamilton, Trans.). New York: Grune & Stratton.

Schrieber, F. R. (1973). *Sybil*. Chicago: Regency.

Schulsinger, F. (1977). Psychopathy: Heredity and environment. In S. A. Mednick & K. O. Christiansen (Eds.), *Biosocial bases of criminal behavior* (pp. 109–126). New York: Gardner.

Searles, H. F. (1959). The effort to drive the other person crazy— An element in the aetiology and psychotherapy of schizophrenia. *British Journal of Medical Psychology*, 32, 1–18.

Searles, H. F. (1961). The sources of anxiety in paranoid schizophrenia. In *Collected papers on schizophrenia and related subjects* (pp. 465–486). New York: International Universities Press, 1965.

Searles, H. F. (1965). *Collected papers on schizophrenia and related subjects*. New York: International Universities Press.

Searles, H. F. (1986). *My work with borderline patients*. New York: Jason Aronson.

Sechehaye, M. A. (1951a). *Autobiography of a schizophrenic girl*. New York: Grune & Stratton.

Sechehaye, M. A. (1951b). *Symbolic realization: A new method of psychotherapy applied to a case of schizophrenia*. New York: International Universities Press.

Segal, H. (1950). Some aspects of the analysis of a schizophrenic. *International Journal of Psycho-Analysis, 31*, 268–278.

Segal, H. (1964). *Introduction to the work of Melanie Klein*. New York: Basic Books.

Shapiro, D. (1965). *Neurotic styles*. New York: Basic Books.

Shapiro, D. (1989). *Psychotherapy of neurotic character*. New York: Basic Books.

Shengold, L. (1987). *Halo in the sky: Observations on anality and defense*. New York: Guilford Press.

Shinefield, W. (1989). Crisis management of patients with borderline personality disorder: A competency-based training module. Unpublished doctoral dissertation. Graduate School of Applied and Professional Psychology, Rutgers University. *Dissertation Abstracts International*, 50, 4787B.

Sifneos, P. (1992). *Short-term anxiety-provoking psychotherapy*. New York: Basic Books.

Silverman, D. K. (1986). Some proposed modifications of psychoanalytic theories of early childhood development. In J. Masling (Ed.), *Empirical studies of psychoanalytic theories* (Vol. 2, pp. 49–72). Hillsdale, NJ: The Analytic Press.

Silverman, K. (1986). *Benjamin Franklin: Autobiography and other writings.* New York: Penguin.

Silverman, L. H. (1984). Beyond insight: An additional necessary step in redressing intrapsychic conflict. *Psychoanalytic Psychology, 1,* 215–234.

Silverman, L. H., Lachmann, F. M., & Milich, R. (1982). *The search for oneness.* New York: International Universities Press.

Singer, M. T., & Wynne, L. C. (1965a). Thought disorder and family relations of schizophrenics: III. Methodology using projective techniques. *Archives of General Psychiatry, 12,* 187–200.

Singer, M. T., & Wynne, L. C. (1965b). Thought disorder and family relations of schizophrenics: IV. Results and implications. *Archives of General Psychiatry, 12,* 201–212.

Sizemore, C. C. (1989). *A mind of my own.* New York: Morrow.

Sizemore, C. C., & Pittillo, E. S. (1977). *I'm Eve.* Garden City, NY: Doubleday.

Slater, P. E. (1970). *The pursuit of loneliness: American culture at the breaking point.* Boston: Beacon.

Slavin, M. O., & Kriegman, D. (1990). Evolutionary biological perspectives on the classical–relational dialectic. *Psychoanalytic Psychology, 7,* 5–32.

Slavney, P. R. (1990). *Perspectives on "hysteria."* Baltimore: Johns Hopkins University Press.

Smith, S. (1984). The sexually abused patient and the abusing therapist: A study in sadomasochistic relationships. *Psychoanalytic Psychology, 1,* 89–98.

Sorel, E. (1991, September). First encounters: Joan Crawford and Bette Davis. *The Atlantic,* p. 75.

Spence, D. P. (1982). *Narrative truth and historical truth: Meaning and interpretation in psychoanalysis.* New York: Norton.

Spence, D. P. (1987). *The Freudian metaphor: Toward paradigm change in psychoanalysis.* New York: Norton.

Spezzano, C. (1993). *Affect in psychoanalysis: A clinical synthesis.* Hillsdale, NJ: The Analytic Press.

Spiegel, D. (1984). Multiple personality as a post-traumatic stress disorder. *Psychiatric Clinics of North America, 7,* 101–110.

Spiegel, H., & Spiegel, D. (1978). *Trance and treatment: Clinical uses of hypnosis.* Washington, DC: American Psychiatric Press.

Spitz, R. A. (1953). Aggression: Its role in the establishment of object relations. In R. M. Loewenstein (Ed.), *Drives, affects, behavior* (pp. 126–138). New York: International Universities Press.

Spitz, R. A. (1965). *The first year of life.* New York: International Universities Press.

Spotnitz, H. (1969). *Modern psychoanalysis of the schizophrenic patient.* New York: Grune & Stratton.

Spotnitz, H. (1976). *Psychotherapy of preoedipal conditions.* New York: Jason Aronson.

Spoto, D. (1993). *Marilyn Monroe: The biography.* New York: Harper Collins.

Stanton, A. H., & Schwartz, M. S. (1954). *The mental hospital: A study of institutional participation in psychiatric illness and treatment*. New York: Basic Books.

Steinberg, M. (1991). The spectrum of depersonalization: Assessment and treatment. In A. Tasman & S. M. Goldfinger (Eds.), *American Psychiatric Press review of psychiatry* (Vol. 10, pp. 223–247). Washington, DC: American Psychiatric Press.

Steinberg, M. (1993). *Structured clinical interview for DSM-IV dissociative disorders (SCID-D)*. Washington, DC: American Psychiatric Press.

Sterba, R. F. (1934). The fate of the ego in analytic therapy. *International Journal of Psycho-Analysis, 15*, 117–126.

Sterba, R. F. (1982). *Reminiscences of a Viennese psychoanalyst*. Detroit: Wayne State University Press.

Stern, D. N. (1985). *The interpersonal world of the infant: A view from psychoanalysis and developmental psychology*. New York: Basic Books.

Stern, F. (1961). *The politics of cultural despair*. Berkeley, CA: University of California Press.

Stewart, J. B. (1991). *Den of thieves: The untold story of the men who plundered Wall Street and the chase that brought them down*. New York: Simon & Schuster.

Stoller, R. J. (1968). *Sex and gender*. New York: Jason Aronson.

Stoller, R. J. (1975). *Perversion*. New York: Pantheon.

Stoller, R. J. (1980). *Sexual excitement*. New York: Simon & Schuster.

Stoller, R. J. (1985). *Observing the erotic imagination*. New Haven: Yale University Press.

Stolorow, R. D. (1975). The narcissistic function of masochism (and sadism). *International Journal of Psycho-Analysis, 56*, 441–448.

Stolorow, R. D. (1976). Psychoanalytic reflections on client-centered therapy in the light of modern conceptions of narcissism. *Psychotherapy: Theory, Research and Practice, 13*, 26–29.

Stolorow, R. D., & Atwood, G. E. (1979). *Faces in a cloud: Subjectivity in personality theory*. New York: Jason Aronson.

Stolorow, R. D., & Atwood, G. E. (1992). *Contexts of being: The intersubjective foundations of psychological life*. Hillsdale, NJ: The Analytic Press.

Stolorow, R. D., Brandchaft, B., & Atwood, G. E. (1987). *Psychoanalytic treatment: An intersubjective approach*. Hillsdale, NJ: The Analytic Press.

Stolorow, R. D., & Lachmann, F. M. (1978). The developmental prestages of defenses: Diagnostic and therapeutic implications. *Psychoanalytic Quarterly, 45*, 73–102.

Stone, L. (1954). The widening scope of indications for psycho-analysis. *Journal of the American Psychoanalytic Association, 2*, 567–594.

Stone, L. (1979). Remarks on certain unique conditions of human aggression (the hand, speech, and the use of fire). *Journal of the American Psychoanalytic Association, 27*, 27–33.

Stone, M. H. (1977). The borderline syndrome: Evolution of the term, genetic aspects and prognosis. *American Journal of Psychotherapy, 31*, 345–365.

Stone, M. H. (1980). *The borderline syndromes: Constitution, personality, and adaptation*. New York: McGraw-Hill.

Stone, M. H. (Ed.). (1986). *Essential papers on borderline disorders: One hundred years at the border*. New York: New York University Press.

Strachey, J. (1934). The nature of the therapeutic action of psychoanalysis. *International Journal of Psycho-Analysis, 15*, 127–159.

Strupp, H. H. (1989). Psychotherapy: Can the practitioner learn from the researcher? *American Psychologist, 44*, 717–724.

Styron, W. (1990). *Darkness visible: A memoir of madness*. New York: Random House.

Suffridge, D. R. (1991). Survivors of child maltreatment: Diagnostic formulation and therapeutic process. *Psychotherapy, 28*, 67–75.

Sullivan, H. S. (1953). *The interpersonal theory of psychiatry*. New York: Norton.

Sullivan, H. S. (1954). *The psychiatric interview*. New York: Norton.

Sullivan, H. S. (1962). *Schizophrenia as a human process*. New York: Norton.

Sullivan, H. S. (1973). *Clinical studies in psychiatry*. New York: Norton.

Sulloway, F. J. (1979). *Freud, biologist of the mind: Beyond the psychoanalytic legend*. New York: Basic Books.

Surrey, J. (1985). The "self-in-relation": A theory of women's development. In J. V. Jordan, J. B. Miller, A. G. Kaplan, I. P. Stiver, & J. L. Surrey (Eds.), *Women's growth in connection: Writings for the Stone Center* (pp. 51–66). New York: Guilford Press.

Symington, N. (1986). *The analytic experience*. New York: St. Martin's.

Tansey, M. J., & Burke, W. F. (1989). *Understanding countertransference: From projective identification to empathy*. Hillsdale, NJ: The Analytic Press.

Thigpen, C. H., & Cleckley, H. (1957). *The three faces of Eve*. New York: McGraw-Hill.

Thomas, A., Chess, S., & Birch, H. G. (1968). *Temperament and behavior disorders in children*. New York: New York University Press.

Thomas, A., Chess, S., & Birch, H. (1970). The origins of personality. *Scientific American, 223*, 102–104.

Thompson, C. M. (1959). The interpersonal approach to the clinical problems of masochism. In M. Green (Ed.), *Clara M. Thompson: Interpersonal psychoanalysis* (pp. 183–187). New York: Basic Books.

Thompson, C. M. (1964). Psychology of women (Part IV) and Problems of womanhood (Part V). In M. Green (Ed.), *Clara M. Thompson: Interpersonal psychoanalysis* (pp. 201–343). New York: Basic Books.

Tomkins, S. S. (1962). *Affect, imagery, consciousness: Vol. 1. The positive affects*. New York: Springer.

Tomkins, S. S. (1963). *Affect, imagery, consciousness: Vol. 2. The negative affects*. New York: Springer.

Tomkins, S. S. (1964). The psychology of commitment, part 1: The constructive role of violence and suffering for the individual and for his society. In S. S. Tomkins & C. Izard (Eds.), *Affect, cognition, and personality: Empirical studies* (pp. 148–171). New York: Springer.

Tomkins, S. S. (1991). *Affect, imagery, consciousness: Vol. 3. The negative affects: Anger and fear*. New York: Springer.

Tomkins, S. S. (1992). *Affect, imagery, consciousness: Vol. 4. Cognition: Duplication and transformation of information*. New York: Springer.

Tribich, D., & Messer, S. (1974). Psychoanalytic type and status of authority as determiners of suggestibility. *Journal of Counseling and Clinical Psychology, 42*, 842–848.

Tudor, T. G. (1989). Field trips in the treatment of multiple personality disorder. *The Psychotherapy Patient, 6*, 197–213.

Tyson, P., & Tyson, R. L. (1990). *Psychoanalytic theories of development: An integration*. New Haven: Yale University Press.

Vaillant, G. (1975). Sociopathy as a human process. *Archives of General Psychiatry, 32*, 178–183.

Vandenberg, S. G., Singer, S. M., & Pauls, D. L. (1986). Hereditary factors in antisocial personality disorder. In *The heredity of behavior disorders in adults and children* (pp. 173–184). New York: Plenum.

Veith, I. (1965). *Hysteria: The history of a disease*. Chicago: University of Chicago Press.

Veith, I. (1977). Four thousand years of hysteria. In M. Horowitz (Ed.), *Hysterical personality* (pp. 7–93). New York: Jason Aronson.

Viscott, D. S. (1972). *The making of a psychiatrist*. Greenwich, CT: Fawcett.

Waelder, R. (1960). *Basic theory of psychoanalysis*. New York: International Universities Press.

Wallerstein, J. S., & Blakeslee, S. (1989). *Second chances: Men, women, and children a decade after divorce*. New York: Ticknor & Fields.

Warner, R. (1978). The diagnosis of antisocial and hysterical personality disorders: An example of sex bias. *Journal of Nervous and Mental Disease, 166*, 839–845.

Weiss, J. (1992). Interpretation and its consequences. *Psychoanalytic Inquiry, 12*, 296–313.

Weiss, J. (1993). *How psychotherapy works: Process and technique*. New York: Guilford Press.

Weiss, J., & Sampson, H., & the Mount Zion Psychotherapy Research Group (1986). *The psychoanalytic process: Theory, clinical observations, and empirical research*. New York: Guilford Press.

Weissberg, M. (1992). *The first sin of Ross Michael Carlson: A psychiatrist's account of murder, multiple personality disorder, and modern justice*. New York: Dell.

Wender, P. H., Kety, S. S., Rosenthal, D., Schulsinger, F., Ortmann, J., & Lunde, I. (1986). Psychiatric disorders in the biological and adoptive families of adopted individuals with affective disorders. *Archives of General Psychiatry, 43*, 923–929.

Westen, D. (1990). Psychoanalytic approaches to personality. In L. Pervin (Ed.), *Handbook of personality: Theory and research* (pp. 21–65). New York: Guilford Press.

Westen, D. (1993). Commentary. The self in borderline personality disorder:

A psychodynamic perspective. In Z. V. Segal & S. J. Blatt (Eds.), *The self in emotional distress: Cognitive and psychodynamic perspectives* (pp. 326–360). New York: Guilford Press.

Wheelis, A. (1956). The vocational hazards of psychoanalysis. *International Journal of Psycho-Analysis, 37*, 171–184.

Wheelis, A. (1966). *The illusionless man: Some fantasies and meditations on disillusionment*. New York: Norton, 1966.

Will, O. A. (1961). Paranoid development and the concept of the self: Psychotherapeutic intervention. *Psychiatry, 24* (Suppl.), 74–86.

Wills, G. (1970). *Nixon agonistes: The crisis of the self-made man*. Boston: Houghton Mifflin.

Winnicott, D. W. (1945). Primitive emotional development. In *Through paediatrics to psycho-analysis* (pp. 145–156). New York: Basic Books.

Winnicott, D. W. (1949). Hate in the countertransference. In *Collected papers* (pp. 194–203). New York: Basic Books, 1958.

Winnicott, D. W. (1960a). Ego distortion in terms of the true and false self. In *The maturational processes and the facilitating environment* (pp. 140–152). New York: International Universities Press, 1965.

Winnicott, D. W. (1960b). The theory of the parent-infant relationship. *International Journal of Psycho-Analysis, 41*, 585–595.

Winnicott, D. W. (1965). *The maturational processes and the facilitating environment*. New York: International Universities Press.

Winnicott, D. W. (1967). Mirror-role of mother and family in child development. In *Playing and reality* (pp. 111–118). New York: Basic Books.

Wolf, E. S. (1988). *Treating the self: Elements of clinical self psychology*. New York: Guilford Press.

Wolf, E. K., & Alpert, J. L. (1991). Psychoanalysis and child sexual abuse: A review of the post-Freudian literature. *Psychoanalytic Psychology, 8*, 305–327.

Wolfenstein, M. (1951). The emergence of fun morality. *Journal of Social Issues, 7*, 15–24.

Wolman, B. B. (1986). *The sociopathic personality*. New York: Brunner/Mazel.

Yalom, I. D. (1975). *The theory and practice of group psychotherapy*. New York: International Universities Press.

Yarok, S. R. (1993). Understanding chronic bulimia: A four psychologies approach. *American Journal of Psychoanalysis, 53*, 3–17.

Young-Bruehl, E. (1990). *Freud on women: A reader*. New York: Norton.

Zetzel, E. (1968). The so-called good hysteric. *International Journal of Psycho-Analysis, 49*, 256–260.

Author Index

Abraham, K., 22, 42, 155, 229, 239
Abrahamsen, D., 158
Adler, A., 23, 37, 168, 178
Adler, G., 52, 65, 81, 95, 113
Adorno, T. W., 113
Aichhorn, A., 138, 155
Akhtar, S., 64, 155, 167, 190, 248, 254, 256
Akiskal, H. S., 249, 254, 318
Allen, D. W., 303, 316, 317
Alpert, J. L., 52
Altschul, S., 233
Aniskiewitz, A. S., 309, 322
Appelbaum, A. H., 63
Arieti, S., 72, 95, 223
Arlow, J. A., 25
Aronson, M. L., 215
Asch, S. S., 258
Atwood, G. E., 20, 36, 39, 81, 132*n*
Aynesworth, H., 158

Bach, S., 36, 180, 188
Bak, R. C., 266
Baker, G., 254
Balint, A., 29
Balint, M., 29, 81, 116, 169, 196
Bateson, G., 59, 76, 194
Batson, C. D., 291
Baumeister, R. F., 259
Beebe, B., 196n
Bellak, L., 70
Beres, D., 289
Bergler, E., 270
Bergman, A., 24
Bergman, P., 177, 208
Bergmann, M. S., 105, 172*n*
Berliner, B., 258, 264, 265
Bernstein, D., 136*n*
Bernstein, E. M., 343
Bernstein, I., 264
Bers, S., 231*n*
Bertin, C., 311
Bettelheim, B., 39, 109
Bibring, E., 231
Bion, W. R., 116, 169
Biondi, R., 151
Birch, H. G., 190, 208
Blakeslee, S., 235
Blanck, G., 5, 39, 41, 66, 81, 135
Blanck, R., 5, 39, 41, 66, 81, 135
Blatt, S. J., 36, 231, 231*n*
Bleuler, E., 189, 195
Bleuler, M., 189, 190, 195
Bollas, C., 159
Bornstein, B., 78
Bowlby, J., 169
Bowman, E. S., 342
Boyer, L. B., 81
Brandchaft, B., 81
Braude, S. E., 324
Braun, B. G., 118*n*, 328*n*, 329, 331, 332
Brazelton, T. B., 190, 208, 236
Brenman, M., 265
Brenner, C., 25, 39, 105, 258
Breuer, J., 146, 325
Brody, S., 3*n*
Brown, R., 113

Buckley, P., 66
Buie, D., 81
Burke, W. F., 90
Bursten, B., 104, 151, 152, 167, 171, 186

Cameron, N., 207
Capote, T., 158
Carr, A. C., 63
Casey, J. F., 337
Cath, S. H., 157
Cattell, J. P., 331
Cattell, J. S., 331
Celani, D., 308
Chase, T.
Chasseguet-Smirgel, J., 136*n*, 255, 282
Chess, S., 152, 190, 208
Chessick, R. D., 39, 194
Chodoff, P., 308, 318
Chodorow, N. J., 136*n*, 194*n*, 239
Cleckley, H., 152, 153, 325
Cohen, M. B., 254
Cohen, R. A., 254
Colby, K., 83, 94
Coleman, M., 79
Coons, P. M., 333*n*, 342
Coontz, S., 333
Cooper, A. M., 228, 267, 278
Cuesta, M. J., 189

Darley, J., 291
Davanloo, H., 70
de Leon, J., 189
de Monchy, R., 258
Deri, S., 200
Des Barres, P., 311
Deutsch, H., 50, 155, 258
Diamond, M. J., 157
Dinnerstein, D., 194*n*
Dorpat, T., 265
Drye, R. C., 50

Easser, B. R., 309
Edelstein, M. G., 242
Ehrenberg, D. B., 34
Eigen, M., 66, 72
Eissler, K. R., 43, 81, 341
Ekstein, R., 34
Ellis, A., 155
Erikson, E. H., 23–24, 35, 41, 51, 54, 55, 69, 169
Escalona, S. K., 190

Fairbairn, W. R. D., 29, 39, 169
Farberow, N. L., 14
Fast, I., 136*n*
Federn, P. 72, 79
Fenichel, O., vii, viii, 48, 66, 78, 83, 138, 142, 144, 229, 249, 256, 258, 281, 283
Ferenczi, S., 29, 103, 105, 282, 311
Fine, C. G., 347
Finell, J., 110
Fisher, S., 4, 282
Fleck, S., 194
Fogelman, E., 177
Fonda, H. 229*n*
Forster, E. M., 169*n*–170*n*
Fraiberg, S., 101
Frances, A., 228
Frank, J. D., 14, 270
Frenkl-Brunswick, E., 113
Freud, A., 28, 109, 117*n*, 144, 232
Freud, S., 19, 21, 22, 25, 27, 31, 38–39, 43, 103, 109, 118, 119, 135, 138, 146, 168, 178, 205, 211, 228, 229, 230, 231, 239, 257, 262, 270, 281, 302, 303, 304, 313, 323, 325, 327*n*
Friedenberg, E. Z., 56
Friedman, R. C., 309
Fromm, E., 31, 169
Fromm-Reichmann, F., 31, 39, 72, 94, 223, 241, 254
Frosch, J., 50
Furman, E., 234

Gabbard, G. O., 18
Gabrielli, W., 152
Gaddis, T., 164
Galenson, E., 260
Galin, D., 303
Gardiner, M., 43, 131
Gardner, M. R., 182
Gay, P., 132*n*, 215*n*
Gaylin, W., 256
Gill, M. M., 18, 90
Gilligan, C., 239
Giovacchini, P. L., 66, 81, 95
Glick, R. A., 278
Glover, E., 296
Goldberg, A., 20, 36, 177
Goldstein, K., 299
Gottesman, I., 190
Green, H., 343
Greenacre, P., 155
Greenberg, J. R., 39, 137
Greenberg, R. P., 4, 282
Greenfield, S., 316*n*
Greenson, R. R., 47, 70, 78, 94, 182, 218, 229
Greenspan, S. I., 5, 236
Greenwald, H., 155, 163, 186
Grinker, R. R., 50, 81
Grossman, W., 258
Groth, A. N., 186

Grotstein, J., 156
Grünbaum, A., 4
Grunberger, B., 282
Gunderson, J. G., 50, 51*n*, 65, 113
Guntrip, H., 39, 191, 193, 204

Hack, R., 207
Haley, J., 59
Hall, C. S., 39
Halleck, S. L., 303
Hammer, E., 83
Hare, R., 83, 199, 200, 218, 219, 223, 244, 273, 296
Harris, D. 207
Hartcollis, P., 66
Hartmann, H. 26
Hecox, W., 151
Hedges, L. E., 94
Hendin, H., 137, 169
Herman, J. L., 115*n*, 309, 333*n*
Herzog, J., 157
Hirsch, S. J., 302
Hoch, P. H., 50
Hoenig, J., 343
Hollender, M. H., 302, 303
Horner, A. J., 6, 10, 43, 78, 94, 302, 303
Horney, K., 20, 31, 136*n*, 169
Horowitz, M. J., 322
Hughes, J. M., 39
Hutchings, B., 152

Isaacs, K., 146

Jackson, D. D., 59
Jacobs, T. J., 90
Jacobson, E., 72, 169, 231, 233
Janet, P., 280, 323
Jaspers, K., 190
Johnson, A., 153
Jones, E., 170
Josephs, L., 66, 296
Jung, C. G., 23*n*, 37, 170, 311

Kael, H. C., 282
Kahn, H., 123
Kalafat, J., 14
Karasu, T. B., 240
Karon, B. P., 9, 60, 72, 73, 75, 95, 161*n*, 193, 198, 209, 211, 215, 223
Karpe, R., 325
Kasanin, J. S., 192
Katan, M., 249
Keith-Spiegel, P., 315
Kernberg, O. F., 5, 9, 18, 20, 24, 32, 35, 50, 51*n*, 52, 62, 63, 65, 81, 95, 98, 110, 113, 122*n*, 146, 153, 156, 160, 166, 172, 177, 178, 181, 182, 183*n*, 184, 185, 186, 187, 188, 227*n*, 228, 247, 252, 253, 254, 255, 258, 260, 267, 302*n*, 320, 327
Keyes, D., 337
Khan, M. M. R., 195
Klein, M., 29, 33, 39, 72, 110, 116, 158, 164, 193, 231, 232, 239
Kluft, R. P., 323, 326*n*, 328*n*, 329, 330, 333, 339, 342, 344, 347
Knight, R., 50
Koenigsberg, H. W., 63
Kohut, H., 5, 35, 39, 169, 171, 173, 178, 180, 181, 182, 183*n*, 184, 185, 188, 267
Kraepelin, E., 43, 65, 190, 198, 318
Krafft-Ebing, R., 258, 260
Kretschmer, E., 190, 191
Kriegman, D., 37
Kris, E., 296
Kuhn, T. S., 34, 328
Kupperman, J., 3*n*

Lachmann, F. M., 42, 112*n*, 169, 196*n*
Laing, R. D., 59, 66, 192, 194, 198
Langness, L. L., 302
Langs, R. J. 82
LaPlanche, J., 258
Larntz, K., 318
Lasch, C., 169
Laughlin, H. P., 98, 117*n*, 144, 228, 232, 247, 256, 258
Lax, R. F., 66, 264, 278
Lazare, A., 314
Lependorf, S., 178
Lesser, S., 309
Levenson, E. A., 39, 137
Levin, J. D., 296
Levinson, D. J., 113
Lewis, H. B., 169
Lichtenberg, J., 115*n*
Lidz, T., 59, 72, 76, 95, 194
Lifton, R. J., 123
Lilienfeld, S. O., 318
Lindner, R., 79, 223
Linton, R., 302
Lion, J. R., 160, 190
Litman, R. E., 13
Little, M. I., 11, 72
Livingston, M. S., 196
Loeb, J., 152
Loewald, H. W., 137
Loewenstein, R. J., 328
Loewenstein, R. M., 78, 261
Long, J., 164
Lothane, Z., 211*n*
Lovinger, R. J., 18
Lykken, D., 152
Lynd, H. M., 169

MacIsaac, D. S., 180
MacKinnon, R. A., vii, 18, 34, 149, 211, 213, 218, 223, 282
Maheu, R., 207
Mahler, M. S., 24, 41, 52, 64, 120, 234
Main, T. F., 50, 113
Malan, D. H., 70
Mandelbaum, A., 52
Mann, J., 70
Marmor, J., 303
Masling, J., 41
Masson, J. M., 305
Masterson, J. F., 14, 35, 50, 52, 64, 82, 88, 89, 95
McClelland, D. C., 287
McDougall, J., 121, 144
McGoldrick, M., 231
McWilliams, N., 52, 128, 134, 157, 178, 213, 238, 274
Mednick, S. A., 152
Meissner, W. W., 66, 137, 171, 205, 207, 221, 226
Meloy, J. R., 151, 152, 156, 159, 160–161, 166, 167, 186, 318
Menaker, E., 30, 258, 265, 271
Menninger, K., 46
Messer, S., 282
Meyers, D. I., 278
Michaud, S., 158
Michels, R., viii, 18, 34, 149, 211, 213, 218, 223, 282
Milgram, S., 109
Milich, R., 42
Miller, A., 36, 171, 172, 175, 188, 236
Miller, J. B., 136*n*, 239
Milstein, V., 333*n*, 342
Mischler, E., 59, 76
Mitchell, S. A., 39, 137
Modell, A. H., 153, 169
Money, J., 140
Morrison, A. P., 169, 171, 188
Mowrer, O. H., 120
Mueller, W. J., 309, 322
Mullahy, P., 194*n*
Murray, H. A., 19, 37
Myerson, P. G., 54, 119

Nagera, H., 280, 300
Nannarello, J. J., 189, 192
Nelson, B., 79
Nemiah, J. C., 66, 131
Newman, R., 18
Niederland, W., 211
Noblin, C. D., 282
Noel, B., 317*n*
Nunberg, H., 46
Nydes, J., 214, 219, 266, 272, 273

Ogden, T. H., 116
Ovesey, L., 209

Panken, S., 258
Paolino, T. J. Jr., 94, 258
Pauls, D. L., 152
Peralta, V., 189
Piaget, J., 103
Pine, F., 20, 24, 39, 81, 94, 145–146
Pittillo, E. S., 325
Polatin, P., 50
Pontalis, J. B., 258
Pope, K. S., 315, 316
Prichard, J. C., 42
Prince, M., 323
Putnam, F. W., 324, 329, 334, 336, 338*n*, 339, 343, 346

Racker, H., 33, 59
Rado, S., 231, 239
Rank, O., 30, 37, 168
Rasmussen, A., 265, 266
Rawn, M. L., 47
Recovering Patient, A., 80
Redl, R., 155
Redlich, F. C., 18
Reich, A., 169
Reich, W., 22, 27, 35, 45, 168, 170, 258, 281
Reik, T., 69, 120, 126, 258, 263, 277
Ressler, R. K., 151, 153
Rhodes, J., 215*n*
Rice, J., 229
Richfield, J., 296
Richman, J., 302
Rinsley, D. B., 52
Robbins, A., 183, 193, 194*n*, 200, 201
Rockland, L. H., 72, 95
Rogers, C. R., 183*n*
Roland, A., 25, 90
Rosanoff, A. J., 318
Rosen, Z. A., 192
Rosenfeld, H., 72
Rosenhan, D. L., 319*n*
Rosenwald, G. C., 282
Ross, C. A., 324, 327, 328*n*, 335, 339, 342, 346, 347
Ross, D. R., 328
Rosse, I. C., 49
Rowe, C. E., 180
Rutter, M., 208

Sacks, R. G., 329
Salzman, L., 211, 259, 264, 280, 300
Sampson, H., 19, 37, 138, 146, 243, 252
Sandler, J., 90, 116
Sanford, R. N., 113

Sass, L. A., 194, 195, 197, 198
Savran, B., 177
Schactman, T., 151, 153
Schafer, R., 94, 109*n*, 258, 267
Scharff, J. S., 107, 116
Schatzow, E., 333*n*
Schneider, K., 190, 239
Schrieber, F. R., 329
Schulsinger, F., 152
Schwartz, M. S., 113
Searles, H. F., 72, 81, 95, 194, 210, 215
Sechehaye, M. A., 343
Segal, H., 72, 136*n*
Selzer, M. A., 63
Shapiro, D., 27, 48, 205, 213, 221, 226, 281, 292, 300, 303, 322
Shengold, L., 282
Shinefield, W., 13
Siegel, M., 3*n*
Sifneos, P., 70
Silverman, D. K., 136
Silverman, K., 124
Silverman, L. H., 42, 222
Singer, M. T., 50, 59, 76
Singer, S. M., 152, 194
Sizemore, C. C., 325
Slater, P. E., 38, 169
Slavin, M. O., 37
Slavney, P. R., 319*n*
Small, L., 70
Smith, S., 316
Sorel, E., 126
Spence, D. P., 34, 305
Spezzano, C., 146
Spiegel, D., 324, 328
Spiegel, R., 328
Spitz, R. A., 169, 236, 264
Spotnitz, H., 37, 79, 223
Spoto, D., 329*n*
Stanton, A. H., 113
Stein, J., 274
Steinberg, M., 331
Sterba, R. F., 26, 30, 55
Stern, D. N., 23, 41
Stern, F., 215*n*, 236
Stewart, J. B., 151
Stoller, R. J., 140, 141
Stolorow, R. D., 20, 36, 39, 81, 112*n*, 132*n*, 169, 180, 183*n*, 267, 278
Stone, L., 260
Stone, M. H., 5*n*, 50, 52, 66
Strachey, J., 296
Strupp, H. H., 31, 137
Styron, W., 229*n*
Suffridge, D. R., 262
Sullivan, H. S., 18, 23, 24, 31, 72, 85, 169, 194*n*, 195, 216, 221
Sulloway, F. J., 257
Surrey, J., 239
Symington, N., 39

Tabachnick, B. G., 315
Tansey, M. J., 90
Thigpen, C. H., 325
Thomas, A., 152, 190, 208
Thompson, C. M., 31, 136*n*, 264
Timmons, E. O., 282
Tomkins, S. S., 19, 37, 128, 146, 208, 211
Tribich, D., 282
Tudor, T. G., 334, 341
Tyson, P., 41, 65
Tyson, R. L., 41, 65

Vaillant, G., 318
Van Valkenburg, C., 318
Vandenberg, S. G., 152
VandenBos, G. R., 9, 72, 75, 95, 161*n*, 193, 198
Veith, I., 302, 322
Viscott, D. S., 187

Waelder, R., 36, 98
Wallerstein, J. S., 235
Wallerstein, R. S., 34
Warner, R., 319
Waxler, N., 59, 76
Weakland, J., 59
Weigert, E., 254
Weiss, J., 19, 37, 39, 138, 146, 262, 275
Weissberg, M., 345
Wender, P. H., 229
Werble, B., 50
Westen, D., 3*n*, 39, 52
Wheelis, A., 196
White, H., 196
Will, O. A., 211
Wills, G., 259
Wineman, D., 155
Winnicott, D. W., 32, 39, 169, 175, 183, 194
Wolf, E. K., 52
Wolf, E. S., 36, 95, 171
Wolfenstein, M., 177
Wolman, B. B., 151
Wynne, L. C., 59, 76, 194

Yalom, I. D., 297
Yarock, S. R., 288
Young-Bruehl, E. 304*n*

Zetzel, E., 302, 302*n*

Subject Index

Abandonment depression, 14, 88–89
Abraham, Karl, 22, 42
Abreaction, 305*n*, 339
Acting out
  description of, 138–140
  in hysterical personalities, 307, 311
  in masochistic personalities, 261–263
  in psychopathic personalities, 155
  versus compulsive actions, 284–285
Adaptive processes
  in compulsive personalities, 283–286
  in depressive personalities, 231–233
  in dissociative personalities, 329–332
  in hysterical personalities, 304–308
  in manic personalities, 249
  in masochistic personalities, 261–264
  in narcissistic personalities, 173–174
  in obsessive personalities, 283–286
  in paranoid personalities, 209–211
  in psychopathic personalities, 153–155
  in schizoid personalities, 192
Advice giving, supportive therapy and, 76
Affect
  compulsive personalities and, 281–283
  depressive personalities and, 229–231
  dissociative personalities and, 328–329
  hysterical lability of, 302
  hysterical personalities and, 303–304
  manic personalities and, 248–249
  masochistic personalities and, 260–261
  narcissistic personalities and, 171–173
  negative, 12–13, 129–130
  paranoid personalities and, 207–209
  psychopathic personalities and, 152–153
  schizoid personalities and, 190–192
Affect block in psychopathic personalities, 153
Aggression
  hysterical personalities and, 307
  psychopathic personalities and, 152, 157–158
  sexualization of, 141
Aggression-inward model, 230
Alcohol abuse, diagnosis of, 8
Altruism, 128, 134, 291
Amnesia, 305, 332
Anaclitic depression, 231*n*
Anal character
  in early psychoanalytic theory, 22
  obsessive personalities and, 281–282
Anal-expulsive, 23
Anal-incorporative, 23
Anal phase, 23, 24, 41
Analyst. *See* Therapist
Analyzability, 70
Anger
  compulsive personalities and, 282
  depressive personalities and, 244
Anhedonia, in clinical depression, 228
Antipsychotic drugs, 44
Antisocial personalities. *See also* Psychopathic personalities
  terminology, 2
Anxiety
  attack, 3
  displacement of, 131
  neurosis, 3
  paranoid personalities and, 212–213
  primitive defense and, 93
  repression and, 28–29, 119

Approach–avoidance conflict, 196*n*
As-if personalities, 50
Attentional deficits, from toxic or organic conditions, 118
Attention-seeking behavior, of hysterical people, 312
Authoritarian personalities, 113
Autistic fantasy, 100
Autistic phase, 24
Autonomic nervous system reactivity, in psychopathic personalities, 152
Autonomy, 23, 51

Balint, Michal and Alice, 29
Basic trust, 23
BASK model of dissociation, 118*n*, 331–332
 in obsessive compulsive psychology, 284–286
Behavioral defenses. *See also* Defense mechanisms
Behavioral treatments, 68
Behavior change versus intrapsychic change, 70
Bipolar disorder, 8, 227
Borderline personality structure
 abandonment depression and, 14
 characteristics of, 61–65
 countertransference with, 65
 defense mechanisms in, 61
 diagnosis of, 49–53
 differential diagnosis of
  versus dissociative personalities, 344
  versus neurotic personality structure, 55–56, 61–65
  versus psychotic personality structure, 61–65
 DSM-III, 51*n*
 expressive psychotherapy for, 94
 impulsivity in, 149
 projection/introjection in, 98
 projective identification and, 112
 psychoanalytic therapy for, 80–91
 stable instability of, 32
 suicidal preoccupation and, 14, 16
 transference with, 64–65
Borderline states, 50
Borderline syndrome, 50
British School of psychoanalysis, 29, 30. *See also* Object relations theory
Bulimia, 10

Caregiver, perceived omnipotence of, 105, 106
Castration complex, 304
Character. *See also* Character diagnosis
 assessment
 pathology versus situational factors, 147–148
 structure versus pathology, 147
 individual patterns, 4
 interaction of maturational and typological dimensions, 91–94
 other psychoanalytic contributions to, 37–38
  rationale for, 145–147
  types of, 145. *See* specific personality types
 rationale for how presented, 145–147
 structure. *See* Personality structure
 use of term, 3*n*. *See also* Personality
 versus responsivity, 147–148
"Character armor," 27
Character diagnosis
 advantages, 7
 categories, in ego psychology, 45–49
 communication of empathy and, 12–14
 consumer protection and, 10–12
 depth versus type distinctions in, 42
 forestalling flights from treatment and, 14–15
 fringe benefits of conducting, 15–17
 historical context and, 42
 interview format for, 349–351
 prognostic implications, 9–10
 rationale for, 7–18
 treatment planning and, 8–9
 utility, limits of, 17–18
Character neuroses, versus symptom neuroses, 45–49
Chief complaints, in diagnosis interview format, 349
Child abuse
 in dissociation, 327, 332, 335
 in masochism, 266–267
 in psychopathy, 334*n*
 sociologic factors in, 332
Classical psychoanalysis, 68*n*
Client, use of term, 3*n*
Cognitive defenses, in obsessive compulsive psychology, 283–284. *See also* Defense mechanisms
"Coitus-interruptus" theory, 119*n*
Compartmentalization, 127
Complementary countertransference, 33
Compulsive personalities, 279–280, 280–281. *See also* Obsessive personalities
 adaptive processes in, 283–286
 affect and, 281–283
 countertransference with, 292–294, 295, 300
 defensive processes in, 283–286
 description of, 129*n*
 differential diagnosis of
  versus hypomanic personalities, 254–255
  versus organic brain syndromes, 299–300
 drive and, 281–283

Compulsive personalities (*cont.*)
object relations in, 286–289
occupations associated with, 280
reaction formation in, 286
self-experience and, 289–292
temperament and, 281–283
therapeutic implications of diagnosis for, 294–298
transference with, 292–294, 300
versus schizoid personalities, 203
Concordant countertransference, 33
Conscience. *See also* Superego
absence of, in psychopathic personalities, 153
development of, 163
harshness of, in obsessive compulsive psychology, 289
Consumer protection, character diagnosis and, 10–12
Control, in families of origin, for obsessive and compulsive people, 287–288
Control–mastery theory, 19, 37, 198, 274–275
Conversion
defensive identification and, 137
versus somatization, 121*n*
Coping
defense mechanisms and, 97–98
methods of, 143–144
Couch, use of, 242*n*
Counterdependence, 14–15, 139
Counterhostility, 139
Countermasochism, 269
Counterphobia, 139
Countertransference
appreciation of, 32
borderline personality structure and, 65, 90–91
compulsive personalities and, 292–294, 295, 300
concordant and complementary, 33
depressive personalities and, 239–241
dissociative personalities and, 336–338, 346
hysterical personalities and, 313–316, 321
manic personalities and, 251
masochistic personalities and, 268–270, 277
narcissistic personalities and, 178–180
neurtoic personality structure and, 56
obsessive personalities and, 292–294, 295, 300
paranoid personalities and, 216–217
primitive devaluation and, 106–107
psychopathic personalities and, 159–160
psychotic personality structure and, 59–60
schizoid personalities and, 197–199
transformation from obstacle to asset, 34
Creative arts therapy, for schizoid personality, 200–201
Creativity, schizoid personalities and, 192
Criminality, sociopathy and, 104
Crisis-intervention model, 13–14
Criticism, 176, 238
Cult abuse, 326*n*
Current mental status, in diagnosis interview format, 350
Cyclothymic personalities, 103, 227, 248

DDNOS (Dissociative Disorder Not Otherwise Specified), 331
Death instinct, 257*n*
Decision-making, obsessive personalities and, 290
Defense mechanisms. *See also* specific defense mechanisms
benign functions of, 97
in compulsive personalities, 283–286
coping and, 97
in depressive personalities, 231–233
developmental prestages of, 112*n*
diagnostic labels and, 96
dissociation, 114–115
in dissociative personalities, 308*n*, 329–332
ego psychology and, 28
higher-order. *See* Secondary defenses
in hysterical personalities, 304–308
insufficient, 97
maladaptive, 97
in manic personalities, 249
in masochistic personalities, 261–264
mature. *See* Secondary defenses
in narcissistic personalities, 173–174
in obsessive personalities, 283–286
in paranoid personalities, 209–211
preferential/automatic reliance on, 97–98
primary or primitive. *See* Primitive defenses; specific primitive defenses
in psychopathic personalities, 153–155
in psychotic personalities, 57
purposes of, 36
in schizoid personalities, 189, 191, 192
secondary. *See* Secondary defenses
splitting, 112–114
terminology of, 96
unconscious nature of, 121
weakening power of, 97
Defensive identification, 135
Defensive processes, 27
Dementia praecox, 43
Demographic data, in diagnosis interview format, 349
Denial
description of, 101–103
disadvantages of, 102
in manic and hypomanic personalities, 249

as primitive defense, 98
versus repression, 98–99
Dependency
idealization and, 106
masochistic personalities and, 265
sexualization of, 141
Depression
mourning and, 109
of psychopathic personalities in therapy, 163–164
terminology for, 3
vegetative signs and, 36–37
Depressive personalities, 110, 255–256
adaptive processes in, 231–233
affect and, 229–231
clinical depression and, 228–229
countertransference with, 239–241
defensive processes in, 231–233
development of, 22
differential diagnosis of, 246–248
versus masochistic personalities, 247–248, 275–276
versus narcissistic personalities, 186, 246–247
drive and, 229–231
object relations in, 233–237
occupations associated with, 238*n*
oral qualities of, 229–230
self-experience in, 237–239
temperament and, 229–231
therapeutic implications of diagnosis for, 241–246
transference with, 239–241
Depressive–masochistic personalities, 260
Derivatives, id and, 26
Detoxification program, 8
Devaluation, 98
narcissistic personalities and, 173–174
psychopathic personalities and, 158
primitive, 105–107
Devaluing transferences, 179
Developmental levels, 40–41, 67
Deviation, sexual, 2
Diagnosis. *See* Character diagnosis
Diagnosis-influenced interventions, 18
Diagnostic and Statistical Manual of Mental Disorders, vii, 10, 45
borderline personalities organization, 5*n*
dependent personality disorder and, 12
dissociative identity disorder diagnosis, 324*n*
histrionic personality disorder diagnosis, 122*n*, 302*n*
hypomanic personalities and, 248
infantile personalities and, 122*n*
obsessive compulsive personalities and, 279
masochistic personality disorder and, 260*n*
mood disorders, 228
narcissistic personality disorder and, 170
paranoid personality disorder and, 205–206
schizoid conditions and, 190
Diagnostic labels, 2–3
Displacement
description of, 130–131
in obsessive compulsive psychology, 283
Dissociation
advantages of, 115
description of, 114–115
hysterical personalities and, 323–324
psychopathic personalities and, 154–155
Dissociative Experiences Scale, 343
Dissociative Disorder Not Otherwise Specified (DDNOS), 331
Dissociative personalities
adaptive processes in, 329–332
affect and, 328–329
countertransference with, 336–338, 346
defensive processes in, 308n, 329–332
diagnosis of, therapeutic implications for, 338–341
differential diagnosis of, 342–346
versus borderline conditions, 344
versus functional psychosis, 343
versus hysterical personalities, 320, 344–345
versus masochistic personalities, 276–277
versus paranoid personalities, 165–166
versus psychopathic conditions, 165–166, 345–346
drive and, 328–329
object relations in, 332–334
range of problems in, 342
with schizophrenia, 343*n*
screening devices for, 342–343
self-experience in, 334–336
temperament and, 328–329
therapy for, 327–328
transference with, 336–338, 346
triggers for, 330
Distrust, 47
Doubting mania, 290
Drive
character organization and, 145, 146
compulsive personalities and, 281–283
depressive personalities and, 229–231
dissociative personalities and, 328–329
hysterical personalities and, 303–304
manic personalities and, 248–249
masochistic personalities and, 260–261
narcissistic personalities and, 171–173
paranoid personalities and, 207–209
psychopathic personalities and, 152–153
schizoid personalities and, 190–192
Drive-based fixation model, 22
Drive theory, 19, 21–25, 41, 97, 148
Drug use, primitive withdrawal and, 100

DSM-II. *See Diagnostic and Statistical Manual of Mental Disorders*
DSM-III. *See Diagnostic and Statistical Manual of Mental Disorders*
DSM-III-R. *See Diagnostic and Statistical Manual of Mental Disorders*
DSM-IV. *See Diagnostic and Statistical Manual of Mental Disorders*
Dynamic processes, in character, 37–38
Dysfunctional family systems, members, boundaries between, 52

Eating disorders, 288
Efficacy, 23
Ego, 26, 28, 31, 59
Ego alien phenomena, 26, 45, 46, 55
Egocentrism, 101, 103
Ego development, 93
Ego psychology
  character diagnosis and, 25–29
  development of, 19
  diagnostic categories in, 45–49
Ego splitting. *See* Splitting
Ego states, 31
Ego strength, 27
Ego syntonic phenomena, 26, 45, 46
Emotional honesty, of therapist, 73–74
Empathy
  communication of, character diagnosis and, 12–14
  psychopathic personalities and, 161
Engulfment, fear of, schizoid personalities and, 193, 196, 197
Envy
  hysterical personalities and, 363–364
  narcissistic personalities and, 172–173
  paranoid personalities and, 208–209
  psychopathic personalities and, 158–159
Erikson, Erik, 23–24, 41, 51
Erotization, 140–142
Erotomania, 211
Evaluative atmosphere in childhood narcissistic personality and, 176
Evaluative versus therapeutic role, and psychopathy, 160
Evolutionary biology model, 37
Exhibitionism
  in hysterical personalities, 312
  in masochistic personalities, 263
  normal, 139*n*
Experiencing ego, 26
Experiential symbiosis, 31
Explosivity, 109
Expressive psychotherapy, for patients with borderline personality structure, 81–91
  getting supervision from patient in, 86–88
  interpreting during quiescence and, 89
  interpreting primitive defenses in, 84–86
  promoting individuation and discouraging regression in, 88–89
  respecting countertransference data in, 90–91
  safeguarding boundaries technique in, 81–83
  voicing contrasting feeling states in, 83–84

Facial expression, 73
Fairbairn, W. R. D., 29
False self, 175
Family romance concept, 30
Family systems therapy, 68
Fausse reconnaissance, 307
Feelings, interpretation of, 78–80
Femininity, 311*n*
Ferenczi, Sandor, 29
Fetishes, sexual, 130–131
Field trips, for dissociative personality therapy, 341
Fixation, 22, 40
Fixation–regression hypothesis, schizoid personalities and, 193
Four-factor theory, of multiple personality disorder, 333
Fraternity hazing, 133
Freud, Anna, 28, 117*n*, 129
Freud, Sigmund
  defense mechanisms and, 96–97
  depression and, 229, 231, 233
  dissociation and, 323–324, 325, 327, 327*n*
  drive theory of, 19, 21–25
  The Ego and the Id, 25
  hysterical personalities and, 304–306, 313
  identification and, 136*n*
  libido and, 140
  love and work as therapeutic objective, 56
  masochistic personality and, 257, 258, 262
  maturational issues and, 323–324
  mother–son relationship, 132*n*
  multiple personality disorder and, 327*n*
  narcissistic personalities and, 168, 169
  object relations theory and, 30–31
  obsessive compulsive personality and, 281–282, 286, 292–293
  paranoia and, 211
  repression and, 118–120
Fromm, Erich, 31
Fromm-Reichmann, Frieda, 31
Fugue states, 307–308
Functional psychosis, versus dissociative personalities, 343

Gardener's hysteria, 321
Gender differences
  in hysteria versus psychopathy, 318–319
  in masochistic personality development, 260–261

in psychopathy, 154*n*
in schizoid personality, 194*n*
Glove paralysis or anesthesia, 306
Grandiose self, 173
Grandiosity, 158, 170–171
Gratitude, narcissistic personalities and, 178
Grief, denial of, 235
Grief reactions, 228
Guilt
compulsive personalities and, 288–289
depressive personalities and, 237
hysterical personalities and, 307–308, 310
masochistic personalities and, 263–264
narcissistic personalities and, 183
obsessive compulsive personality and, 287–288
paranoid personalities and, 209
versus shame, 172

Hatching, 24
Healthier patients
conventional therapy modes for, 69–70
other therapy approaches for, 70–71
Higher-order defenses. *See* Secondary defenses
Histrionic personalities, 3, 302*n*. *See also* Hysterical personalities
Homosexual preoccupations, paranoid personalities and, 215
Honesty, of therapist, 162
Horney, Karen, 31
Human imperfections, acceptance of, 182
Humanistic counseling, 68
Humor, in therapy of paranoid personality, 218–220
Hungarian School of psychoanalysis, 29, 30
Hypnosis, for dissociative personalities therapy, 340
Hypochondria, 122, 149
Hypomanic personalities, 256. *See also* Manic personalities
borderline personalities and, 227*n*
definition of, 102–103
depression and, 248
diagnosis, therapeutic implications for, 251–253
differential diagnosis of, 253–255
versus compulsive personalities, 254–255
versus hysterical personalities, 253–254
versus narcissistic personalities, 254
flights from treatment, forestalling, 14–15
Hysterical personalities, 301–302, 321–322
acting out and, 140
adaptive processes in, 304–308
affect and, 303–304
boundaries of, 9
countertransference with, 313–316, 321
defensive processes in, 304–308
development of, 22
diagnosis, therapeutic implications for, 316–318
differential diagnosis of, 318–321
versus dissociative personalities, 320, 344–345
versus hypomanic personalities, 253–254
versus narcissistic personalities, 187, 319–320
versus psychopathic personalities, 318–319
drive and, 303–304
manipulation and, 13
object relations in, 308–310
occupations associated with, 302
repression and, 119
self-experience in, 310–313
temperament and, 303–304
terminology for, 3
transference with, 313–316, 321
Hysterical psychosis, 302

Iatrogenic hypothesis, dissociation and, 328*n*
Id, 25–26, 28, 31
Idealization
dependency and, 106
depressive personalities and, 233
narcissistic personalities and, 173–174
primitive, 105–107
dependence on, 106–107
and mature forms of, 99
Identification
advanced levels of, 51
with aggressor, 109
defensive, 135
description of, 135–138
drive theory and, 23
as neutral process, 136
nondefensive, 135
oedipal situation and, 136
with therapist, 137–138
use of term, 109*n*
Identity
integrated sense of, 54
integration, 61–62, 93
Imagery, in communication with schizoid personalities, 200–201
Imperfections
human, acceptance of, 182
in self, 105–106
Impulsive personalities, 139–140
Impulsivity, 109, 149
Incest
borderline dynamics and, 52
dissociation and, 332
Individual therapy, 8–9
Individuation, promotion of, 88–89

Infantile grandiosity. *See* Infantile omnipotence
Infantile omnipotence, 103–104, 109, 154
Infantile personalities, 122*n*, 149
"Inheritance"
  of character structure, 176
  of narcissistic personalities, 176
  of paranoid personalities, 212
  of psychopathic personalities, 157
  of vulnerability to depression, 229
Initiative, versus guilt, 23, 51
Insanity
  historical context and, 42
  versus sanity, 42, 49
Instinctualization, 140–142
Intellectualization
  description of, 123–124
  isolation and, 123
  obsessive personalities and, 283
  schizoid personalities and, 192
Interpersonal psychoanalysis, 19, 31
Interpersonal task, 51
Interpretation upward, 78, 200
Interview, structured, 8
Introjection. *See also* Projective identification
  in borderline personalities, 98
  definition of, 108
  description of, 107–112
  mourning and, 109–110
  pathological, 108–109
Introjective depression, 23*n*
Introjective identification, 98
Introjects, 32
Inversion, 2
Isolation, 122–123, 283

Jealousy, delusional, in paranoia, 211
Joining the resistance, 79
Judgmental meanings, of psychoanalytic terms, 2

Klein, Melanie, 29
Kohut, Heinz, 35–36
Kraepelin, Emil, 43–44

La belle indifférence, 307
Language, psychodiagnostic abuse of, 7
  nonstigmatizing, 2
Libido, 140
Loss, early, depression and, 233–234
Lust, displacement of, 130–131

Mahler, Margaret, 24, 41
Malignant grandiosity, 153
Malingering, 121–122
Manic-depressive psychosis, 43. *See also* Bipolar disorder
Manic personalities, 227, 248, 256. *See also* Hypomanic personalities
  adaptive processes in, 249
  affect and, 248–249
  countertransference with, 251
  defensive processes in, 249
  denial and, 102
  differentiation from schizophrenia, 255
  drive and, 248–249
  object relations in, 250
  self-experience in, 250–251
  temperament and, 248–249
  therapeutic implications of diagnosis for, 251–253
  transference with, 251
Manipulation
  conscious, 86*n*
  in psychopathic personalities, 157
  use of term, 154*n*
Manipulative clients, 13
Masculinity, 31*n*
Masochism, 2, 139*n*
Masochistic personalities, 277–278
  adaptive processes in, 261–264
  affect and, 260–261
  countertransference with, 268–270, 277
  defensive processes in, 261–264
  depressive personalities and, 260
  diagnosis, therapeutic implications for, 271–275
  differential diagnosis of, 275–277
    versus depressive personalities, 247–248, 275–276
    versus dissociative personalities, 276–277
  drive and, 260–261
  moral masochism and, 258–259
  object relations in, 264–267
  self-experience in, 267–268
  temperament and, 260–261
  transference with, 268–270, 277
Masturbation, 126
Maturational stages, 22–23, 24–25
Megalomania, in paranoia, 211, 264–265
Melancholia, vegetative signs and, 36–37
Memory deficits, from toxic or organic conditions, 118
Minority groups, identification, sensitivities to, 3
Misdiagnosis, fear of, 15
Mistrust, versus trust, 51
Modeling, 135
"Modern psychoanalysis," 37, 79
Money exchange, psychotically vulnerable people and, 74
Mood disorders, 228

Moral insanity, 2, 42. *See also* Antisocial personalities
Moralization
 description of, 125–127
 in masochistic personalities, 263
 modeling of, 288
 in obsessive compulsive psychology, 283
 of psychoanalytic terms, 2
 splitting and, 126
Moral masochism, 126, 258–259
Moral standards, 28
Mother
 distorted responsiveness of, 212–213
 good versus bad, 99
Mourning
 depression and, 109
 introjection and, 109–110
MPD. *See* Multiple personality disorder (MPD)
Multiple function principle, 98
Multiple personality disorder (MPD). *See also* Dissociative personalities
 clinical features of, 323–326
 core beliefs in, 335
 diagnosis of, therapeutic implications for, 338–341
 dissociation and, 114, 115*n*
 four-factor theory of, 333
 Freud and, 327*n*

Narcissism, primary, 103
Narcissistic defense, 185
Narcissistic extensions, 172*n*, 173–174, 175–176
Narcissistic personalities, 35–36, 148, 168–171
 adaptive processes in, 173–174
 affect and, 171–173
 defensive processes in, 173–174
 definition of, 168
 diagnosis, therapeutic implications of, 181–184
 differential diagnosis of, 184–187
  versus depressive personalities, 186, 246–247
  versus hypomanic personalities, 254
  versus hysterical personalities, 187, 319–320
  versus narcissistic reactions, 185
  versus obsessive compulsive personality, 186–187, 298–299
  versus psychopathic personalities, 166, 185–186
 drive and, 171–173
 envy and, 172–173
 idealization and, 106
 object relations in, 174–177
 perfectionism and, 174, 177–178
 self-acceptance, development of, 169
 self-experiences, 177–178
 shame and, 172, 208
 sociopathy and, 49
 temperament and, 171–173
 transference with, 178–180, 184
Narcissistic reactions, versus narcissistic personalities, 185
Nazism, 215*n*
Neuroses
 character versus symptom, 45–46
 versus psychoses, 43–44
Neurotic paradox, 120
Neurotic personality structure
 characteristics of, 53–56
 classical psychoanalysis for, 67
 clinical ramifications of, 44
 psychoanalytic therapy with, 69–71
 uncovering therapies for, 94
 versus neurotic symptoms, 47–48
 working alliance and, 47
Neurotic symptoms, versus neurotic personalities, 47–48
Nondefensive identification, 135
Nonverbal communication, 24
Normalization, patient education and, 76–77

Object constancy, 24, 99
Object relations
 in borderline psychopathology, 49–53
 in compulsive personalities, 286–289
 in depression, 233–237
 in dissociative personalities, 332–334
 in hysteria, 308–310
 in mania, 250
 in masochism, 264–267
 in narcissism, 174–177
 in obsessive personalities, 286–289
 in paranoia, 211–214
 in psychopathic personalities, 155–157
 in schizoid personalities, 193–195
Object relations theory, 19, 29–34, 30*n*
Observing ego, 26, 45
Obsessive compulsive personalities. *See also* Compulsive personalities; Obsessive personalities
 diagnosis of, 43
 versus narcissistic personalities, 186–187, 298–299
Obsessive personalities, 22, 129*n*, 279–281. *See also* Compulsive personalities
 adaptive processes in, 283–286
 anality and, 281–282
 countertransference with, 292–294, 295, 300
 defensive processes in, 283–286

Obesessive personalities (*cont.*)
  differential diagnosis of, 298–300
    versus narcissistic personalities, 298–299
    versus organic brain syndromes, 299–300
    versus paranoid personalities, 224–225
    versus schizoid personalities, 203, 299
  object relations in, 286–289
  prognosis for, 9–10
  reaction formation in, 286
  self-experience and, 289–292
  therapeutic implications of diagnosis for, 294–298
  transference with, 292–294, 300
Oedipal level of personality, 25. *See also* Neurotic personality structure
Oedipal phase
  as cognitive developmental milestone, 31
  description of, 22, 23, 136
  hysterical personality development and, 303–304
  time frame for, 41
Omnipotent control
  description of, 103–104
  fantasies of, 128, 285–286
  as primitive defense, 98
  in psychopathic personalities, 153
  self-esteem and, 103
  undoing and, 127–128
Oral character, dependent versus aggressive, 22
Oral-explorative, 23
Oral-incorporative, 23
Oral phase, 23, 24, 41
Organic brain syndromes, versus obsessive personalities, 299–300

Panic disorder, 3
Paradigmatic psychoanalysis, 79
Paradoxical intervention techniques, 79
Parallel process, 34
Paranoid personalities, 93, 225–226
  adaptive processes in, 209–211
  affect and, 207–209
  attributions of, 206–207
  countertransference with, 216–217, 220
  defensive processes in, 209–211
  diagnosis of, 205
  differential diagnosis of, 224–225
    versus dissociative personalities, 225
    versus obsessive personalities, 224–225
    versus psychopathic personalities, 165, 224
  drive and, 207–209
  masochism, relation to, 266–267
  object relations in, 211–214
  political/social movements and, 207*n*
  psychoanalytic definition of, 108*n*
  reaction formation and, 132–133
  self-experience in, 216
  self-representations in, 214–216
  temperament and, 207–209
  therapeutic implications of diagnosis for, 217–223
  therapeutic split and, 55
  transference with, 210–211, 216–217
Paranoid stare, 216
Parataxic distortions, 131
Parent(s)
  abuse from, in dissociative personality development, 332–333
  control from, in obsessive compulsive personality development, 286–288
  criticism from, in depressive personality development, 235–236
  depression of, in depressive personality development, 236
  humiliation from, in paranoid personality development, 211–212
  inadequacy and narcissism of, in hysterical personality development, 309
  overinvolvement and deprivation from, in schizoid personality development, 194–195
Parental-impingement theory, 194
Parental modeling, 157
Parenting
  drive theory and, 21–22
  empathic, 54
  overinvolved, 194
Passive aggressive personalities, 149
Passive-into-active transformation, 133
Pathological character. *See* Personality disorder
Patient, use of term, 3*n*
Patient education, supportive technique and, 76–78
Patty Hearst phenomenon, 307
Pedophiles, 296*n*
Penis envy, 304
Perfectionism, narcissistic personalities and, 106, 174, 177–178
Persona, 170
Personal history, in diagnostic interview format, 349–350
Personality
  assessment. *See* Character, assessment
  change, limits on, 148–149
  developmental dimensions, 92
  developmental levels of organization, 40–66
  problems, depth/extensivity of, 9–10
  structure. *See* Personality structure
  typological dimensions, 92
Personality disorders, 47, 49, 147. *See also* specific personality disorders

Personality structure, 143
  appreciation of, 10
  assessment of, 18, 147
  borderline-level. *See* Borderline personality structure
  dimensions of, 40. *See also* Defense mechanisms; Developmental levels
  neurotic-level. *See* Neurotic personality structure
  psychotic-level. *See* Psychotic personality structure
Personology, 19, 37
Perversion, 139
Phallic character, 22
Phallic narcissistic character, 35
Phallic phase, 22
Pharmacological treatments, 68
Phobia, character diagnosis and, 10
Physiological conditions, versus hysterical personalities, 320–321
Pine, Fred, 20
Pleasure principle, 21
Pollyana-like individuals, 101
Posttraumatic stress reactions, repression and, 118
Practicing, 24
Primary dependency issues, 51
Primary egocentrism, 103
Primary gain, 306
Primary motivation, sexuality as, 140
Primary narcissism, 103, 169
Primary process thought, 25
Primitive defenses, 98, 99–100
  in borderline personality structure, 61
  denial, 101–103. *See also* Denial
  devaluation, primitive, 105–107
  dissociation, 114–115. *See also* Dissociation; Dissociative personalities
  idealization, primitive, 99, 105–107
  interpreting, in expressive therapy for borderline-level patients, 84–86
  introjection, 107–112. *See also* Introjection; Projective identification
  in neurotic-level personality structure, 54
  omnipotent control, 103–104. *See also* Omnipotent control
  projection, 107–112. *See also* Projection; Projective identification
  splitting, 112–114. *See also* Splitting
  withdrawal, 100–101. *See also* Withdrawal
Primitive envy, in psychopathic personalities, 158–159
Primitive idealization, 98
Primitive projection, 135–136
Prognosis, character diagnosis and, 9–10
Projection, 98. *See also* Projective identification
  definition of, 108
  malignant forms of, 108
  mature, versus projective identification, 110–111
  in paranoid personalities, 219–220
Projective identification, 54, 98
  borderline personality organization and, 112
  description of, 107–108, 110
  maintaining empathy and, 111
  in paranoid personalities, 210
  in psychopathic personalities, 154–155
  as self-fulfilling prophecy, 111
  versus mature projection, 110–111
Provocation, in masochistic personality, 263
Pseudoerotic transference storms, in paranoid personalities, 222–223
Pseudologia fantastica, 307
Pseudoneurotic schizophrenia, 50
Psychic numbing, 123
Psychoanalysis
  with neurotic-level patients, 69–71
  object relations viewpoint in, 49–53
  for psychologically advantaged people, 67, 68
  terminology, 68*n*
Psychoanalytic theories other than drive, ego psychology, object relations, and self psychology, 19–20
Psychological testing, 8
Psychopathic personalities, 2, 43, 151–152
  acting out and, 155
  adaptive processes in, 153–155
  affect and, 152–153
  countertransference with, 159–160
  defensive processes in, 153–155
  diagnosis of, 151–152
    therapeutic implications for, 160–165
  differential diagnosis of, 165–166
    versus dissociative personalities, 165–166, 345–346
    versus hysterical personalities, 318–319
    versus narcissistic personalities, 166, 175*n*, 185–186
    versus paranoid personalities, 165, 224
  dissociation in, 154–155
  drive and, 152–153
  object relations in, 155–157
  range of, 151
  self-experience and, 157–159
  temperament and, 152–153
  transference with, 159–160
Psychopharmacology, for depressive personalities, 240
Psychoses
  hysterical, 302
  overt, 57
    versus neuroses, 43–44
Psychosexual stages, 23

Psychotic personalities, 50
Psychotic personality structure, 56–65
 countertransference with, 59–60
 psychoanalytic therapy for, 72–80
Psychotic–symbiotic personality structure. *See* Psychotic personality structure
Pursuer–distancer paradigm, 196*n*

Racker, Heinrich, 33
Rage, psychopathic personality, and, 153
Rank, Otto, 30
Rapprochement, 24, 120–121
Rational–emotive therapy, 68
Rationalization, 99, 102, 124–125
Reaction formation
 description of, 131–133
 in obsessive compulsive personalities, 283, 286
 in paranoia, 211
Reality
 distortion of, withdrawal and, 101
 neurotic-level people and, 54
Reality principle, 21, 98
Reality testing, 62, 210
Reconstruction upward, 78
Referral by self or others, significance, 45
Regression
 description of, 120–122
 discouraging, in borderline clients, 88–89
 fears of, 78
 in hysterical personalities, 315
 somatization and, 121
Reich, Wilhelm, 22
Religion
 omnipotent caregiver and, 106
 undoing and, 128
Religious clients, 17–18
Remorse, narcissistic personalities and, 178
Repetition compulsion, 262
Repressed memory, in hysterical personality, 305–306
Repression
 anxiety and, 28–29, 119
 description of, 118–120
 essence of, 118
 in healthier people, 54
 hysterical personalities and, 305, 306–307
 problematic, 119
 trivial, 119
 versus denial, 98–99
Responsivity, versus character, 147–148
Reversal, 133–134
Rigidity of personalities, 27
Ritual abuse, 326*n*, 330
Rogers, Carl, 35

Sadism
 as countertransference to masochism, 269
 defense mechanisms and, 109
 normal aspects of, 139*n*
 in psychopathy, 149
 against self, 230
Sadness, depression and, 230–231
Safeguarding boundaries for borderline clients, 81–83
Same-sex closeness
 delusional paranoid person and, 211
 paranoid personalities and, 215
Sanity, versus insanity, 42, 49
Scapegoating, 131
Schizoid personalities, 189–190
 adaptive processes in, 192
 affect and, 190–192
 countertransference with, 197–199
 defensive processes in, 189, 191, 192
 degree of pathology in, 202–203
 diagnosis, therapeutic implications for, 199–202
 differential diagnosis of, 202–203
  versus compulsive personalities, 203
  versus obsessive personalities, 203, 299
 drive and, 190–192
 DSM-III criteria, 190
 self-experience in, 195–197
 sex ratio for, 194*n*
 temperament and, 190–192
 transference with, 197–199
 vocations associated with, 189
 withdrawal into fantasy and, 100, 189
Schizophrenia
 with dissociative personalities, 343*n*
 historical aspects of, 43
 versus mania, 255
Script theory, 19, 37
Searles, Harold, 32
Secondary defenses, 54, 93, 99
 absence of, 54
 acting out, 138–140. *See also* Acting out
 compartmentalization, 127
 diagnostic labels and, 134
 displacement, 130–131, 283
 identification, 135–138. *See also* Identification
 instinctualization, 140–142
 intellectualization, 123–124, 192
 internal boundaries and, 98
 isolation, 122–123, 283
 moralization, 125–127. *See also* Moralization
 rationalization, 99, 102, 124–125
 reaction formation, 131–133, 283, 286
 regression, 120–122. *See also* Regression
 repression, 118–120. *See also* Repression
 reversal, 133–134
 sexualization, 140–142, 304
 sublimation, 142–144

turning against self, 129–130, 232–233
undoing, 127–129, 283, 284
Secondary gain, 306
Secondary process thought, 26
Seduction theory, 327
Self-defeating personalities, 3, 260n. *See also* Masochistic personalities
Self-disclosure, supportive therapy and, 76
Self-esteem, 35–36, 148
based on unrealistic goal, 177
in compulsive personalities, 291
defensive behavior and, 97
in hysterical personalities, 311
in manic personalities, 250–251
in neurotic-level people, 69
in obsessive personalities, 291
omnipotence and, 103
problems of maintaining, 168
in schizoid personalities, 196–197
selfobject transferences and, 180
Self-experience
in compulsive personalities, 289–292
in depressive personalities, 237–239
in dissociative personalities, 334–336
in hysterical personalities, 310–313
in manic personalities, 250–251
in masochistic personalities, 267–268
in narcissistic personalities, 177–178
in obsessive personalities, 289–292
in paranoid personalities, 216
in psychopathic personalities, 157–159
in schizoid personalities, 195–197
Selfobject transferences, 180
Self psychologists, 9, 35–37, 180–182
Self psychology, 19, 34–37
in character diagnosis, 34–37
narcissism and, 180–182
Self-referral versus referral by others, significance of, 45
Separation–individuation process
borderline personalities and, 25, 64
depressive dynamics and, 234
devaluation and, 105
developmental failures in, 52
rapprochement subphase of, 120–121
secondary issues, 51
Sexuality, schizoid personalities and, 193
Sexualization, 140–142
Sexual orientation, 2, 77, 309, 311
Shame
compulsive personalities and, 283, 288–289
narcissistic personalities and, 172, 183
obsessive personalities and, 288–289
paranoid personalities and, 208
versus guilt, 172, 288–289
Shoplifters, 296n
Short-term analytic therapies, 70
Short-term individual therapy, for depressive personalities, 243
Short-term therapy, 11–12
Sick role, regression to. *See* Somatization
Situational factors, 147–148
Social learning theory, 158
Sociopathy. *See* Psychopathic personalities
Somatization, 98, 121n
Sour grapes rationalization, 124–125
Splitting
description of, 112–114
moralization and, 126
as primitive defense, 98, 99
Stage theories, post-Freudian advances in, 22–24
Stage theory of development, 22–23
Sterba, Richard, 30
Stockholm syndrome, 307
Stress
identification and, 136–137
interpretation of, 78–80
Structural theory, 25, 28, 29
Structured Clinical Interview for DSM-IV Dissociative Disorders, 342–343
Sublimation, 142–143
Suffering, masochistic personalities and, 258
Suicidal ideation, 16–17
Suicidal intent, assessment of, 13–14
Sullivan, Harry Stack, 31
Superego, 27–28, 31, 289. *See also* Conscience
Supportive technique
interpretation of feelings/stresses, 78–80
patient education and, 76–78
providing psychological safety and, 72–76
for psychotic-level patients, 72–80
Sweet lemon rationalization, 125
Symbiotic–psychotic personalities. *See* Psychotic personality structure
Symbiotic relatedness, 24
Symptom neuroses
description of, 47–48
versus character neuroses, 45–49

Temperament
character organization and, 145, 146
compulsive personalities and, 281–283
depressive personalities and, 229–231
dissociative personalities and, 328–329
hysterical personalities and, 303–304
manic personalities and, 248–249
masochistic personalities and, 260–261
narcissistic personalities and, 171–173
paranoid personalities and, 207–209
psychopathic personalities and, 152–153
in schizoid personalities, 190–192

Terminology, 1–3
Therapeutic alliance, 47–48
Therapeutic frame, 82
Therapeutic nihilism, 160–161
Therapeutic relationship
  diagnostic process as a good start for, 15
  settling in process for, 15–16
Therapeutic split in the ego, 26, 55
Therapist(s)
  classical treatment and, 7*n*
  consistency of, 163, 222
  educative role of, 46
  empathy conveyance and, 12–14
  honesty of, 73–74, 162
  incorruptibility of, 161–162
  independent strength verging on indifference of, 164
  offering direction and, 76
  "outpsyching the psychopath" and, 163
  patient level of character organization and, 68
  self-esteem of, 16
  trustworthiness of, 72–76
  versus evaluator, 160
  willingness to take position on behalf of patient, 75–76
Thompson, Clara, 31
Toilet training, compulsive personalities and, 281–282
Tone of therapist's interventions, 4
Transactional analysis, 37
Transcendental meditation, 242*n*
Transference
  benefit of, 16
  borderline personality structure and, 64–65
  compulsive personalities and, 292–294, 300
  depressive personalities and, 239–241
  dissociative personalities and, 336–338, 346
  Freud and, 31
  hysterical personalities and, 313–316, 321
  manic personalities and, 251
  masochistic personalities and, 268–270, 277
  narcissistic personalities and, 178–180, 184
  neurosis, 54
  obsessive personalities and, 292–294, 300
  paranoid personalities and, 216–217
  parataxic distortions and, 131
  psychopathic personalities and, 159–160
  schizoid personalities and, 197–199
  tests, 198
Trauma
  relationship to dissociation, 114–115, 332–333
  self-initiated sexualizations of, 141
  terminology, 3
Treatment planning, character diagnosis and, 8–9
Trust, versus mistrust, 51
Trustworthiness, demonstration of, 72–76
Turning against self
  in depressive personalities, 232–233
  description of, 129–130
Twelve-step programs, 297
Type A personalities, 279

Undoing
  compulsive personalities and, 283, 284
  description of, 127–129
  as lifetime project, 128

Vegetative disturbances, in clinical depression, 36–37, 228
Voicing contrasting feeling states, in expressive psychotherapy for borderline personalities, 83–84
Voyeurism, 139n
Vulnerability, defenses against, in psychopathic personalities, 156, 161

Will, Otto, 31
Windows of diagnosability, in dissociative conditions, 330
Winnicott, D. W., 32
Withdrawal
  advantage of, 101
  disadvantage of, 100–101
  primitive and mature forms of, 98–101
  schizoid personalities and, 192, 194
Working alliance, 15*n*. *See* Therapeutic alliance

Yawning, during therapy, 219